HOW TO HAVE A MAGNIFICENT MIDLIFE CRISIS

HOW TO HAVE A MAGNIFICENT MIDLIFE CRISIS

RETHINK, REBOOT, REVIVE – AND THRIVE.

KATE MUIR

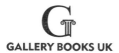

GALLERY BOOKS UK

London · New York · Amsterdam/Antwerp · Sydney/Melbourne · Toronto · New Delhi

First published in Great Britain by Gallery Books,
an imprint of Simon & Schuster UK Ltd, 2025

1 3 5 7 9 10 8 6 4 2

Simon & Schuster UK Ltd
1st Floor
222 Gray's Inn Road
London WC1X 8HB

www.simonandschuster.co.uk
www.simonandschuster.com.au
www.simonandschuster.co.in

Simon & Schuster Australia, Sydney
Simon & Schuster India, New Delhi

The authorised representative in the EEA is Simon & Schuster Netherlands BV,
Herculesplein 96, 3584 AA Utrecht, Netherlands. info@simonandschuster.nl

A CIP catalogue record for this book is available from the British Library

The stories provided in this book should not replace medical advice.
Always consult a healthcare professional.

Hardback ISBN: 978-1-3985-2550-4
eBook ISBN: 978-1-3985-2551-1

Typeset in Stone Serif by M Rules
Printed and Bound in the UK using 100% Renewable Electricity
at CPI Group (UK) Ltd

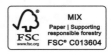

Contents

Introduction   1

MIND

1 Navigating the Mental Health
  Maelstrom   13

2 The Midlife Brain Reboot   37

3 Could I Be Neurodivergent?   53

4 How Not to Disappear at Work   71

5 How to Dodge Dementia   87

6 The Power of Wild Swimming   106

BODY

7 Ageproof Yourself with HRT   127

8 Reclaiming Testosterone   149

9 The Importance of Being Cliterate   176

10 Viva la Vulva 194

11 Pumping up Your Muscle and Bone 209

12 Avoiding the Midlife Muffin Top 225

SPIRIT

13 Women and Wine 249

14 Digital Detox 268

15 Divorce, the Moneypause and the
   Couplepause 283

16 Renovating Relationships and
   Friendships 304

17 Creative Awakening 326

18 The Psychedelic Adventure 341

   Conclusion 362

   Acknowledgements 369

   Further Resources 371

   Notes 373

   Index 397

I have been to hell and back, and let me tell you, it was wonderful.

LOUISE BOURGEOIS

Introduction

This is the book I wish I'd read in my forties before I fucked up. If you, too, are being sucked down into the midlife vortex, I'm keen to pass on some hard-earned wisdom and box-fresh research – from my own experience and the stories of the many women I spoke with who shared their experiences from the other side of the Midlife Crisis.

To start, let's be clear on what we mean by crisis and why it's so essential we all have one – and a magnificent one at that. This crisis is not merely a chance to be your own bomb disposal squad, but a positive turning point where you actively choose the future direction of your life. Midlife is not a time of decline, but of transformation and re-formation. This often involves an initial act of destruction, and if we don't want to completely crack apart, or explode, we need to make change in midlife, but it has to be intentional, not just something that we fall into. As one of my friends said when I started writing this: 'We are always becoming.' Let's own that.

Historically, men have owned the midlife crisis, as both a joke and a life stage. Women haven't really had a look-in, until recently. I found the perfect quote on this from

Miranda July's deliciously perverse perimenopause novel *All Fours*. Her female narrator ponders: 'Maybe midlife crises were just poorly marketed. Maybe each one was profound and unique and only it was a few silly men in red convertibles that gave them a bad name. I imagined greeting such a man solemnly: "I see you've reached a time of great questioning. God be with you, seeker."' Well, now it's our turn. Women have reached a time of great questioning, of ourselves and those around us, and maybe some are seeking something deeper and more spiritual. We need a new, grand story of midlife.

I can't pinpoint when the need to change and adapt starts, but it often seems to be somewhere between your late thirties and your sixties. Inevitably the midlife crisis boils up and bursts messily when you least expect it: an emotional stealth bomber. For some people, there can be two or even three midlife crises; for others it is more of a transition: a subtle, secret series of sleeping policemen, bumps to overcome on the road to somewhere calmer, more creative and fulfilling. For the mad ones like me, the crisis took on epic and messy proportions. More revolution than gentle evolution. More scorched earth.

How to Have a Magnificent Midlife Crisis is about new ways to understand and own this turning point and ensure it is a transition into a bigger, better, more magnificent future. In order to do this, we need to arm ourselves with the necessary knowledge. We also need to uncover the unconscious rules we've been following as women for millennia – and enjoy breaking them extravagantly at this midpoint in our lives. This book investigates everything, from taking a life-altering psychedelic trip to having better, possibly pansexual sex, and explains the art of the comeback, from divorce to leaving your job, with a whiff of justified revenge. It is not vague, 'woo-woo' self-help, but a guided trip through life experience, science and research. Having passed through the midlife crisis myself, having taken that magic mushroom trip, done the divorce, left the job, I am offering to be your test pilot, or perhaps crash-test dummy, in the midlife maze.

Obviously, it is important to pay attention to the four pillars of health – nutrition, exercise, sleep and stress reduction – and there are plenty of books and podcasts out there covering that in detail. That's not my job here. I am digging deeper into psychotherapy, into careers, into relationships, and into mind-altering substances, from hormones to psilocybin. We are going to open windows on mental healthiness, creative renaissance, vanquishing the midlife muffin top, editing your friends, ditching anxiety and addiction, and the surprising reassurance of discovering later-life neurodiversity. I take a deep dive into the vaginal microbiome, make a case for the powers of the female hormone testosterone, and learn how we can make our sexspan last longer and defeat the growing male–female orgasm gap as we age. I solicit advice on how to avoid osteoporosis and Alzheimer's disease, along with discovering extremely promising news around longevity. Inevitably, there is also icy wild swimming and tasteful nudity – because what's a midlife crisis without those?

We're packing a lot in because the more you know, the more you're going to flourish through your own midlife crisis.

There's so much to look forward to, but it's also tough out there, and you need to be fully equipped. Divorce, anxiety and depression all peak in the doldrums of midlife. When life is full and we are running on empty, the fallout can be catastrophic. I managed to cover a fair few of the fallout possibilities in my own midlife crisis: within a couple of years, I left my home and marriage, had an affair with a married man, got divorced, lost my memory, lost my job, and lost my mother to Alzheimer's. Also, the dog died after a tick bite. There were profound losses, but there was also healing, and I'll talk about how that took place as we wander through the chapters. I emerged on the other side with a new direction, and now bounce joyously out of bed in the mornings into a quite different life in a different house with a new partner and career – and a scruffy dog I found one night on Gumtree.

Everyone's midlife moment is unique – the partner, house, job and dog might stay exactly the same, but how you relate to them might feel completely different. For some, it will be a period of freedom and empowerment, for others past trauma can resurface; grief is quietly always with us, and issues we assumed had faded away, like body image or addictions, can come slinking back. For most, it will be a combination of both. Then there's The Rage; when the loving, protective hormonal padding of estrogen and progesterone disappears around perimenopause, a roar of long-suppressed anger can emerge. As women, we have subsumed so much of ourselves in work and household duties, and doing the right and polite thing, that we no longer remember who we really are. When we have time at last to think, freed from constant domestic burdens, or

Introduction

when a seismic event like the death of a parent or the end of a relationship cracks open our lives, we are confronted with this, and that realisation can bring with it a lot of (justified) anger, which is hard to process. We try anything: turning to CBD and cannabis, leaping into affairs, testing psychedelics to help with depression, or self-medicating with alcohol or prescription drugs. Over the course of researching this book, I asked psychotherapists and doctors where this anger comes from, what actually works in terms of handling it, and how to take preventative and positive action. I learned a lot – somewhat after the event in my case. Hindsight is absolutely terrific.

I deeply regret the emotional damage I caused to those I love during my own crisis; however, it did me a huge amount of good to be pared down to the basics and to live by myself for the first time in thirty years, except when my teenage daughter was staying part of every week (my two older sons were away at university by then). I had discovered I just couldn't hold a family, a full-time job and all those demands and expectations and institutions on my shoulders anymore I couldn't turn the supertanker, so I jumped off. I didn't find out why until later.

My rented flat was a lifeboat, a safe space, but inside it I was achingly lonely and full of shame. Obviously, I pretended all was well. All I had to sit on was four £10 IKEA garden chairs, but I invited lots of people to dinner parties, and often had to ask them to bring their own chair. Everyone thought this was funny, but like the flat, I felt completely bare, like a tree that had been brutally pruned, all the deadwood cut out.

By way of decoration for the flat, I had a poster I'd been given after interviewing the veteran French New Wave film director Agnès Varda on the re-release of her black-and-white 1962 film *Cleo from 5 to 7*. Radically for then, the fictional film appears to be two hours of documentary footage, tracking the elegant Corinne Marchand as Cleo, a singer, who goes around Paris killing time as she waits for a yes-or-no diagnosis of cancer. 'It's a film about living life in the shadow of death, about how viewing the world without sunglasses lets in the light, and shows us the truth,' goes the blurb. At one point Cleo consults a Tarot reader, and when the Death card is inevitably played, the fortune teller says it can also indicate a profound change in the person's life, rather than the end. Cleo panics, and goes hat shopping, as you do. She buys a glamorous black fur number. You need to watch the whole film, but it ends with hope, as Cleo gets a better-than-expected diagnosis and meets a soldier who himself is staring into the future, as he is sent back to the Algerian War. To me, the movie was about facing change and loss and keeping right on walking, staying open and alive to everything – as well as having the right accessories. I put the poster up above the mantelpiece in the empty flat.

It is ten years since my life imploded so spectacularly – and since I started to rebuild it. It took a while, but after a couple of years and some bracing psychotherapy, I rebuilt my friendships and the relationships with my adult children took new shape. My body, career and purpose all began to slowly recover. I felt small green shoots begin to grow. I was half a century old, and I was sprouting. Becoming me again. The poster of Cleo is properly framed, overseeing the kitchen of my new house.

And, surprisingly, this latest decade has turned out to be the most creative, entertaining, sexy and politically active time since my twenties. I wish someone had told me this. When I talk to women in their thirties, forties, fifties and sixties, often their main emotions around midlife are the three Fs: frazzlement, frustration and fear of the future. They see perimenopause, menopause and the long years stretching out afterwards as impending darkness, a shroud falling, the beginning of decrepitude. That's just bollocks. I know, because I've been there, and come out the other side. It's important that we share these stories and experiences, because that's one thing that women do so well. The tales women have so generously told me of their reinvention are lyrical, wise, painful, and often eccentric. Storytelling is our lifeforce. Women learn from listening to other women. Then we say, 'Thank you for your story. This is my story . . . ' Sometimes we find the matching narrative and that provides enlightenment; sometimes we learn from stories that are so very different to our own. So this book is a group effort: my own story and those of women who have handed me – and you – access to their inner lives. Lots of people have allowed me to use their full names, and their truth. (The few who remain anonymous here do so mostly for legal reasons: those who have been on an illegal psychedelic trip with me, and others who have been sacked in midlife and made to sign silencing NDAs, non-disclosure agreements, a tool the notorious Harvey Weinstein used a lot.)

*

I've divided this book into three sections: Mind, Body and Spirit, and in keeping with the unconventional content, you can read them in any order you fancy. Pick and mix what you need, or gather knowledge to pass on to your friends, but I hope this book will help you handle the incoming change fearlessly, as well as learning from the experts that I've met over the last five years. Consider the experts I've interviewed here to be a special advisory committee, just for you. What we need to do is gird our girdles for the midlife crisis and reclaim it as our own, not just the territory of men. After all, women experience the greatest midlife changes: becoming untethered from mothering, losing our hormones and fertility, being rendered invisible by the patriarchy – for what? What's next? That's the juicy question we'll be investigating. The wider journey I'm taking you on is less *Eat, Pray, Love* and more *See It, Say It, Sort It*, as you handle the unexploded bomb of midlife.

So let's dig further into embracing this time of transformation, and reject boredom and convention. Let's lean in to recalibrating the next stage of our lives. We are still culturally habituated to our parents' traditional life stages of child-rearing ending around the age of 50, nests emptying, retirement arriving at 60 or 65, and a pension providing a safety net as the horror of golf and Zumba classes loom, followed by frailty and death in the seventies or eighties. But that's not what's going to happen to us. 'If we are going to live to a hundred, it's time we get a better grip of what to expect – and how to navigate – longer lives. And why the extra decades that science has gifted us this past century changes the shape of life as a whole.' These are the words of Avivah Wittenberg-Cox, an author on gender and generational balance at work, who is advocating new ways of looking at maturing, rather than ageing. Life expectancy for women in the USA is predicted to be 83 in 2030, and in the UK it's higher at 85. If that's the average, women in good health may be heading towards 100. Life expectancy for men is three years lower. So Wittenberg-Cox has come up with an engaging proposition: that we divide our lives into four quarters with encouraging names. Quarter 1 up until 25 years old is 'Grow', Quarter 2 up to 50 is 'Achieve', Quarter 3 up to 75 is 'Becoming', and Quarter 4 up to 100 is 'Harvesting'. 'There is a yawning midlife and post-midlife gap that we have not thought through in terms of fulfilment, work, pleasure and economic survival,' she said, and now we can look upon that fruitful, future time as 'Becoming'. I like that.

Reframing life stages is exhilarating for women and men. What if I am going to work until I am 80? What if I go back to university or art school at 90? Where will a psychedelic trip take me? What if I become a politician? What if I have a second career? Or a third husband? Frankly, what's not to like? I want you to navigate this time of change and rebellion with joy. I want you to be glorious rather than notorious, magnificent rather than insignificant. I want you to throw crockery with purpose, and to be armed with practical knowledge, philosophical resilience and hormonal superpowers. Let's go.

MIND

CHAPTER 1

Navigating the Mental Health Maelstrom

Midlife is a maelstrom. I was in a small boat being drawn towards one of the most powerful maelstroms in the world – the Corryvreckan whirlpool off the island of Jura in Scotland – when I had an epiphany about my mental health. You expect a whirlpool to look like a spinning plughole, violently sucking in objects within its radius, but nearing the Corryvreckan, the water had a suspicious flat, mirrored surface in the sunlight. Our skipper explained that invisible beneath the navy-blue water was a dramatic landscape of rocky mountains and ravines. Suddenly a huge wave erupted out of the glassy calm. More white-topped breakers crowded behind, pushed up by the jagged underwater cliffs. Towering waves plunged down into black holes that appeared unbidden in the sea. Here, the tides of the Atlantic and the Sound of Jura clash in opposing directions, and the maelstrom erupts. In storms, the Corryvreckan has dragged ships down or smashed them against the rocks. We felt the magnetic pull, then revved up the engines and motored round the chaos.

The whirlpool was less a draining plughole and more a boiling cauldron, caused by forces beneath that we could not comprehend or see. Welcome to the midlife crisis. My midlife was like this – glassy and well organised on the surface, wild and unpredictable below, with hidden mountains of pain and resentment, unresolved tides of grief and incomprehension. At my point of crisis, I jumped out of that boat and swam into the maelstrom. I was so desperate, it was the only way forward.

So many of us find that the perfect storm of midlife erupts when we least expect it and when we are least ready to cope with the fallout. But the multitasking midlife cliché is true for so many of us, male and female: working full time for demanding bosses, caring for carnaptious, aged parents, placating teenagers oozing horrible hormones. At the same time, we are holding together a partnership or marriage or friendships that are rusty and uncared for. For women in their forties (and some non-binary or trans people), there is also the double whammy of unpredictable hormonal highs and lows that will eventually result in a serious crash as progesterone and estrogen drain away at menopause. The crossing into midlife is made all the more treacherous by the intersection of these biological, psychological and social elements – 'biopsychosocial' chaos is the technical term, or more colloquially, a shitstorm.

I was convinced I would ride through that shitstorm by running 10Ks, doing yoga, writing an (imaginary) best-selling film and socialising wildly, on top of my other weighty responsibilities. Wrong. Luckily, I had the wisdom and support of others who had been there before me to draw on. I was eventually rescued from my own manic mental maelstrom by a combination of therapies: the return of my natural hormones through hormone replacement therapy (HRT) and, just as importantly, eighteen months of psychotherapy with a therapist who was feminist, prescriptive and bracingly direct. Over many weeks and even more tissues, she ushered me gently out of my uptight Scottish Presbyterian lifeboat and into the deep waters beneath. With her help I explored the shadows of my life and relationships, looking at the mountains of unresolved emotion beneath the water's surface.

I had absolutely no idea I was bottling anything up, or that I deserved any credit for working and mothering and fighting on, or that I'd carried a literally unspeakable burden as an only child with parents with dementia, and I could no longer hold it. As I cleared out my dying mother's flat in Glasgow, I ran off into an affair with a married man on my way out of my own marriage, but that was a symptom and not a solution to my problems. It was only after I had been living on my own for three years – with various older children appearing part-time – that I began to see myself clearly, be kind to myself, and atone for some of the damage I had caused when divorcing and escaping. The therapist sat there with her searing intelligence and comforting floral dresses and handed me a set of psychological tools for coping with life, as well as the insight and self-compassion that I had lacked before. It had only taken half a century to find out about these things. I wish someone had told me earlier.

Of course, some people are rather more evolved and in tune with themselves than I was, but I'll bet that for the majority, midlife pressure releases some of these underwater volcanos. But it is the combination of these pressures with the hormonal onslaught of the menopause that can really trigger a mental health crisis for some. Professor Jayashri Kulkarni, an Australian psychiatrist at Monash University who is perhaps the foremost thinker on mental health, hormones and midlife right now, told me that, 'What's happening in a woman's life and work at this time often doesn't explain the sudden onset of severe anxiety, change in mood and difficulties with cognition that occur all too commonly. We have women experiencing serious mental ill-health for the first time ever in their mid-forties, while others with previously well-managed depression suddenly find their mental health falls apart.' She believes the menopausal transition is the tipping factor that causes a significant change in mental health. In a groundbreaking paper, 'Menopause depression: Under recognised and poorly treated', Professor Kulkarni and her team created the MENO-D rating scale to detect depression in perimenopause. It's meant for professionals, but you could also google it and get a sense of what's going on in your head and hormones before a consultation by doing the survey online. It asks about low energy, paranoid thinking, self-esteem, irritability, isolation, anxiety, physical symptoms, sleep disturbance, weight gain or loss, sexual interest, memory and concentration, and gives a points scale afterwards from mild to severe perimenopausal depression. Data on your mood always helps if you're thinking of visiting the doctor.

I am professionally obsessed by the way women and their doctors and psychiatrists still fail to recognise hormonal symptoms in perimenopause and menopause, resulting in unnecessary mental carnage; in particular, depression, anxiety, brain fog and rage. I'll talk more about how your brain completely rewires during menopause in the next chapter, but in terms of the impact on mental health, it's important to understand the basis of what is happening physiologically. During menopause, the production of potent neurosteroids (hormones) decreases, in a jagged way over a number of years, and they are crucial to our well-being. While estrogen, progesterone and testosterone have traditionally been described as 'sex hormones', that's just one part of their function, and in fact much of their work is done in the brain. Estrogen regulates neurotransmitters like serotonin and dopamine. Serotonin controls happiness, focus, mood and appetite, and dopamine is released when you do something that feels good, like eating, drinking or competing, affecting motivation and rewards. Estrogen is also a major regulator of brain circuits and memory functions. Testosterone is involved in drive and libido, although as we'll see in its own chapter, it has multiple other, lesser-known functions. Meanwhile, progesterone enhances the activity of our GABA receptors, which are in many parts of the brain and regulate our central nervous system, including increasing calm and sleep. So when progesterone levels drop, anxiety can ramp up. Together, these hormones form an orchestra in your brain that suddenly becomes out of tune in midlife.

For some this triggers a crisis point, like my own

whirlpool moment, but lots of women have told me about 'just feeling flat' around menopause; the technical term for this is 'anhedonia' – lack of interest and enjoyment in life's pleasures. As a result, we are seeing the large-scale use of antidepressants by midlife women experiencing mental health problems for the first time, but medicating in this way fails to take account of the hormonal changes in the brain. It could be personal circumstances and other mental health problems, or it could be hormones, or both – but why not check? The official Diagnostic and Statistical Manual of Mental Disorders (DSM), the gold standard for doctors, astonishingly doesn't include perimenopausal or menopausal depression as a diagnosis. Yet we know from the leap in use of antidepressants in women in the 45–55 age group to a high of around 16 per cent in the UK and 20 per cent in the US (compared to 6 to 8 per cent in men of the same age) that peri/menopause is a huge invisible player in collapsing mental health. When many doctors stopped prescribing HRT after a safety scare in 2002 (which I'll debunk in Chapter 7, Ageproof Yourself with HRT), one significant study in Canada of over 50,000 women showed that as hormone prescriptions went down, antidepressant prescriptions rocketed up, indicating that HRT had been a major player in psychological healthcare. In the survey I did with the Fawcett Society of 4,000 women, 69 per cent reported psychological changes around menopause, including increases in low mood, anxiety and depression.

Anxiety is a huge spanner in the midlife works, and when I go to workplaces to give menopause talks, it's that and brain fog that women bring up most. They speak of an inexplicable, creeping anxiety that stops them doing tasks they found easy before: speaking at a meeting, delivering a PowerPoint, reading a spreadsheet, working on a tight deadline. What should be smooth operating suddenly becomes mired in procrastination, muddle and fear. 'Around the time the anxiety started, I was working as a teaching assistant, my husband was on the road working, and I was doing everything for our two kids, and I just stopped doing things: no more dinner parties, no keep fit, no meeting friends and I cancelled holidays,' said Rachael, who lives in a village in South West England, and found her anxiety building in her early forties, soon after she'd started having occasional night sweats. 'I started having panic attacks. One morning I was driving to work, it was freezing, and I had a hot flush and I started panicking. I could hardly breathe and had palpitations and chest pains. I stopped the car in the village, and a doctor there helped me through the panic attack.' That rising fear came to her again at a Christmas dinner party in Bristol: Rachael anxiously moved place cards so she could sit at the end of the table near the door, ready to escape, 'and then I panicked and realised I couldn't do it at all and walked out.'

Her anxiety peaked again when she was heading to her school reunion. 'I had to take the train to Paddington and then the tube to East Putney, and I suddenly didn't know how to do it. I couldn't work out how to get another tube, but a friend from Bristol met me at the station and was able to show me where to go. I felt really self-conscious.' Once she was at the event, she found she couldn't take part in any of the conversation. 'It was all a fuzz of noise, everyone talking about their successes, all looking well, slim and glamorous, and I felt I was an absolute wreck.'

Throughout her forties, Rachael's symptoms got worse, particularly heavy bleeding, along with low mood, anxiety, headaches and joint pain in her fingers. Still no one identified all this as the result of low hormones. 'Then, one morning in 2012, I sat up in bed and I said to my husband, "I want to top myself."' Her husband was shocked and encouraged Rachael to see her GP. 'He's a lovely doctor – very kind and caring – but essentially, he didn't recognise my menopause symptoms because he hadn't been trained. When I told him of my suicidal thoughts, he instantly diagnosed depression and said I needed antidepressants. I tried to argue as I didn't think I was; I've never been depressed before and felt certain it was hormonal and linked to my cycle. But he insisted, so I left the surgery with a prescription for antidepressants. Two nights later we had to call paramedics because my heart was racing at 140 beats a minute. I could barely breathe or speak and was in a terrible state. So I stopped taking the antidepressants and hoped things would get better. I just thought I'd struggle on and it would work itself out and I'd be fine … But it really didn't.'

An appointment for stomach problems with a different GP led to Rachael being offered HRT patches in perimenopause. (At that time, perimenopause wasn't even mentioned on the NHS website.) 'Little by little, things started to improve. First the anxiety subsided and the brain fog lifted. I could think more clearly. I started to feel more confident about myself. I could stand up for myself and I could defend myself.' But she still had dangerously heavy bleeding, and eventually ended up having a hysterectomy with her ovaries removed, which put her into full surgical menopause in 2015. Since then, Rachael has been on estrogen-only HRT, vaginal estrogen and more recently testosterone, is still working in special needs education, with additional responsibilities, and is feeling great. 'I'm a different woman. I'm out walking, I'm learning new things, I'm strong and life is good. And that's what I want for all women. I want women who come after me to know what to expect and to have doctors who support them, and not have to diagnose themselves.' She still raises awareness on her Instagram account @not_your_usual_menopause.

Rachael's anxiety was on an epic scale, but there is also 'good' anxiety, the kind that used to have us listening out for predators at night, the kind that keeps us alive. This form of anxiety is like a warning light on a car – do something about it now, take action if you can, and you won't crash or run out of fuel – and this is more easily handled. Loads of women complain to me about waking up with pre-dawn anxiety, and this is the moment to write in a notebook by the bed in the dark, deposit your fears and get back to sleep. Tackle it in the morning. My dentist, Sunita Daswani, found she was so plagued with sleeplessness and related anxiety around menopause that she considered giving up the work she loved – until she went for a two-day meditation course with her husband. Since then, she has meditated with recorded chanting for twenty minutes every morning to calm herself before going to the surgery, and says, 'If I get a hot flush that disturbs my sleep in the middle of the night, I just put in my headphones and do a sleep meditation, which helps me get back into a deep sleep.' She's brilliant, and does her very best with my Glasgow teeth, raised on full-strength Ribena and Mars Bars.

There's no predicting how each woman's menopause or midlife changes will play out, and many, like Rachael, might have had no previous history of depression and anxiety. Professor Kulkarni said: 'Destabilisation varies widely between individuals – some women experience debilitating mental health changes, but others have compensatory mechanisms that mean there's minimal or no impact on their mental health, and that might depend on biological or social factors.' She also said that routine blood tests of hormones will not provide details of brain fluctuations or neurochemistry, and the best way to find out what's going on is to take a comprehensive clinical history of the patient. 'And listen.'

This kind of help can seem hard to come by, and we're often still expected to 'sail through the menopause transition' without help. When we do seek out help, the menopause is often ignored as a potentially contributing factor, as was the case for Rachael. But the previous system of treating peri/menopausal mental health in the same way that all mental health is managed might be missing a trick. While there are media suggestions that menopause is being 'over-medicalised' or 'pathologised', Professor Kulkarni believes that hormones can often be the missing link and should be considered. She said that HRT is 'an important part of the treatment options available for menopausal mental health issues, particularly in the early perimeno-pause timeframe', as well as advice on lifestyle. Professor Kulkarni learned about the surprising power of hormones in the brain when she was training in women's psychiatric wards years ago in Australia. She saw a number of mothers who had been perfectly well in pregnancy, high on huge surges of estrogen and progesterone, until the hormonal crash of severe post-natal depression, and others whose breakdowns came around menopause. She got permission from the hospital and the women to do a pilot study on topping up natural estrogen in eleven patients with severe psychosis, while they remained on their anti-psychotic med-ications. Many, but not all, recovered their mental health very quickly. One patient in her forties had continuous auditory hallucinations ('voices in her head') for years after giving birth, but they stopped after four days on estrogen, and the woman was eventually discharged and found a job and a new relationship.

Knowing that in earlier life you were very sensitive to hor-monal change, such as during pregnancy or post-partum, can be a clue to what your journey through midlife and menopause might hold. Dr Hannah Ward has seen repro-ductive depression from both sides, as a physician and a patient. She had always felt fantastic during pregnancy, but the aftermath was getting harder with each child. After having her third baby, she had the typical struggles with sleep and fatigue, but she was also very anxious, particularly when she returned to work part-time. 'My doctor thought I needed an antidepressant, but when I started it, I developed paranoid thoughts, sweats at night and my sleep became much worse. Those weeks of taking the drug sertraline were honestly the worst three weeks of my life.' She read up professionally about the work of Dr Katharina Dalton, who started treating post-natal women with progesterone for mood problems and had published a book on it back in 1980 – which had been largely ignored until recently. Dr Ward got hold of some progesterone pessaries, and 'within twelve hours I went back to normal'. She came off hormones for a few years, but realised the same symptoms were welling up as she headed into her mid-forties and perimenopause, and went happily back on HRT. She is now a GP and menopause specialist with Newson Health.

When hormones fluctuate and crash causing premenstrual dysphoric disorder (PMDD), post-natal depression and perimenopause, why is the first-line treatment antidepressants? Why can't most doctors see the bleeding obvious or at least look into combining antidepressants, therapy and hormonal treatment? Of course, mental health is complex, but when will experts see the whole woman, including her hormones? I recently looked through a four-year curriculum for a psychotherapy qualification, and I was gobsmacked to see there was nothing on the intersection of hormones and menopause with mental health. Similarly, when I was asked to give a speech to the Royal College of Psychiatry about women's experience of menopause in 2024, I was surprised. Weren't they across the subject, the biggest hormonal change since puberty and pregnancy? 'No,' said the psychiatrist inviting me. 'We don't even have a module on menopause in our training yet.'

*

As well as the more common mental health issues of anxiety and depression, we must consider the clash of menopause and midlife chaos with rarer, serious mental health disorders. The prevalence of suicidal ideation is seven times higher in perimenopausal women and we know from a survey of 1,000 women by the charity Bipolar UK that more than 55 per cent of respondents over 40 said perimenopause or menopause had affected their bipolar symptoms and more than a quarter of these said the impact was significant. Bipolar disorder, formerly called manic depression, is a mental health condition that causes extreme mood swings. I spoke to psychiatrist Professor Arianna Di Florio. 'My professional passion is bipolar disorder,' she said. 'There is this moment in which, all of a sudden, the world changes: there is either a light switching on, or a light switching over. I became interested in the experiences of women who develop bipolar disorder for the first time really late in life, when the textbooks said the onset was generally in your twenties.'

Thanks to Di Florio's work with her team at Cardiff University, which appeared in the journal *Nature Mental Health* in 2024, we now have evidence showing that perimenopause is associated with an increased risk of developing bipolar and major depressive disorders for the first time. 'During perimenopause, approximately 80 per cent of people develop a variety of symptoms, but the impact of perimenopause on the onset of severe mental illness was unknown until now,' said Professor Di Florio. They studied 128,294 women in the UK Biobank population database and found a 112 per cent increase in incidence of bipolar at perimenopause. Onsets of major depressive disorder increased by 30 per cent, but incidences of schizophrenia (a major mental illness affecting feelings, thoughts and behaviour, often accompanied by hallucinations and delusions) did not seem to be affected. 'We've expanded our knowledge of the mental health changes associated with perimenopause, and can help provide explanations for women who have previously been left in the dark about what's happening to them.'

Untangling existential and menopause symptoms is difficult around mental health, and Professor Di Florio is also cautious about 'perpetuating the stereotype that hormones make women crazy'. She pointed to the early diagnoses of hysteria blamed on the 'wandering womb', and recalled the famous painting by André Brouillet in 1887 of the French neurologist Jean-Martin Charcot demonstrating hysteria in a hypnotised patient at the Salpêtrière, in which doctors surround a young, décolleté woman, who seems to be falling into a rather erotic reverie. There is so much going on for women at this point in their lives that pinpointing a 'cause' for worsening mental health is virtually impossible. 'Is it hormones, the 2024 version of hysteria, or is it also because women are expected to lead impossible lives, working forty-plus-hour weeks, using their screens late into the evening, becoming sleepless, and raising families?' She ended by saying that at this point, we simply don't know enough. 'For one group of women there is a distinct hormonal trigger, and for another substantial proportion it is mostly psychosocial. So you know you need to consider all these factors. We need to be really humble about what we understand. You know, I don't see many people being humble in this.'

I met the engaging Professor Di Florio in person months after I'd interviewed her over Zoom, when I was getting an honorary fellowship for my menopause work at the science faculty in Cardiff. I know it's not entirely humble to mention that, but I was really delighted to have the recognition of the degree, wear the silly velvet hat, and speak to over a thousand young people about the coming menopause revolution. Because sometimes you just feel like a punchbag in the women's health arena, when you fight and fight, and the medical establishment continues to bury its gender-biased institutional head in the sand and ignore the profound effect of hormones on women in midlife. So I'm very pleased to be able to share a peek into Di Florio's pioneering work.

Of course, the story *is* much bigger than just hormones at menopause, and I wanted to gain a wider psychological and social picture of this midlife time of change, so I interviewed a fantastic psychotherapist, Dr Kalanit Ben-Ari, who specialises in relationship therapy and has observed the vicissitudes of midlife in her individual clients for decades. I love how so many smart women flow serendipitously into my life, and I met Dr Ben-Ari through a friend, Lorraine Candy, host of the Postcards from Midlife podcast, when swimming in the cold slow lane at Parliament Hill Lido. For our first chat, Dr Ben-Ari and I returned there and swam in the slightly warmer 16-degree water, before heading into the public sauna and then the café. It's amazing how quickly you can get to know and trust someone in extremes of hot and cold, and there's something thrillingly gladiatorial about a therapist and an investigative journalist asking each other questions, revealing layers. We decided to do a proper interview a few weeks later, and this is some of what I learned from her:

'I think many people feel that shift in midlife, but it's also important to say not everyone feels it. For those who do, it might be because of the physical symptoms: the hot flushes and other things that create confusion. But there's more. We create the identity of who we think we are in our thirties and early forties, and then it alters. It's a mishmash of the psychological part, the changing body and hormones, the ending of youth and of the ability to have children. There can be a huge sense of loss, worse for people who had difficult losses and trauma in the past. It's all going to surface.'

When your last period goes, and you are officially infertile, there is huge relief at escaping the hormonal hassle, the cramping and the flooding. It's often the thing women cite as the best part of menopause. Miranda July describes the last unpredictable and gruesome periods of perimenopause perfectly in her novel *All Fours* as 'thick black blood eels' and 'ghost cycles with cramps but no bleeding'. But there is also a reorienting that is not altogether comfortable. As my periods receded into the distance at 52, I had a sudden, piercing sense that I was no longer facing in the direction of birth. I was looking out towards death, which is not necessarily a bad thing. It was time to get on with living, right now, with purpose and pleasure. That moment is often physically clear-cut around fertility for women, less so perhaps for men who experience a far less abrupt change in fertility as they age. Dr Ben-Ari sees the resultant maelstrom as potentially positive, as people can pause and ask: 'Who am I? What do I want to do?' In middle age, people are searching for meaning. The loss of a parent, a body change, an affair ... Whatever it is, ask yourself, 'What is the meaning of this?' It's a very worthwhile self-inquiry, and one that can be deeply spiritual.

Midlife can feel like a time of loss in many ways – of fertility, of parents, of time. When our children leave home, that's another loss, and although I'm not covering parenting here (that's another vast subject), journalist Lorraine Candy has written books about parenting teens and midlife, so she is very much across empty nest syndrome as a mother with kids going off to university, and said: 'This is a form of grief, a form of living loss, your whole life has changed, your parenting has changed, your family dynamic has changed.' The silence at home can be devastating, particularly if your life centred around your children. Lorraine suggests, aside from luxuriating in the lack of dirty unpaired socks, that you create a list of things you can do now you have more time and space, and that you don't electronically hover, but arrange to phone your offspring once a week. 'They do come back a lot and you have a whole new relationship to look forward to.'

The end of parenting sheds a klieg light on the remaining relationship at home, and Dr Ben-Ari specialises in couples therapy, as well as individual work, and has noticed that suddenly women are cutting their losses as they hit this change. 'Life is short. They don't want to waste it. One of the things that I see clinically is that between ages 49 to 50, there's a huge jump in a woman asking for divorce. It's like a switch has gone off. She's not interested in couples therapy anymore.' That correlates with the official statistics with the divorce rate at its highest between the ages of 40 and 49 for lesbian and heterosexual couples, and 62 per cent of divorces in heterosexual relationships are initiated by the woman. I'll talk more about that in Chapter 15, on divorce.

Women often look to divorce after a parent has died. Dr Ben-Ari said: 'The first year when people lose a parent makes them very vulnerable. Midlife and losing parents, those two together, create a huge, maybe internal crisis that requires change. Sometimes, the end makes people want to live life to the fullest. But sometimes it's also a way out of grief, not knowing what to do, and thinking and projecting the problems onto the relationship.' I squirmed a bit listening here: my mother Ella died in June 2015, and by October that year I had separated from my former husband. Then his mother died a few weeks later. The pain and grief was raw and on the surface for both of us. Dr Ben-Ari continued: 'So usually I tell people, don't make decisions in the first year of grieving a parent.'

She sees men having more of a crisis around the age of 40, and women later. But she said men in their fifties and sixties often become more dependent on the woman, unless they have a relationship outside of the marriage. 'It seems that men mostly leave a marriage because they have another relationship, but women often leave just to have time for themselves. They want to find a partner eventually, but they don't want to compromise.' Many women also seem to care less about what people think of them. 'They can let that go and think instead, what brings me joy?'

There is also that loss of sexual visibility, the end of heterosexual flirting when men subconsciously know you are no longer fertile, because previously their testosterone took a little leap when a fertile woman entered the room. Whatever your wit or intellectual abilities, pheromones are pheromones, and there's nothing we can do to change that, and that invisibility might feel like a loss. Dr Ben-Ari has an interesting take on that: 'I think that men also look for other things, and they're looking for depth and an opportunity to be in touch with something else. They find something else inside of you. That makes it super attractive.' As someone who met her new partner at the age of 54, and is still with him at 60, I get that.

One of the most serious disruptions at midlife is the re-surfacing of trauma from long ago, often triggered by overwhelm or health issues. Cortisol, the stress hormone made by the adrenal glands, often remains imbalanced in people with PTSD. 'Living with that embedded trauma can leave us constantly stressed,' said Dr Ben-Ari. 'If there was a trauma, if there are things that weren't settled in the early years of growing up or later on, if our nervous system didn't recover, then we're always in a state of alarm, alarm, alarm. We can't concentrate when our nervous system is always on the alert for danger.' Looking inside and doing the psycho-therapeutic work is the only way out.

Karen Arthur – who tells her story about going from being a teacher to a fashion designer, @MenopauseWhilstBlack campaigner and podcast creator in the coming Creative Awakening chapter – brought up this question of trauma when we talked. She walked out of her teaching job in London in 2015 and was signed off with depression around the time of perimenopause, after a build-up of circumstances that included leaving her emotionally abusive partner, raising her two girls mostly on her own and the daily microaggressions of racism. There was a lot of trauma, but it can be hard to recognise this when you're in the thick of everything that midlife throws at you. 'It wasn't until I left teaching and went into therapy that I started to pull down walls,' says Karen.

She was seriously depressed, so much so that she didn't bother fixing her boiler, not feeling she was worth it, 'and I was eating fish-finger sandwiches practically every night. I wasn't dressing the way that I love dressing, and I was in bed a lot'. At the peak of her depression, she went away to Eastbourne in the wintry depths of February. 'I put a pin in Airbnb. I needed some space.' She found herself standing on the cliffs above the sea at Beachy Head, an infamous suicide spot, thinking: 'I've got my office in order. I've written all my passwords down, got my will in order, so everyone will be able to find them. So I was ready, but not ready.' Karen paused, and added, 'It's extraordinary how women think of other people, and even organise things when they're at their lowest ebb.' And then she described looking over the edge of the cliff, and thinking: 'Oh no, I'm not doing that. So I went to a pub across the way, on the South Downs. It was fucking freezing. I just remember I was like, what was I thinking? I needed some chips and some hot chocolate and some calm. And I thought then, I'm staying, but I'm going to curate the rest of my life the way I want to do it.'

Karen went to a psychotherapist for three years, and thinks it is one of the best investments she ever made. The therapist was also Black and lived seven minutes away from her house. Sometimes she was the only person Karen saw in a week. Some therapists say that depression can be caused by anger that is repressed or not processed and is turned inwards, towards the individual. The burden and anger Karen was carrying included the trauma of an emotionally abusive relationship, as well as racial discrimination. She also explored the weight of 'women's work': 'Before I started therapy, I didn't have any boundaries. I was the fixer. I was the doer. I'm the oldest child, the girl child. I'm the one who does all the things, organises all the things. And I felt resentment, but I didn't feel I had a choice.'

As time, and healing, went on, Karen also began looking at the big picture for Black women in menopause – they tend to start a year or so earlier than white women. 'I was aware of racial weathering, although I didn't know that was the term then, and the negative effects that racism has on Black bodies and our health outcomes. I knew that racism was a form of stress, and I knew that menopause could be brought on by stress. So I'm just thinking where are my Black women now, where are my Black menopausal women, how are they coping?' She started her @MenopauseWhilstBlack Instagram when she didn't see anyone in midlife who looked like herself on social media, and a podcast, as well as doing a survey of Black women's experiences. Only 6 per cent of Black women use HRT in the UK, compared to 23 per cent of white women. 'I'm also transparent that I'm a Black woman who takes HRT because it just doesn't sit right with my audience.

They've got sharp eyes, and I understand what's still going on with medical racism and unconscious bias and not being believed and being distrustful of the doctors. I get that. But I'm also honest about how it's helped me, along with life-style changes and therapy.'

Karen has used therapy to move forward and reframe her life, but her past experience still determines the battles she chooses to fight, and the creative decisions she makes. I was listening to psychotherapist and author Julia Samuel speak at a menopause and longevity event, and she mentioned 'post-traumatic growth' (PTG). Some people may struggle with post-traumatic stress disorder for life, but Samuel explains how we can also, to some extent, heal from trauma and even grow as a result of it, by exploring it, engaging in therapy and finding self-compassion. The brain is malleable. On her website she wrote: 'Post-traumatic growth never denies the devastation of the traumatic event, which needs to be processed, but it shows that for some people the experience can lead to growth, where the person's perception of what matters changes – more about love and connection, less about aspiration and success. People who have experienced PTG may well feel that they not only survived, but also grew from what they thought would break them.'

But it's hard to grow without help, and how many people can afford weekly therapy at £60 to £100 a session right now? If you have the resources, perhaps it is a case of prioritising therapy over other 'luxuries'. Dr Ben-Ari points out that 'people will pay a lot for make-up, a lot for coffee, a lot for the gym, a lot for a cream for their face. So you put your money on what you think is important and what you value.'

If you don't have the resources, talking therapy is available on the NHS, although the chances of getting an appointment are slim, with a long waiting list, and often the best they can offer is a six-session online Cognitive Behavioural Therapy (CBT) course, which they say will help you 'manage your problems by changing the way you think and behave'. But there are other options. If you want affordable in-depth therapy, you can get it at cheaper or even pro-bono rates from trainees, who are carefully supervised, at many of the major psychotherapy schools; look out for BACP or UKCP approved courses. And if you don't get on with the first therapist or trust them, think of it as speed dating – you need to find the right one. As Dr Ben-Ari said, 'You're paying for a good conversation. Think of it like going to a supermarket. You want a pasta. You know exactly what you buy. You know exactly how it's going to taste. You know exactly what you're paying for. But you don't with psychotherapy. Let's talk. Let's play. Let's see where it will lead you.' She finds that midlife women start to ask different questions, look for different meanings. 'Philosophical questions. Spiritual. Everyone understands spirituality differently. It is something bigger than us. There is a longing for something different. I love it, I love working with them, because this is exactly the opening that fascinates me.'

If therapy isn't for you, you can strike out on your own. Daily journalling is often a kickstarter of insights. Just sitting down for five or ten minutes in the morning and filling a blank page or two or three with your stream of consciousness and repressed emotions is like taking the re-cycling out for your brain. Proper notebooks and pens are the way forward, not screens. You can express thoughts and feelings without worrying about grammar or structure – this is a private space where you can let it all out and behave appallingly if you want. You can clarify your thoughts and plans, dump your stress, and often discover more about who you are becoming.

We are woefully undereducated about how to handle our needs and emotions, and understanding that is such a useful tool as we proceed through life, a new lens to see through. These are changing times for women, and time changes us too. I've come out the other side after ten years, battered but better, with more insight into my own and other people's struggles. I also went back to the Corryvreckan whirlpool on a glorious May morning in 2024, and much had been resolved for me: a new life, a new house, a new career, a new partner, a new dog and a ton of trouble offloaded with a great therapist. On the boat, we motored feet away from rocks packed with fat, flopping, pregnant seals and white cubs sunbathing, and spotted a sea eagle's nest as we passed a thicket of trees on the edge of Jura. Through binoculars I saw the parent eagle observing regally from a branch; the brown and cream chick was in a nest that looked to be about the size of a double bed. This was indeed the case – the birds have an eight-feet wingspan, like a small plane. The vast bird took off, and so did we, riding into the waves, riding into the best natural rollercoaster in the world, the Corryvreckan, no longer fearing what was beneath.

CHAPTER 2

The Midlife Brain Reboot

Why has no one informed women that their brains completely rewire up to three times in life and that we are miracles of plasticity? Or that this transformation is one of our female superpowers? The three Ps – puberty, pregnancy and perimenopause – are times of neurological deconstruction and rebuilding to achieve new goals, and all are kickstarted by hormones. For women, the three big hitters are estrogen, progesterone and testosterone, but all hormones are crucial messengers between the brain and body, influencing everything from metabolism to mood, growth, sleep and sexual function. They're made all over our bodies, from our brains to our thyroid and adrenal glands and ovaries. Estrogen, progesterone and testosterone are part of a hormonal orchestra which includes serotonin, dopamine, insulin, thyroxine and cortisol. And when one of those hormones is off-key, the whole symphony can fall apart.

Hormones in our heads really matter, at every stage of our lives. It's not rocket science – it's neuroscience, and the female branch of neuroscience has been criminally neglected by medicine and academia. Because women have long been treated, medically and culturally, as mere vessels for reproduction, most research until now has focused on hormones in the ovaries, rather than their profound effects on the brain. Dr Lisa Mosconi, director of the Women's Brain Initiative at Weill Cornell Medicine, and author of *The Menopause Brain*, describes the bias as 'bikini medicine' – women have been medically considered as small men, but for their breasts and vaginas. 'Women's brain health remains one of the most under-researched, under-diagnosed and untreated fields of medicine. Not to mention underfunded,' she said. The majority of the clinical data on neurology, psychology and neurobiology focuses on men, and women, non-binary and trans people barely get a look in. We're almost in uncharted territory.

We have always known that brains change in our teenage years during the Puberty Reboot, as hormonal eruptions send emotions haywire. Because girls and boys have been studied together, we know quite a lot about this first major rewiring. In the early teenage years (or younger, as girls now get their periods at an average age of 11 or 12 in the UK and US), the brain undergoes a 'synaptic pruning' as the new tide of hormones, including testosterone, estrogen and dehydro-epiandrosterone (DHEA), alter brain structure and influence neuron growth. It's fairly simple: neurons are grey matter, which deals with processes like movement, memory and emotions. Synapses are pathways, the junctions between neurons. Triggered by increases in estrogen and testosterone, those synapses are gradually pruned throughout adolescence until around 40 per cent are lost, mostly in the regulatory frontal lobes. Obviously, this process is messy, and the emotional and risk-taking parts of the brain often alter ahead of the more sensible frontal lobes, hence door slamming and drug taking may well occur, along with unfortunate fashion and tattoo choices. But ultimately, when the chaos subsides, this leaves the teenage brain trimmed, focused and ready for adult life.

The Pregnancy Reboot is also a time of fascinating change, and the rather infantilising term 'Baby Brain' fails to convey the usefulness of these adaptations. During pregnancy, estrogen and progesterone hit between 15 and 40 times their normal level – hence that floaty maternal glow as the hormones increase blood flow and collagen in the skin, and at the same time, grey matter volume goes down by around 4 per cent in the run-up to giving birth. Most of that grey matter pops up afterwards in different places, usually within a year, particularly in areas related to social cognition and processing other's emotions and intentions. Basically, the changes make women smarter, better parents – and that specialised emotional understanding can help in other areas of life, including the workplace. The memory loss is temporary, as the brain's memory bank, the hippocampus, regains the volume that it lost in pregnancy. So within a few months, the capacity for memory is back, but those of us who have children know a lot of 'Baby Brain' confusion and memory loss can be blamed on exhaustion due to chronic lack of sleep. Hormonal and physical recalibration and recovery takes months, and this is also the time, often due to the overnight crash of hormones after giving birth and other factors, that post-natal depression appears in some mothers. That usually changes when hormones return to normal levels, but the grey matter changes remain, so much so that you can identify a 'mother brain' on a scan. These alterations are not a loss of function. Indeed this neuroplasticity may be an upgrade, a refinement of neural connections to support the demands of motherhood.

Once you've finished having children, that post-partum brain – or the original version – will head into the Perimenopause Reboot, the third and perhaps the most radical rewiring most women will undergo, a seismic neuro-endocrinological event that continues for up to a decade. When women are in their forties, the brain starts erratically losing two of its essential chemical messengers, the hormones estrogen and progesterone, which disappear almost completely when most women's periods stop around the average age of 51. (Premature ovarian insufficiency (POI) and surgical menopause create a much earlier deficit.) Female testosterone also slowly descends from our late twenties onwards, though it can linger for some women in small amounts in the brain and body into their sixties and seventies. A minority of women cope with this brilliantly, the ones who declare they 'sailed through' menopause. But for most of us, the major hormonal losses of midlife feel like puberty-gone-backwards – the tsunami of hormones that arrived as we entered our teens pulls back, leaving us high and dry, like fish flopping around and asphyxiating on a beach after the water suddenly disappears. No wonder our minds and bodies behave badly. Fear not, however. There are natural ways, including replacing your own, natural hormones, to survive this human climate change, but it's no wonder the medical term for menopause used to be 'The Climacteric'.

The Perimenopause Reboot can be extremely disruptive, with a long period of hormonal chaos leading to the loss and later recouping and redistribution of grey matter, which I'll explain in more detail later. What's particularly devious – and it's why I call perimenopause 'menopause's dastardly little sister' – is that hormones in our mid-to late forties are extremely erratic, and we don't necessarily know what's going on with them until our periods stop. We blame ourselves and our circumstances for failings, when the reality is that our hormones are often the culprits. You may have seen Pixar's *Inside Out* film, where the cartoon characters Fear, Anxiety, Joy and Disgust jockey for position in a girl's brain. Well, imagine the Midlife version of *Inside Out*, as the key characters joyful Estrogen and calming Progesterone mess around with each other for years and then storm out of the brain for ever, leaving mighty Testosterone, stressed-out Cortisol and dwindling Oxytocin and a few dregs of other hormones coping with the resulting chaos. It's not quite that simple, but understanding what happens when hormones leave your brain, and taking action, helps you to stay sane in the midlife transition.

In terms of how this manifests at the time, if you think of how mood disorders affect most women during Premenstrual Syndrome when progesterone and estrogen crash just before a period, then scale this up and you get a sense of what menopause might feel like; in particular, when estrogen goes from erratic to almost non-existent in the brain's hypothalamus, which regulates temperature in the body – hot flushes increase and night sweats disrupt sleep. However, as mentioned, hormones at this time are unpredictable, and there are also unprecedented estrogen highs that can cause energetic and creative leaps, or for some, the enjoyable 'perimenopausal sex surge' – all followed by sudden lows. The reason for this is that estrogen affects the 'feel-good' neurotransmitter serotonin, by increasing the enzyme that creates serotonin, and slowing down its resorption, so we stay happier for longer. When serotonin peaks, the brain is flush with joy and effervescent energy, and when it packs up, depression or low mood can take its place. Meanwhile, progesterone helps us sleep and stay calm, as it can enhance the activity of GABA, a neurotransmitter known for its relaxing properties. When progesterone goes into a grumpy downward slump, anxiety increases and the quality of our sleep decreases – it's harder to fall asleep and stay asleep. Progesterone is also the hormone that regulates the build-up of our womb lining, so its wayward behaviour is partly responsible for those flooding extra-heavy periods that turn up unexpectedly in perimenopause.

These hormonal shifts within the brain can leave us feeling physically and mentally diminished – I certainly did. Most alarming for me was when my memory went and I couldn't remember the names of people I knew well, or would sometimes forget why I had begun a sentence. 'Brain fog', reported by 73 per cent of women around menopause, is real. Estrogen is fuel for the brain, maintaining good blood flow, connectivity and neuroplasticity, and low estrogen means lower hippocampal (memory bank) activity. The phone-in-the-fridge trope pervades the perimenopause conversation online, and the Postcards from Midlife podcast even has a regular confessional for 'Brain-Fog Bloopers'. In Bridget Christie's brilliant midlife comedy series *The Change*, there's a rambling, foggy conversation between a group of women that ends with one saying: 'I couldn't remember what toes were called the other day. I called it a foot finger.' In my own neuroscientific nosiness, I asked women on my @menoscandal Instagram to send in their worst or funniest brain fog moments and I was inundated: 'Taking the dog's health supplements', 'Throwing my credit card and specs in the bin', and 'Going out with one black boot on and one brown one'. One woman confessed: 'Couldn't remember what a bicycle was called. Said to my son "one of those things you sit on and push the pedals".' Another revealed: 'Most recently it was sudden panic that I'd lost my mobile ... whilst I was talking to my friend on it.' The messages poured in. 'Forgot my own husband's name at a party.'

Car-related brain fog is in a special terrifying category of its own. I used to get sick with fear when I had to drive during perimenopause; I have never been good at knowing my left from my right under pressure and it took me three shots to pass my driving test, so it was reassuring to realise I wasn't alone: 'Not knowing which side of the road I should be driving on', is common, as well as 'Forgetting how to change gears', and 'Memory loss while driving – couldn't remember which was the brake and which was the gas pedal. Had to leave foot hanging in the air above them for about a minute on the autobahn!' There was a flurry of instances of 'Couldn't remember where I parked the car'. (You can track your car on your phone. Just a tip.) One woman kept 'Slowing down for green traffic lights', and another went to the petrol station to fill up, and 'instead of opening the petrol cap, I opened the back door and poured the petrol on to the seat'.

But while these mental aberrations might be joked about afterwards, at the time they often leave women feeling irresponsible and inadequate, and in unwarranted fear of impending dementia. Some of this loss of confidence, however temporary, plays out in the workplace, where one in ten women between 45 and 55 leave their jobs due to menopausal symptoms. For some, this is because they worried about the risks they might pose to others; one healthcare professional confided: 'I forgot which drug to prescribe to a patient. Used it all the time, for twenty years. Had to look it up.' Another woman reported how brain fog left her 'missing exits and turns in a city I've lived in for decades. Had to take months off work because between migraines and brain fog, I couldn't remember what my clients were telling me or articulate helpful feedback – and I'm a mental health therapist.'

Brain scans in perimenopause and menopause have recently and radically changed the way we think about brain fog and midlife memory, and groundbreaking research is being done by a team led by Dr Mosconi. Scans of a woman with a normally functioning brain in pre-menopause at 43 and postmenopause at 53 show in shocking full colour that average brain activity reduces by around 30 per cent over those ten years. The bright red and yellow patches indicating energy in the premenopausal brain turn to lower-energy green and blue in the postmenopausal brain later. 'The change in luminosity reflects a drop in brain energy,' said Dr Mosconi. 'Men of the same age do not exhibit similar changes.' The reason for this is a change in how our brains are having to fuel themselves. Before menopause, the brain is largely fuelled by glucose, with estrogen assisting in the process of converting that glucose to energy; when estrogen levels drop, the neurons still have access to glucose, but without estrogen transporters to help, they are not burning it as fast. As a result, the brain has to look elsewhere. While the brain ran on glucose before menopause, after menopause we have to pump up the blood flow to our brains instead. 'The menopause brain is in a state of adjustment, even remodelling, like a machine which once ran on gas is switching to electricity.' This change in the type of fuel is discombobulating. Brain energy levels stabilise a few years postmenopause, almost to previous levels due to increased cerebral blood flow, but that's no consolation if the disruption has shattered your career or relationship.

'It's not just brain energy that changes during menopause but that the brain's structure, regional connectivity and overall chemistry are also impacted,' said Dr Mosconi. Studies of women's brains, as opposed to men's of similar age, show that grey matter goes down in perimenopause, but, in better news, then makes a roaring comeback postmenopause, sometimes to even higher levels, according to biomarkers tracked by Dr Mosconi. (If you like a geeky read, her team's seminal article is in the journal *Nature* (9 June 2021). 'Menopause impacts human brain structure' is terrific, with literally mindblowing scans.) White matter, the communication network between different areas of grey matter, goes down from perimenopause onwards, seemingly levelling out postmenopause. We need more research into what happens in the decade after menopause, but at least we do know there is this bounceback of grey matter. 'Many lines of evidence indicate that women's brains have the remarkable, much underestimated, yet-to-be-celebrated ability to adapt to menopause,' said Mosconi. The message is that we are resilient – it's just the changeover that hurts. And at least the science confirms we are absolutely justified in having a massive midlife crisis, even becoming different people, and that the changes start long before periods end in menopause. This is scientific proof of what women have been saying for decades.

Generally speaking, most women handle this mental and physical chaos remarkably well, considering. Perhaps because we have always handled hormonal ups and downs in our monthly cycles, and got used to keeping calm, shutting up and carrying on. Society has a high cultural tolerance of women's suffering, particularly that of older women, and in some ways we have internalised that. Women have a long history of 'making the best of things', and that includes the postmenopausal brain changes, which many women see in a positive light. Perhaps there is a lingering feeling that it would not be feminist to do otherwise, but this is also backed up by the fact that grey matter seems to make a comeback for most after the chaos. Many people genuinely have a postmenopausal renaissance and report more contentment and greater intellectual clarity when hormones no longer play their erratic game. This could be partly because we no longer have so much emotional and physical labour to do looking after families, colleagues or ageing parents, but Dr Mosconi also wonders: 'It is plausible that possibly as the brain approaches menopause it gets another chance to become leaner and meaner, discarding information and skills it no longer needs while growing new abilities.'

Anthropologist Margaret Mead is often quoted as saying: 'The most powerful force in the world is a menopausal woman with zest,' and talking about PMZ – postmenopausal zest – in her later career during the 1960s and 1970s. She said: 'I think estrogen makes us willing to take big bites out of life, to take on problem-solving.' It should, of course, be noted that Mead, who was born in 1901, was cheerily topping up her estrogen with the pills available in the 1950s, long before hormone replacement therapy became part of everyday medicine – and, of course, for the majority of women who do not take HRT or indeed get the chance to, it still isn't. But whether HRT is an option for you or not, there are many encouraging examples of later-life female power: think of Diana Ross giving a magnificent performance at Glastonbury in 2022 aged 78, or Simone de Beauvoir tracking every stage of her life philosophy in her books, from *The Second Sex* at 49 to *The Coming of Age* when she was 70, or Jane Fonda executive-producing and starring in the sitcom *Grace and Frankie* in her eighties, or Ruth Bader Ginsburg who died at 87, still serving on the US Supreme Court.

In her 2006 book *The Upgrade: How the Female Brain Gets*

Stronger and Better in Midlife, neuropsychiatrist Dr Louann Brizendine said: 'Women's brains are reshaped, for the better, in a way that creates new power, a bracing clarity, and a laser-like sense of purpose if you know how to seize it.' For the first time ever, we are not acting on myths and hunches about our changing minds in midlife, but science and truth. Seizing that knowledge and using it for what we want to achieve is essential for the next act. You will be a different person, so how are you going to embrace that?

There is still so much we need to know about what is happening to our brains at this time, physiologically, and there's very little research going on, especially into the later post-menopause years. Brains scans are expensive, and studies of patients over a decade are even more so. However, some grants have gone into another hopeful project, MsBrain, led by Rebecca Thurston, chair in Women's Health and Dementia at the University of Pittsburgh. Her study looks at menopausal symptoms like hot flushes, cardiovascular health, sleep, cognition and brain ageing across ethnicities, and it seems that high levels of hot flushes are associated with poorer verbal memory, and night sweats with increased white matter hyperintensities, lesions which carry a dementia risk. Poor sleep and hot flushes seemed to pose more of a risk to the brain than mere low hormones,but then, as we've seen, low hormones can be contributing factors to both these symptoms – it's something of a chicken-and-egg scenario and more research is urgently needed to understand and mitigate the effects of shifting hormonal levels on the brain. We are, for example, lacking decent data on what testosterone does in the female brain, a potentially thrilling area of research, and I investigate that hormone further in Chapter 8, Reclaiming Testosterone.

Dr Mosconi's groundbreaking books *Brain Food* (2018), *The XX Brain* (2020) and *The Menopause Brain* (2024) unfurl an investigation over the years which focuses increasingly on hormones, including the positive possibilities for the brain of replacing them with HRT. Dr Mosconi and other neuroscientists have not yet been able to research what the brain on HRT looks like over decades, and I am part of the first generation to use the safer body-identical replacement hormones into our sixties and seventies. No one is scanning our brains yet, year on year, but I'll bet they look very different from those who have a permanent hormone deficit. What about the HRT users in the Gen X and Millennial cohort? How do their brains function on the better body-identical HRT? Will this generation be a new kind of human that didn't exist before, and lead a different, healthier and more engaged later life?

The UK government's Women's Health Ambassador Professor Dame Lesley Regan is 68 and on HRT, which she credits for her daily energy in a tough job. Oprah Winfrey is 70 and uses body-identical HRT, along with Michelle Obama, Naomi Watts, Kathy Lette, Davina McCall and Angelina Jolie. The UK's first female prime minister Margaret Thatcher stayed on the contraceptive pill right into her late fifties and then changed to an HRT patch. Make of this what you will, but I also hear from sources in the medical community that Queen Elizabeth partook of HRT, which might explain her upbraiding prime ministers and even riding a horse at 96. How important or unimportant are hormones for female power and longevity? Is taking HRT a no-brainer?

However, for those for whom HRT is not an option, there are lifestyle factors that can promote brain health during this transitional period and beyond. Aside from hormonal rewiring, there are other ways the brain changes, like responding to daily events, or trauma, or exercise, or the stomach microbiome. Dr Mosconi advocates the Mediterranean diet, for example, which improves brain health and decreases the biomarkers for Alzheimer's disease. Eating vegetables, fruit, berries, nuts and seeds and oily fish helps, as well as lashings of olive oil, which basically acts like WD40, lubricating the brain and body from within. Conversely, the scans show an American diet of fast and ultra-processed food diminishes brain health. (We'll talk more about this in Chapter 5, How to Dodge Dementia.) When you exercise, you pump blood to the brain and you make nerve growth factor (NGF), a special protein that helps brain cells grow, survive and work better, rather like a fertiliser. NGF helps regulate neurons in the brain and supports myelin, the neuroprotective sheath which can degenerate with age.

In terms of other preventative action, there is good scientific backing around meditation and mindfulness and how they don't only help improve mood and promote calmness, but also change the shape of the brain for the better in the long term. Again, we now have proof from brain scan measurements. For instance, after at least eight weeks of meditation, yoga or mindfulness, the amygdala, which helps with emotional processing, often reduces in volume: as stress levels lower, you chill, and it doesn't have to work so hard. These practices also seem to reduce recovery time for the amygdala, which returns more quickly to normal after negative experiences. After regular meditation, the brain areas regulating memory, self-reflection, spatial reasoning and decision-making also show increased activity, connectivity and volume. Whether it is a religious or secular practice, meditation or mindfulness, results are much the same: better emotional regulation and often an increased sense of well-being. As you know, you can download free apps or videos, and the meditation habit is a brain bonus that everyone might want to add to their midlife survival pack.

Dr Mosconi calls menopause 'a renovation project on the brain', and as we know, Grand Designs are far from straightforward, and it's hard to live among that hormonal remodelling for years, however improved the outcome. While the builders smash down and renovate around you, there's a lot of dust, noise and disruption, and it can be difficult to envisage the final spectacle. I lived on a building site for a year after my divorce, when I renovated an old, mushroom-filled, damp, sinking house into loveliness. That domestic chaos perfectly reflected my midlife brain; the house and I suited each other. And in some ways I don't regret being battered emotionally and physically by perimenopause and bareknuckling it, because I think the challenges and the failures and the falling changed me and my trajectory through life, made me more resilient – and empathetic.

Afterwards, when the house was finished – with gleaming floorboards, Farrow and Ball paint in colours like 'dirty sock', the sun pouring into the extension, and my cheeseplant growing like a triffid – I felt calm within its walls, and within my own psychological walls. Every morning I get up and I know what to expect of myself, and of my renovated mind: no surprises, no mood swings, no memory loss, no fog. My brain used to feel like a clapped-out banger, but now I feel like a brand-new electric car. I've got work to do in the world, and feeling mentally sharp and physically whole again has helped clarify exactly what that is.

CHAPTER 3

Could I Be Neurodivergent?

'Think of neurodiversity like biodiversity. There are different life forms of diversity across human brains, and environments that suit different brains. People think differently and interact differently. Being neurodivergent is not an illness but a lifelong difference, part of who you are.' That's how psychologist Dr Rachel Moseley explained neurodiversity to me. She is working with Professor Julie Gamble-Turner on a much-needed research project at Bournemouth University on the confluence of perimenopause and menopause with autism. People who struggle with being restless and finding it hard to concentrate sometimes find Attention Deficit Hyperactivity Disorder (ADHD) also gets diagnosed at this time. Around menopause it's a double whammy: those who have already been diagnosed on the neurodivergent spectrum often find perimenopause and its cognitive and hormonal chaos hits them like a truck. Other women discover as their hormones disappear in midlife that it leaves them with a stark clarity, or a chaotic crash, which often leads to a late-life diagnosis of neurodiversity. A diagnosis at this stage is a lightbulb moment for many women I've talked to, retrospectively making sense of a complicated past, and hopefully leading to better ways of coping in the future.

I don't identify as neurodivergent myself (although I did one of those 'Do you have ADHD?' quizzes online for research, and scored quite highly) but the subject came up time and again over the course of interviewing many women about their midlife experiences, and clearly merited further investigation. There has undoubtedly been an upsurge of diagnoses of autism and ADHD in recent years, particularly in women, often in later life. This is in part due to an increase in visibility and acceptance of neurodiversity; there is much self-diagnosing of neurodivergence on TikTok, with influencers explaining traits, and the hashtag is sometimes the celebratory #neurospicy. The often-surprising official or self-diagnosis of autism or ADHD or other forms of neurodivergence in women (and some trans and nonbinary people) in midlife, rather than in childhood, comes late because the screening tools were originally based on male models and female and other presentations remained invisible, or at least unobserved. 'From its very conception, autism described male cases,' said Dr Moseley, 'and it's a "young" diagnosis – Baby Boomers, Gen Xers and even Millennials wouldn't have been picked up early or in school. To generalise a bit, autistic girls look more socially normal, and somehow a shy, anxious little girl is seen as OK, whereas a withdrawn or disruptive, noisy boy gets attention. Often non-autistic children help hide the autistic ones, girls take them under their wing in primary school.' In secondary school there is an uptick in diagnoses for girls, when differences often stand out, and there can be a 'Mean Girls' moment where social life gets complicated and mental health problems begin. But many neurodivergent women fly under the radar until well into middle age – or even for their whole lives. And while we are finally seeing an increase in later-life diagnoses for women, it is still a struggle for many to get the recognition and acceptance of what this means. As women, we have become sadly accustomed to people (often men) having opinions on how we should present. Introducing neurodivergence into the mix can often amplify this barrage of unsolicited opinions.

Australian comedian and writer Hannah Gadsby was diagnosed as autistic aged 38, but it took a while: 'I was told I was too fat to be autistic. I was told I was too social to be autistic. I was told I was too empathic to be autistic. I was told I was too female to be autistic. I was told I wasn't autistic enough to be autistic. Nobody who refused me my diagnosis ever considered how painful it might have been for me, and it got really boring, really fast,' she wrote in the *Guardian*.

But even if other people might struggle to accept a diagnosis, it can be a vital step in the clarification of self-knowledge that many women experience in midlife. It's interesting to note that two years after her diagnosis, Gadsby shot to fame with the Netflix stand-up comedy show *Nanette*, which tackled and validated her lesbian, neurodivergent and gender non-conforming experience. 'It was difficult to believe that I wasn't entirely to blame for my life being such a painful struggle, because I was so used to assuming I was a bad person. It took me a long time to get brave enough to simply share my diagnosis. My experience did not match the popular understanding of autism, and I knew I had to become an expert in neurobiology in order to untangle the myriad myths surrounding autism – just to beg permission to claim that piece of my identity.' To do that in public is hugely encouraging for other women on the cusp of their own discoveries.

Gadsby found that people had strong opinions on what autism 'looks' like, many of which did not apply to her. But what is autism in its 'female' form, and is this a helpful question to ask? Labels are simultaneously redefining and confining, and it is important to challenge ourselves on why we feel the need to label something. In the case of autism, it can present very differently in males and females, and until this was understood, neurodivergent women were being chronically misunderstood.

In basic terms, Autism Spectrum Disorder involves 'challenges in social communication and interaction, along with restricted and repetitive behaviours'. In women, the signs can be more internal than external, so were traditionally less diagnosed. Autistic people prefer straightforwardness and clear communication. Sometimes there's avoidance of eye contact (but women are often very good at masking that by constantly forcing themselves to connect), and there can also be difficulty understanding others' feelings, the confusion making it harder to form friendships and relationships – or read the room at work. Gadsby has described being on the spectrum as feeling like an alien dropped in from outer space who can never quite belong and is constantly trying to translate the world around them: 'My neurobiological situation makes it hard for me to "see" all the networks of undercurrent connections that drive the interactions of the more typical thinkers, which in turn makes it incredibly difficult for me to intuitively reflect peer group behaviours.'

Some autism traits are of course shared across the genders, such as sensitivity to sensory stimulation, intense noise or vision. Many autistic people find that routine and consistency often help, whereas unexpected change can cause serious anxiety. This need for familiarity can also result in an obsession or expertise in a particular subject or activity. Repetitive body movements or constantly fiddling with something, known as 'stimming', are often soothing, as is the need for solitude and quiet to recharge after being in intense and busy social and work situations. Part of the exhaustion comes from masking in public, the effort of seeming as 'normal' as possible, when people with autism often feel they cannot truly be themselves.

Add perimenopause or menopause or the burdens of midlife to the complexities of autism, and you have a dangerous combination. 'People who are just managing to hold down a job and function suddenly find everything falls apart when hormones in the brain change.' It's a sort of electrical storm. 'They face job losses, lack of self-worth and sometimes even have to move back in with elderly parents,' said Dr Moseley. 'When the hormones estrogen and progesterone fluctuate and decrease, that influences the neurotransmitters involved in cognition and emotion like GABA, dopamine and serotonin. When we've got low levels of estrogen, we're more reactive to cortisol, the stress hormone that's heightened in people who have already had a lot of trauma and adversity. So neurodivergent people are more likely to struggle in menopause.'

The Bournemouth University survey of neurodiverse midlife women, entitled 'Autism research is "all about the blokes and the kids": Autistic women breaking the silence on menopause', revealed women talking about 'crushing tiredness and suddenly feeling I had the cognitive function of a 12-year-old', finding it harder to meet deadlines and plan, and sometimes falling into financial arrears. Burnout was prevalent, as well as anger and feeling overwhelmed. They reported a much higher level of distress around menopause than neurotypical people experience. People talked about depression and even suicide attempts. One autistic woman described menopause as 'life threatening'. GPs should be on high alert as neurodiverse patients, who are quite likely unaware of this, head into perimenopause in their forties – and sometimes, due to lifetime stress exposure, those patients have an earlier menopause. A diagnosis long before midlife's disruptions seems a good plan.

Rose Matthews from Durham discovered they were autistic at the age of 58, and also identified more recently as nonbinary. Rose has had a wide-ranging career as a police officer, a social worker, an academic and is now working part-time as a children's librarian and researching autism, loss and grief. But hormonal changes were a frightening wake-up call for them. 'I went through perimenopause with undiagnosed autism, and I was diagnosed in menopause. It got a heck of a lot worse immediately after my diagnosis. The two years post diagnosis were probably some of the hardest.' As a child, Rose was given the not always useful label of 'gifted and talented', and got a scholarship to a leading girls' school; Rose's academic ability may have been one of the reasons why no one spotted their autism-related struggles.

Rose has written a powerful essay in the journal *Adult Autism* about their midlife low point, 'The Night I Lost My Freedom, and Got It Back Again', worth reading in full on Rose's website, in which they explain how they ended up spending a night in a police cell: 'I should feel more frightened than I do. I am in shock. I think back to answering the door at home to find two police officers standing there. I did not think they were there because I had done something wrong,' Rose wrote. 'They told me it had to do with their domestic abuse policy, but I did not understand how that related to me.' Rose recounts sitting in a cell trying to unravel what had happened, knowing only that they had been 'overcome by a surge of emotion so strong I could not hope to control it. It terrified both me and my partner.' What exactly had happened following that loss of control that had led to them winding up in a police cell?

Rose was led to an interview room in the police station, where they asked to speak to the duty solicitor. After discussing their earlier outburst with the solicitor – and their confusion as to why all the kitchen knives had mysteriously disappeared from the house – Rose was able to fill in some of the gaps. Eventually, no charges were brought, and Rose was allowed to go home to their partner. 'He was frightened by my outburst and tried to get support. He did not want me to be arrested, but he had no say once the police got involved.'

Later, Rose went to see their GP and explained what happened, asking what could have caused this catastrophic loss of control. 'It must be more than stress at work. But she has no answer. A few weeks pass, and I go back again. "I'm having terrible problems with the menopause," I say.

'"There is something that might help," my GP responds. I wait expectantly.

"Time travel."

'It takes me a while to register the joke. I am crushed.'

That made me so angry. It's a tribute to Rose's extraordinary resilience that they fought on, and got HRT, which helped calm their mood swings. They didn't have the energy to persuade their GP to refer them for an autism assessment (this can take years on the NHS), so Rose went private and was seen in just three months. 'I sit in a high-ceilinged office, watching leaves dancing on a tree outside as a psychologist explains why autistic meltdowns happen, and how to keep myself safe,' they wrote. 'I think back to my arrest and wonder whether it would have been framed as "domestic abuse" if I had been known to be autistic? Would I have been diverted from custody and helped?'

Following a diagnosis of autism, Rose realised that aspects of their life had always been mystifying: 'Frequent job changes, few friends, sensory differences, meltdown, burnout, and being targeted by bullies and abusers were all finally explained when I discovered that I was autistic after unravelling in my fifties due to cumulative trauma.'

The 'autistic meltdown' Rose is referring to is very specific and can often involve uncontrollable responses and acute distress due to overwhelming sensory or emotional experiences. Rose continued, 'It's no exaggeration to say that the discovery of autism was life-saving. I've spent the last six years getting to know myself better, unlearning unhelpful habits I had developed trying to fit in. I live life autistically now, prioritising self-care and maintaining healthy boundaries.'

Discovering neurodivergence as an adult can be both an intense relief and a moment for grieving over past, previously unexplained, struggles. Dr Jay Watts is a consultant clinical psychologist and psychotherapist in London, and neurodivergent herself. She told me: 'I believe it's crucial to acknowledge and mourn the losses associated with being misunderstood, particularly for individuals who receive a late diagnosis. At the same time, I encourage my clients to celebrate and protect what makes them unique.'

As Rose told me their complicated life story, what kept coming up were moments where they questioned practices, or called out corruption or abuse at work, which ended in them being sidelined or having to move on to another job. They were often the whistleblower, ignoring norms of politeness and fitting in. 'So often my life was about getting new jobs, trying to be optimistic, thinking it'll work out this time, I'll avoid the office politics. I'll be much more circumspect.' Rose spotted past patterns more clearly when they got their diagnosis, and started seeing a psychotherapist who was himself autistic. 'I said I was trying to fathom out why I had changed jobs so frequently, why I had not persevered in these jobs. And he said what struck him was how I had stayed so long, given what I'd been through. So it gave me a different perspective.' This is a struggle for many; for another chapter, I interviewed my friend Zelda Perkins, who runs the not-for-profit Can't Buy My Silence, campaigning to end the use of employers' misuse of Non-Disclosure Agreements (NDAs) to buy victims' silence at work. Zelda said: 'I would say 80 to 90 per cent of the people coming to me who are unhappy about being forced to sign an NDA at work are neurodivergent in some way. They're often the whistleblowers, and they're much more black-and-white in their thinking on what's right and wrong. Because they're not reading emotional signals so easily, they'll call out something without thinking of the effect. There's integrity there.' In a way, that's an autistic superpower – but one largely unrecognised by society, where it is often perceived instead as 'being difficult'.

Rose also had other struggles: around toxic relationships, divorce and separation from their children. 'I suffered a lot of trauma, whereas if I'd had better self-esteem and self-confidence, and awareness of what constitutes a healthy relationship, that might have been different.' Rose is now happily married, and began to change their trajectory some time before they got their autism diagnosis. 'I actually set out in quite a deliberate way to find somebody who shared my values, who treated me respectfully, who wanted the same lifestyle.' The diagnosis has also been healing in their relationships with their adult children. Rose lives close to their daughter, and their son was also recently diagnosed with autism, which often has genetic links.

In another tale of late-life neurodivergence, Emma Heathcote-James, who lives in the Cotswolds, had no idea she had a combination of ADHD and autism until she had a breakdown in her mid-forties. Usually she needed a week or so to recover and could get through it but this one was exceptional – trying to juggle running a large business and team, she desperately researched how to help herself get better. She went privately for an ADHD diagnosis (something she'd always presumed she had), thinking an actual diagnosis could provide help and understanding of why she kept 'breaking' every few years. She also advocated to get HRT and went to therapy – it was only here, unmasked and at rock bottom, her autism was picked up. Emma said: 'For me the last few years have been a journey of self-discovery as I've navigated not just the onset of perimenopause symptoms but an ADHD diagnosis – which, let's face it, was not a surprise – but then a totally unexpected autism diagnosis to boot. Both having been hugely amplified by all the raging hormones. It's all been a learning curve and rollercoaster to say the least.'

Nothing's simple when it comes to how our brains work – least of all when they're rewiring during the midlife hormonal shift – and autism can involve just a few of the traits mentioned above, or it can overlap with Attention Deficit Hyperactivity Disorder (ADHD), resulting in AuDHD. But first, let's look at ADHD in more detail. As with autism, this has often gone undiagnosed in girls and women. In recent decades, while boys were getting diagnoses and stimulants like Ritalin at school to help control attention and behaviour, girls were once again camouflaging their symptoms. ADHD generally involves inattention, hyperactivity and impulsivity, which affects people's ability to focus and control impulses. For women, the traits often show up as forgetfulness and disorganisation, being 'scatterbrained' or overwhelmed, sometimes unable to concentrate on a conversation. The hyperactivity can be more verbal in girls and more physical in boys, although lots of women do find it hard to sit still, or keep engaged with a task.

On the upside, for some there is also the ability to hyperfocus intensely on a particular project for a time, which in Emma's case might explain her extreme and successful focus on the creation of her business, The Little Soap Company, which went from her kitchen table and farmers' market stalls to become the first all-natural organic soap in all the main supermarkets like Waitrose and Morrisons. (She sent me the Eco Warrior Shampoo Bar – no plastic bottles to recycle – and I use it after swimming at the Lido.) Emma won accolades like 'Top 50 Most Ambitious Business Leaders', 'Scale Up Business', 'Best Rural Retail Business'. 'My AuDHD brings an ability to super hyperfocus when I'm interested in something, and I can block out everything else if it's rewarding. In my twenties, I worked as a researcher in TV, film and radio and at the same time I did a PhD and published four books. Later on, I found similar stimulation and intensity around scaling the soap business.'

Emma was shocked when she got her diagnosis two years ago: '"I can't be autistic!" I said, when they told me.' But the cliché of rocking-in-the-corner autism is being blown apart by a more nuanced understanding of the different ways that autism and ADHD can present, particularly in women who are more accomplished at masking. 'What I've learned is that neurodiversity is like a colour wheel on a Mac,' and no one was looking for a complex manifestation years ago. 'We masked it so highly that we are a lost generation discovering we are ADHD or autistic.' Once she accepted her diagnosis, Emma realised that some of her difficulties – being so sensory sensitive, her extreme dyscalculia – meant her brain sometimes gets really overwhelmed and overstimulated, and she is stressed and unhappy in crowds. All were part of her neurodivergence, and understanding this meant that she could now find ways to work around these problems.

Emma's diagnosis came at a classic time for many women: the onset of perimenopause. Emma had always been hormone-sensitive; the contraceptive injection and pill made doctors question if she had 'borderline personality disorder' (something many autistic women are incorrectly diagnosed with) and she had raging migraines until she went on HRT. The hormonal shift that came in perimenopause exacerbated some of her ADHD and autistic traits. 'In perimenopause, I had no filter,' she says. 'That's when I really knew.' Professor Julie Gamble-Turner, a health psychologist working with the Bournemouth project, said that menopausal stress on the brain was a huge problem: 'Autistic people struggle with hormonal transitions ... They are more sensitive and easily dysregulated, dealing with strong emotions.' The load can be overwhelming when these changes come at a time when women are under a lot of mental pressure, caring for young families or ageing parents at home and fighting against the invisibility of menopausal women in the workplace. One thing we can do to lighten this load is to share it. Emma wrote about her double-neurodiversity diagnosis and perimenopause on LinkedIn: 'We all know it can be bloody hard at times working and juggling mental health and having weird things going on inside you that you have no control over, so I just wanted to put it out there and share in case this post helps you or anyone you know. It is a thing – you're not alone.'

Emma thinks there's probably an LGBTQI+ autistic crossover too – she divorced her husband and in 2016 married conservationist Dr Sharon Redrobe. Similarly, Rose was brought up female but some time after their diagnosis realised that they prefer to identify as gender fluid, neuroqueer, or non-binary. They felt a reconnection with their childhood 'when I asked to be called Jack, and in my teenage years, when I enjoyed wearing men's shirts and ties and waistcoats. I never identified with femininity.' Dr Jay Watts talks about looking into your past after a neurodivergent diagnosis as 'retroactive backgammon', examining the previous moves and seeing how they played out – and considering how the results might have been different with more self-knowledge. Her practice is proudly LGBTQI+ affirmative, and she modifies psychotherapeutic techniques to fit with the uniqueness of her clients. 'I focus on affirming neurodivergent identities and working with the challenges and strengths that each client brings. Diagnosis can be a retroactive assessment of life, and there's often a presumption that labels are good or bad. But isn't this emancipatory? A chance to unshackle oneself from expected scripts and stories.'

For Kristina Snell, a wedding make-up artist from Chelmsford, Essex, the possibility of having ADHD has rumbled on beneath the surface of her life since she was a teenager. At school in the 1980s, a teacher suspected she had attention deficit disorder, 'but I think they thought that I'd grow out of it. Being female, it was different, and it's been a lifelong struggle.' Aged 40, she now has feelings that remind her of being in puberty again, particularly those elements of being inattentive and hyperactive. 'I find it very difficult to stay in one place. I'm very up, down, up, down. Pacing around. Fidget, fidget. Squirming around. Different. I can't sit properly most of the time. I struggle to focus on anything that's mildly boring. The only thing that I can focus on is anything that's hands on. Anything that's practical, creative or rewarding. I can do a wedding job, and get through seven or eight people's make-ups because I'm hyperfocused. But anything else? I just feel like my brain is going to explode.'

I was actually interviewing Kristina about alcohol in midlife, and changing to better habits around that, when we got into a discussion about neurodiversity. She's planning to seek a professional diagnosis, but even now she questions whether she will be believed, a fear that many women struggle with. Then there's the difficulty of even getting an appointment. 'I'm probably going to go private, just because I don't have the strength to go through all the waiting,' says Kristina. I looked up the waiting times for ADHD assessments on the NHS, and the average wait in 2024 was approximately thirty to forty-four weeks, but it varies wildly around the country: from twelve weeks in Dorset to over ten-plus years in Herefordshire and Worcestershire. And while getting a private diagnosis is an option for some, the expense excludes many, particularly those who are already struggling with combinations of trauma, abuse, poverty, discrimination or disability.

Rose said they were aware it was 'a privilege' to get private help, and they spent an initial £150 to see a psychologist who then recommended a full autism diagnosis, which can cost between £1,000 and £2,500. They explained what it involved: 'Questionnaires for me, questionnaires for my parents, my siblings, my partner. They took a full history, everything I could remember from infancy onwards, and I was observed by two clinicians doing a series of tasks. One of them is to read a book that has pictures but no words. Another one was to be given three random objects and to make a story using the objects.' They found the testing exhausting. After a multi-disciplinary team meeting, psychologists concluded Rose was autistic. They felt intensely relieved, liberated, but it has taken a few years to write and talk about their autism in public and to overcome previous 'guilt and shame. It has taken me all this time to accept that I really was not to blame.'

I get the impression that for those who embrace their diagnosis, there is a cathartic moment when they question everything, and often set new boundaries with families, colleagues and friends. Or just do the things they have always wanted to do. 'I spend hours alone at home rearranging my little piles of bric-a-brac because it's really fun,' wrote Hannah Gadsby. 'I only wear blue clothes because blue makes me feel calm. I listen to the same music, watch the same shows, and eat the same foods over and over again without any qualms. I find joy in my life where once I couldn't because I was too busy trying to do the "right" thing.'

Could I Be Neurodivergent?

The dawning of neurodiversity can mean major changes not just for the autistic person but their partner too. Rose realised they were in a state of metamorphosis, no longer camouflaging themselves, and said to their partner, 'I think it's only fair to give you a kind of opt-out clause.' But he said he wanted to still be married, and they have been together for eighteen years. 'He bought me a unicorn cake to celebrate my diagnosis,' Rose laughed. They have negotiated other difficulties, like when Rose started getting the urge to live on their own, and didn't understand why. 'I can easily get dysregulated if I don't have enough solitude. If I go to a social event, I sometimes have to come and sit in a darkened room for several hours to recover.' After some counselling, the couple worked out Rose didn't want to leave, they just wanted more space within the relationship, practically and emotionally. So that meant they gave up having a separate study and a bedroom, and made each room into a study-bedroom, so they have their own private space.

Towards the end of our interview, Rose, now 64, gave a beautiful speech on her new-found freedom. 'I don't mess around trying to do everything in a non-autistic way. Now I just communicate authentically as myself. I'm autistic. I don't have autism, I am autistic. You know, it's just the way I am, and I love it. I wouldn't swap it. I have more sensory intensity. I have more joy. I'm constantly stopping to photograph things. I've become completely unembarrassed. When I'm on a train, I'm different from most other people. I can't understand why everybody else isn't at the window, just amazed at the sky.'

*

If this chapter raises questions for you, a relative or a friend, there are good resources out there for self-diagnosis, professional help or just to get a sense of the myriad forms neurodiversity can take. The National Autistic Society or Autistica are useful, as is the ADHD Foundation in the UK and *ADDitude* magazine online, as well as neurodivergent-led initiatives like the Square Peg Community. In terms of the chaotic crossover of hormones and neurodiversity, the National Autistic Society's 'Autism and Menopause' downloadable guide offers insights, coping strategies and treatment options. But thinking about what Emma said about neurodiversity being like 'a colour wheel on a Mac', I feel we need greater understanding and compassion for the extraordinary ways in which other people's brains might work – and we need to protect and nurture our own at this time of transition.

CHAPTER 4

How Not to Disappear at Work

It's carnage out there in the midlife working world, but you don't hear much about it. A combination of burnout, brain changes and boredom leaves women lost, itching for change, and walking out of their jobs. Female employees of a certain age tend to go quietly, but in a 4,000-strong Fawcett Society UK poll, one in ten 45–55-year-olds admitted they had left their jobs due to menopause symptoms. The decimation comes less as women are sacked, and more as they self-censor, go part-time, take early retirement or eschew promotion, and many are sidelined for younger colleagues as ageism takes a further toll. Others question whether they want to slog in the same old role for the next two decades. Midlife also seems to be the time when women get 'performance managed' out of their jobs too, given a set of not-always-achievable goals that are regularly tracked by bosses. All this might explain why, despite decades of supposed legal equality at work, in 2024 only eleven of the leading CEOs in FTSE 100 companies are female. Just as we reach out for the top, we are shot down by the triple whammy of menopause, ageism and gender bias.

We are the disappeared generation, and here I'm investigating one of the invisible contributors to that silence, particularly at executive or managerial level: the NDA or non-disclosure agreement. NDAs are often part of end-of-employment settlement agreements after a dispute or some kind of discrimination, and there's usually a pay-off. Of course, there are women who want to be able to leave employment under conditions of privacy and rebuild their lives, but for many the long tail of consequences of signing an NDA can be disastrous: a loss of career, a loss of confidence, a loss of business contacts, a loss of potential, and a sense of shame and failure. Because the dastardly thing about NDAs is that they are gag orders. Once you've signed an NDA you can't ever disclose that the NDA exists, in a brilliant piece of corporate and legal doublethink. You can never explain honestly why you left your last job, or you could be sued for significant damages. So the two women I've interviewed for this chapter remain nameless – an executive in a tech company and a GP, who were forced out of their jobs in midlife, and made to sign NDAs.

The infamous habitual issuer of NDAs was Harvey Weinstein, the Miramax film executive now in prison, who used the legal armour of NDAs to cover up rape and sexual assaults on colleagues in the movie business. Reaction to his trial helped grow the #MeToo movement, and my friend Zelda Perkins was the first former Weinstein employee to break her NDA in 2017. Her courageous whistleblowing helped to bring down Weinstein's whole sleazy house of cards, exposing years of bullying and sexual abuse of women. I met Zelda back when I was involved in the campaigning groups Women and Hollywood and Time's Up. Since the Weinstein legal case, Zelda went on to set up the not-for-profit Can't Buy My Silence, which campaigns to end the misuse of NDAs to stifle victims. This isn't just about sexual harassment, but wider issues too. 'NDAs were created to protect trade secrets,' said Zelda, 'but when they're used wrongly, they become secret settlement contracts used to buy the silence of a victim or whistleblower. They've become the default solution for organisations to settle cases of sexual misconduct, racism, pregnancy discrimination and other human rights violations.' And, of course, the heinous crimes of being over 50 or menopausal.

'Women sign NDAs at a much higher rate than men – biologically we're hit with NDAs twice in our life, at pregnancy and menopause,' said Zelda. 'One of the biggest misuses of the NDA is over maternity discrimination. Discrimination is unlawful, but most people don't realise that they can break their NDA in that case and speak out. Ninety per cent of people who come to us after signing an NDA say it has a catastrophic effect on their mental health, as well as their personal and professional confidence.' There is also a huge power imbalance: compare the lone employee with no legal aid to the corporate and legal might of banks, supermarkets, tech companies and big firms like Deloitte, KPMG and PwC, the triumvirate that recently featured in a *Financial Times* article exposing the misuse of NDAs. Zelda was also surprised to discover that the majority of those coming to ask for help from Can't Buy My Silence were probably neurodivergent in some way. 'It makes sense when you think about it, because people who are neurodivergent tend to not read emotional signals so easily, and they're much more black-and-white in their thinking of what's right and wrong. They don't worry about the effect of speaking up about something that's wrong. Because it's just wrong.' There's more in the chapter on neurodiversity on this.

The two women I interviewed had successful careers, and then faced health problems, which turned out to be surmountable, but showing even a sliver of weakness caused their employers to turn on them and push them out. There is also the complexity for many women in midlife of identifying what's going on in their heads, bodies and impossibly busy lives. Is it burnout or is it menopause, or a combination of the two? Obviously, for legal reasons we can only know one side of these NDA stories, but this is the lived experience of some very smart women, and it's worth listening to what they have to say.

Tasha (a pseudonym) left her job as an executive in an international tech company when she was 51, took a payoff, and had to sign an NDA agreement which included a clause preventing her from discussing the circumstances surrounding her departure. So here goes. Tasha was promoted to director level in her mid-forties, travelling around the world and making presentations, but she started experiencing menopausal symptoms shortly after her promotion. 'I still felt I could do the job, but I had really bad sleep. And

I remember waking up jetlagged in the US, getting terrible, terrible migraines, and having to do a major presentation early in the morning, to a big group of people and feeling, "I'm not going to be able to do this". So I had to be very disciplined.' The only thing that stopped the migraines was coffee, not conducive to sleep. 'Sometimes I couldn't focus, couldn't get words out, and had to write everything down. In the mornings, after constant loss of sleep, I was wrung out and filled with anxiety. But I still did the job.' I know what you're thinking – these are classic perimenopause symptoms, but just a few years ago no one knew what that meant, and the word perimenopause wasn't even on the NHS website at the time. Tasha went to her GP, who said it wasn't menopause and hormones at all, and suggested her life – two children, a busy husband, a major job – might be to blame. 'It was a tough ride to keep going with these changes in my ability to assimilate and retain information. I thought I was crap at my job. I suddenly started feeling absolutely terrified. It was a high-pressure environment, and I was losing confidence.' She did some research and began to think she was in peri-menopause. She tried herbal remedies, yoga and meditation. She also started HRT but found that she was progesterone intolerant so had to stop taking it. She realised she would have to battle through until her health improved.

But mention of menopause was taboo in a youth-skewed company that had just brought in some tech bros to run the show. 'These guys came in and they completely changed the culture, and it didn't feel like a safe space to talk about those kind of things because it was all about hitting the numbers. There was no room for emotional chat.'

Tasha held it all together for over a year in menopause, but her workload built up under the new aggressive regime, and there was shouting and bullying behaviour from her bosses, even online during Covid, and mostly directed at some of her younger male colleagues who were considered 'weak'. She eventually lost her temper at work. 'That was what in the end destroyed me. I was working so hard at not losing it. I was bottling it up so hard, and my husband was great at handling that at home, but at work it was a pressure cooker.' Her reputation for calm crashed. 'The company culture has become really toxic and was just not aligned with my values anymore.' Her husband suggested she left – it just wasn't worth the daily battle. 'I told the company I want to leave, and I deserved a package and they said yes. I said I was exhausted. I didn't make any mention of menopause – of course.' She took the compensation and signed the 'silencing' agreement. Clearly, the company knew something wasn't right in their treatment of her.

But the break and payout did give Tasha a chance to spend more time with her mother, who was in the final stages of Alzheimer's. 'I was really glad to do that. But it's like sniper's alley at this time in our lives at work and home, because it comes at us from all angles, doesn't it?'

Some months later, after her mother had died, Tasha found herself in a sort of limbo, questioning what happened. 'The impact the whole job loss had on me was only in hindsight,' said Tasha. 'It's so obvious to me now that the loss of confidence, the sense of myself disappearing, my fear of public speaking might have been to do with hormonal changes. The question I ask myself every day, which torments me, is how much of this was menopause and how much was everything else?'

Despite working for a major company, as is so often the case, menopause was not part of their private healthcare, and ageism was rife. Most of her colleagues were younger than her, and male, so she never asked for support, especially as she was managing a large team. 'Overall, it felt very isolating. I wanted to talk to other women at work and I didn't feel shame – more like I felt uneasy about talking openly about it. I didn't want to appear weak. If only I'd understood – at the age of 50, I'd freed myself from young children and I felt in my prime in so many ways, I was ready to work hard. You lose a bit of your identity at a time when you should be feeling in control.'

A short-term payoff does not replace a long-term career, and it takes resilience and guts to get back into the job market, especially when you can't say publicly why you left your previous post. But there's good news – Tasha got a new job for a few years at a tech startup, and her energy and drive came back. She's now feeling much better and considering the next steps for her revamped career. She's a survivor, but many are not.

Making a zinging comeback at this time of life is hard, and the Fawcett Society poll revealed that 61 per cent of women said that they had lost motivation at work due to their symptoms, and 52 per cent had lost confidence. Almost a quarter took time off work due to menopause symptoms, but the majority didn't admit to their employer that was why, with many citing anxiety and depression instead. Meanwhile, 14 per cent had gone part-time, and 8 per cent had not applied for promotion. For women in ethnic minority groups, the figures are worse, and those living with disability left work at double the rate of other women. Henpicked: Menopause in the Workplace reports that a quarter of employers have menopause policies now, so there may be some improvement, but anecdotally they say that even employees who are aware of menopause symptoms still struggle to get help from their doctors. When I'm out and about doing menopause talks, I always find that employees who work at companies with private health insurance seem to have a much better experience.

You'd think doctors would be brilliant at handling their own health – 'physician heal thyself' – but for Nadia (a pseudonym) a combination of ageism, gender bias and illness left her out in the cold, signing an NDA, with a tiny payout, after working as a GP at the same practice for thirteen years. She was taken on as the first salaried doctor by the partners who ran the surgery, and combined a successful career with raising two children. 'But when I was 42, I started to get anxious about stuff, and having weird migraines. It took a while for the penny to drop and I realised I needed HRT.' Things felt better. A few years later, the practice started the process of recruiting a new partner to join them. Nadia expected to be asked, but one of the other partners said: 'You're not interested, are you – you've got two kids at school.'

Then another blow came – Nadia found a lump in her breast and waited two weeks, worrying, for a biopsy. It looked borderline, and for eight weeks she came off HRT, including testosterone. 'I felt myself going backwards,' she said. But she applied to be a partner anyway, hoping the interview process would be delayed until after the medical tests were done. 'Instead, the interview and presentation were conducted quickly while I still hadn't got the all-clear on the breast lump, and I was trying to manage the "cold-turkey" coming off my HRT.' After the interview, she was invited into the partners' meeting, full of hope, but they said: 'We need someone younger for our financial security.' The partnership was offered to Nadia's much younger male colleague whom she had trained. Nadia went home in tears. 'It was hugely traumatic and humiliating, and I went on sick leave for four months. I didn't have it in me to fight, so they paid me off, just three months' salary, and I signed a gagging order so I couldn't talk about it.' She lost her NHS career and any further pension, and is now a self-employed (and brilliant) menopause specialist. 'My overwhelming emotion was grief. I walked out of the building one day and left my poor patients and colleagues, never to say goodbye. No one told them what was wrong with me.'

Nadia felt what had happened had left her with post-traumatic stress disorder, and she went to see a counsellor to explore the issues, and try to heal the damage inflicted on her self-worth. It's not just the economic loss of a job; suddenly becoming self-employed or freelance means women lose routines, workplace colleagues, their work email address, and their sense of purpose and identity can be obliterated. Work is where we spend the largest part of the day, often where we wield our power, and by the time we're in midlife what we do is sewn into our personalities and lives. Taking those stitches out can be incredibly painful, particularly when our tolerance for pain is undermined by hormonal changes. We expect new opportunities after our children leave home, and when that doesn't always happen, we lose status. One woman described her feelings as 'like reading your obituary over and over again'.

I got the lowdown in NDAs from Georgina Calvert-Lee, a barrister and employment lawyer at Bellevue Law in London, who specialises in employment litigation and deals with employer–employee settlement agreements, some of which may include a confidentiality clause. I asked her what employees should do when an NDA is inserted into their settlement. 'It's always possible to resist an NDA. You don't have to sign it. However, in reality there is a disparity of power between an employer and an employee. If you're about to lose your job and your employer is offering you a bit of money to ease the pain until you find another job, and they threaten not to carry through the settlement agreement if you don't sign the NDA, then that's hard. It's up to you as an individual to weigh up the risks.'

It's not easy to take a claim to an Employment Tribunal if you feel you've been wrongly dismissed, because there is no legal aid available. 'Access to justice is so incredibly difficult for individuals who are not already wealthy, although you can represent yourself,' said Calvert-Lee. 'You occasionally hear these amazing stories of people who have gone through four years of employment tribunal litigation and done it themselves. But it's not very consumer-friendly or easy to navigate. And employment law has become incredibly technical, just like any area of law.' The system is unfairly biased towards the might of the employer, although there have been a few successful claims for menopause discrimination, but they are rare, and often only go through with financial backing by trade unions. What often happens in settlement agreements is that the employer provides the employee with a 'fair' fee for a consultation with an independent lawyer. 'But it's maybe £350 or £500, which doesn't get you very much advice.' Calvert-Lee said she often has extensive conversations when her clients are working out a settlement, getting their entire employment history, and advising them on any possible claims against the employer, plus, 'Sometimes reading the settlement document properly takes an hour in itself.' A decent legal consultation will probably run into thousands of pounds, but it might be worth it in the long run for a better settlement, and to avoid a confidentiality clause, which makes the next career steps hard to take. 'Sometimes a client is prepared to accept an NDA, so long as they are able to say something authentic about why they left their job, and so I help advise them on what they might want to say going forward, what their public story is going to be, and then see if it can be agreed with their employer.'

While NDAs became normalised, part of the contract template, that habitual use by big companies may be changing, said Zelda. 'I think, thanks to media coverage, NDAs are increasingly seen from the outside as a red flag.' The recent use of NDAs to cover up the UK Post Office scandal and the sexual assaults on employees at Harrods in the Mohammed Al Fayed case are salient examples. The NDA and pay-off system also enables ageism – invisible but rife. 'I think ageism is one of the last protected characteristics that people are ashamed of, so often they don't mention it,' said Calvert-Lee. 'It's amazing how people don't acknowledge age, and it will take me to point that out – look at the facts: there's a younger person coming in. Employers are not even ashamed of saying, "we need younger faces" because they feel that's great.'

Then there is the fact that if you're older, it's often harder to get another job because of the societal pressure. We know the prejudice around ageism is worse in certain industries, like television, film and the media, particularly for reporters, actors and presenters. I was giving a speech on the menopause at Newcastle University and at dinner afterwards I met the engaging and revolutionary Professor Karen Ross, who has been studying age discrimination against women at work, particularly in the media. In her paper 'Gendered ageism in the media industry: Disavowal, discrimination and the pushback' in *The Journal of Women and Ageing*, Professor Ross wrote: 'There was a clear recognition that women who work front-of-house as presenters or actors are significantly more vulnerable to the unrelenting and socially pervasive myths about beauty and age, than women who mostly work behind the scenes in the newsroom or in production.'

The 'past your sell-by date' problem only seems to affect women. Professor Ross cites the case of Miriam O'Reilly, the *Countryfile* presenter whose contract was cancelled at the age of 53, while her equally mature male co-presenters stayed on. Miriam subsequently took her case to an employment tribunal on the grounds of sexism and ageism and was awarded an estimated £150,000 in damages against the BBC. The BBC had offered her a smaller compensatory award, around £80,000, but she would have had to sign an NDA and she wanted her case to have a public airing. In the end only the ageism claim was upheld. Afterwards, Miriam said: 'I won my case, but I lost my career. I had some work afterwards but not very much. I regret that the BBC behaved in the way it did. But I don't regret my behaviour. I would do it again in a heartbeat because it was the right thing to do. It was absolutely the right thing to do.'

Women also lose out if they're on a final salary pension scheme, and we're in a worse position on retirement as our pots are on average half the size of men's (£12,000 p.a. versus £26,000), and many of us have taken a career break due to family responsibilities without realising the long-term financial impact it would have on a private pension.

As Professor Ross points out, gendered ageism is 'scarcely a new phenomenon', and while there are a few women over half a century old thriving on screen, including their patron saint, historian Mary Beard, there are thousands more who have 'crashed and burned at the hands of their (often younger, often male) managers, not because of a sudden loss of professionalism, experience, competence, expertise or audience pulling-power but because they are deemed to no longer look the part'. Often this is a conscious decision made by (male) managers, but sometimes not. It is possibly that there is a subliminal difference between the way men react at work to women who are still fertile, and those who are postmenopausal; we know a man's testosterone rises a tad when he is near an ovulating woman, whether or not she's their partner. It could be that this evolutionary trait plays out invisibly and unintentionally in the office.

There's also the fact that when women are no longer flooded by the cheerful, caring hormone estrogen and the calming hormone progesterone, they might become tougher decision-makers, more likely to get straight to the point without smiling. A bit like men. Interestingly, research into academics' long-term employment assessments in the journal *Organizational Behavior and Human Decision Processes* showed that both men and women are perceived as more capable or effective as they get older, but only women are seen as less warm as they age – causing them to be judged more harshly. They found that male professors' evaluations for teaching performance by students remained consistent over time, but evaluations for female professors quickly declined from their initial peak in their thirties, hitting a low point around the age of 47. After that, they steadily increased again, achieving parity with men by their early sixties. 'At that point, there are different stereotypes of women, and they may benefit from being seen as more grandmotherly,' said the researchers. Lover, mother, grandmother – those still seem to be the subliminal perceptions of women at work, and hard to overcome.

It's not all negative. Awareness and attitudes are shifting – even if not fast enough or radically enough. Being frank and direct with your employer about mental and physical health issues and menopause may be a much easier approach than it was in the past. Acceptance of menopause is changing; a taboo is now a conversation, just as happened for mental health at work. I've done some brainstorming around menopause at the huge international company Accenture in London with executives Jill Ross, Leigh Walters-James (a male ally!) and Sarah Garton, who are all members of the company's MenoWarriors group. Recently, Sarah, who's a managing director now working in India, appeared on the Middling Along podcast with the confession: 'I outed myself as menopausal – and my career took off.' Instead of ruining Sarah's career, it supercharged it. 'Being open about my struggles – brain fog, hot flushes, the lot – opened doors. It strengthened relationships, built trust, and showed me that vulnerability isn't just brave – it's transformative.' We need that kind of honesty to bust the culture of shame and secrecy at work, so women in midlife can thrive.

Even if we do find ourselves leaving a job – by choice or otherwise – it is not the end of the road. Being forced out sometimes forces us to metamorphose. I was the film critic at *The Times*, and within a few years of leaving aged 53, I became a documentary filmmaker and women's health campaigner and writer, and this year I'm starting a novel. Why the hell not? My reckoning is if you keep zig-zagging, they'll never catch you. (On the other hand, I'll probably never have a full-time job with a pension again.) My partner Cameron has given up being a barrister and is retraining as a psychotherapist, and his course is full of people who have pivoted career in midlife. I know so many people in my generation who have retrained, re-aimed and rebooted their careers in completely different directions as caregiving and domestic labour gets out of the way and they look to the future. And it turns out that 50-plus women are also 'the new entrepreneurial superpower', according to a recent *Forbes* article, as the magazine launched the '50 Over 50' list of women entrepreneurs, leaders, scientists and creators in an eruption of power suits.

Striking out in your career in your forties or fifties might seem scary, but there are ways to manage it. You have built up massive resilience over the years, and networks of colleagues and friends rich in advice and connections – ask for support and propulsion. To make the great leap forward, it's often worth doing one of those career quizzes, getting a session with a career coach, or visualising yourself in five years' time doing something phenomenal. If not now, when? As someone once said: 'Your shit is your superpower', and everything you've been through in the last half century probably makes you wiser and stronger.

CHAPTER 5

How to Dodge Dementia

This chapter is deeply personal for me. I'm a daughter of Alzheimer's on my mum's side, with a heightened risk of getting the disease, and a daughter of vascular dementia on my dad's side. It's a double whammy, so my job right now is to get hold of the best, evidence-based information – and share it with those at risk. Of course, there are no guarantees, but in this chapter I've compiled some damn fine advice – backed by the latest science on hormones, exercise, supplements and nutrition – on how to avoid Alzheimer's disease and dementia, or at least reduce the risk. Don't flip to the next chapter thinking this is not a midlife issue. It is, doubly, for those of us looking after relatives with Alzheimer's, and for women in their late forties onwards, because perimenopause is Alzheimer's ground zero. Midlife is precisely the time when we need to take action to avoid Alzheimer's. Any tiny brain changes and memory loss you notice now are a wake-up call for the future. The two most common kinds of dementia are Alzheimer's disease and vascular dementia, which is caused by a clogged-up circulatory system reducing blood flow to the brain. Both dementias sow their seeds of destruction early, long before we are even aware of any changes. But there is good news – many of these risks are often preventable, as we shall see.

I spoke with Professor Roberta Diaz Brinton of the Center for Innovation in Brain Science at the University of Arizona. She told me, 'Alzheimer's disease risk begins in midlife during the menopausal transition.' The fall of the hormones estrogen and progesterone in perimenopause is associated with an increase in amyloid plaques and tau tangles in some women's brains. Imagine plaque coating your teeth (amyloid plaques) and add a messy tangle of used dental floss (tau tangles), and you can get a sense of what's slowly happening inside your head if you're at risk of Alzheimer's, years before any symptoms appear. Or perhaps it's easier to think of it as your brain failing to clean up and take out the recycling at night. This may sound alarming, but you can take some comfort in the fact that you are in the first generation that has scientific information on how to take action on all fronts – medical and holistic – to prevent or slow down future dementia.

Alzheimer's disease and vascular dementia are the biggest cause of death for women in the UK. Two-thirds of Alzheimer's patients are female. Look round a roomful of your female friends or colleagues and know this: one in five of them will get Alzheimer's, unless we radically change medical and nutritional advice right now. Black women are nearly twice as likely to get Alzheimer's as white women, probably due to long-term racial and economic inequalities. Hormone-starved women in early menopause or younger women who have their ovaries removed are more prone to early dementia unless they start hormone replacement therapy. The staggering and continuing growth in female Alzheimer's coincides with our growing post-reproductive lifespan, the many years we spend deprived of hormones, added to bad lifestyle choices. This is a massive economic and public health issue. The costs of care and the emotional burden on carers means that whole families suffer for years, not just the patient. Recent studies indicate that more than four million Americans are affected by Alzheimer's. The annual cost of caring for these patients is estimated to be over $100 billion. By 2050, at least 14 million Americans will suffer from this disease, and two million in the UK.

The fact that billions of pounds has already gone into research on Alzheimer's without looking at the hormonal component in our brains is not merely shortsighted, but perhaps the prime example of egregious gender bias in medicine right now. Only now are we beginning to see relatively tiny amounts of funding going into research specifically on women and their hormones. As is so often the case in medicine, the focus of Alzheimer's research up until now has been on sickness-care rather than preventative health-care, but this is finally starting to shift. Research into the hormonal component of Alzheimer's is one of the most exciting and hopeful areas of medicine, as pioneering female scientists take up the challenge and bring the conversation to tipping point. And this research is already throwing up ways that we can take action in midlife to protect ourselves in later life.

Before I go into detail of the ways women – and men – can massively reduce their risk, I want to tell you a story about Ella Muir, my mum. She worked as a fur-coat buyer for Universal Stores (when fur was still a thing and her squirrel bolero jacket was not only acceptable but covetable) before becoming a personnel manager in Stirling Glens department store in Glasgow. Then, in retirement, she trained as an advisor in the Clydebank Citizen's Advice Bureau. So Ella was always sharp as a stiletto, and she walked so fast on her high heels that people knew she was coming just by the sound. Tiny and energetic, she was somehow the last person you would expect to get Alzheimer's. But she did, in her early eighties, and in the initial stages when she knew her mind was failing, she started drinking heavily for the first time in her life. Conversations became like Möbius strips, her worried questions repeating ad infinitum, time losing its meaning as she paced round the flat in the night. Ella was deeply unhappy, though she wouldn't discuss what was happening. Eventually, she no longer understood. It was awful.

The next few years were spent rolling from crisis to crisis, with me on emergency flights up to Glasgow as Ella ended up in hospital after falls or due to illness, increasingly muddled and frail. While she had lots of genteel mini wine bottles from Marks & Spencer's in her recycling, I was necking football-sized glasses of Chardonnay in the airport bar on the way home to take away the stress of visiting. The local authority care system was byzantine, and a different carer turned up every day to check on Ella and make sure she'd washed and eaten. Naturally, my mum couldn't remember who on earth these strangers were and often wouldn't let them in the door. Eventually, I got a direct payment from the council, topped it up, and recruited a newly retired professional carer, Helen, who was brilliant and came every day, with a substitute at weekends. Helen looked after my mum and helped her stop drinking – or forget about it altogether – and all was as well as it could be until Ella had a final hospital emergency with a urinary tract infection, and was so disorientated she refused to eat, and sometimes walk, so we had to arrange for a place in a nursing home. There, Ella seemed contented, perhaps knowing no better.

Like many other children of Alzheimer's, I searched desperately for a solution, for any information, for my mum – and for my future self. Over the years, I read academic papers, interviewed doctors and researchers, and examined everything the internet spewed out on Alzheimer's and women. Eventually, in a too-late moment after my mum had died, I realised that hormones were probably the villains – and could have been the saviours – in the story. Fixing the hormones, along with other midlife health changes that I will also address, might help protect against Alzheimer's even if you're in the quarter of the population that is a carrier of the late-life Alzheimer's gene variant known as APOE4. Carriers of one APOE4 variant have three times the risk of Alzheimer's of those without, and two copies of the variant raise the risk to eight times or more. But all is not lost.

I wrote briefly about the leading role of hormones in Alzheimer's disease in my previous book *Everything You Need to Know About the Menopause,* but excitingly, even in the three years since I wrote *Menopause,* there's a raft of new research. Major work is being done at Weill Cornell Medicine in New York by neuroscientist Dr Lisa Mosconi, who is director of the Alzheimer's Prevention Program there. Not coincidentally, her grandmother and her two great-aunts all suffered from Alzheimer's. Her great-uncle did not. Understanding why women have a higher risk than men has become Dr Mosconi's life's work, and her revelatory 2024 book *The Menopause Brain* investigates it all.

Quite simply, hormones keep your neurons up to speed, enhancing cognitive function and preventing inflammation. Dr Mosconi says estrogen is a 'master regulator' in the brain, playing a key role in our use of glucose as fuel for the mind. When that energy goes, chaos can ensue. There's good news for some men too – low testosterone is also implicated in male Alzheimer's, so it's worth men topping up their testosterone as a protective measure. Dr Mosconi's team undertook a meta-analysis of the effects of HRT on dementia published in the journal *Frontiers in Aging Neuroscience* in 2023. They looked at a huge data set compiled over several years: six randomised controlled trials where either the HRT drug or a placebo was given to over 40,000 women, and 45 observational reports, which contained over 750,000 patient cases. The results overall were a 32 per cent reduced risk of dementia for women who used estrogen-only therapy, and 23 per cent reductions for those who used estrogen and progestogen therapy. Late life use of HRT had a tiny statistically non-significant increased risk of dementia, but it's worth noting that the majority of those studies were on the older, synthetic, oral HRT taken by older generations. Dr Mosconi explained: 'What I find interesting is that in all of the studies we examined that found a negative association ... the women were on a synthetic form of progesterone [progestin],' Dr Mosconi said. 'There is some evidence that bioidentical progesterone is safer, and that synthetic progestins are what's driving the increased risk.' The new body-identical or bio-identical HRT contains progesterone and has shown good results in some big observational studies, but as Professor Brinton points out, not enough women have been on the better transdermal HRT for long enough, as it is a relatively new preparation, so there should be more news in the next decade.

Dr Mosconi also says timing really matters, the optimum 'window of opportunity' is in perimenopause or early menopause when the estrogen, progesterone and testosterone receptors in the brain are still healthy and hungry for hormones. She did brain scans of over fifty women and discovered that the perimenopausal and postmenopausal brain (when not on HRT) grew more estrogen receptors than before – perhaps out of hormonal starvation – and the biggest increases in receptor density correlated with worse memory. 'Hormones work best for the brain when taken in midlife, in presence of menopausal symptoms,' she told me. Starting body-identical HRT later won't reverse damage that has already occurred, but as soon as it is started it will help prevent those nasty amyloid plaques and tau tangles from building up any further, and will also improve your sleep, which is brain-protective in itself.

There's an interesting MsBrain study in 2024 in *The American Journal of Obstetrics and Gynecology* which showed the more night sweats women had in menopause due to low hormones, the more likely they were to have harmful amyloid plaques in their brains. The findings were not explained by varying age, ethnicity, education, body mass index, APOE4 status or sleep, although sleep is also key to brain health. Sleep allows the brain to clear out toxic waste, flushing out those amyloid plaques, and it also helps consolidate memories. But even if you were tackling all the other possible lifestyle changes to encourage sleep and good health, why wouldn't you want to stop those insidious night sweats and daytime hot flushes clogging up your brain? (And if you can't take hormones, it's worth considering the other flush-lowering options like CBT and CBD, or the new drug fezolinetant detailed in the Ageproof Yourself with HRT chapter.)

There's an important observational study of the effect of HRT on the risk of Alzheimer's, done by a team in 2021 which included Professor Brinton, who has been studying the effects of estrogen on the brain for over thirty years. The study took the health insurance records of nearly 400,000 women in Kentucky over the age of 45, comparing those on HRT to those without, over the course of almost a decade. Women on HRT were up to 58 per cent less likely to develop neurodegenerative diseases including Parkinson's and Alzheimer's, and those taking it for six years or more were 79 per cent less likely to develop Alzheimer's. The longer women stayed on HRT, the better for their brain health. 'The key is that hormone therapy is not a treatment, but it's keeping the brain and this whole system functioning, leading to prevention. It's not reversing disease; it's preventing disease by keeping the brain healthy,' said Professor

Brinton when the study came out. 'With this study, we are gaining mechanistic knowledge. This reduction in risk for Alzheimer's disease, Parkinson's and dementia means these diseases share a common driver regulated by estrogen, and if there are common drivers, there can be common therapies.' There is also a tiny study over three months of forty-three women in the early stages of Alzheimer's which showed that transdermal estrogen improved cognition in naming and visual memory.

More research is needed into the use of HRT in midlife for reducing the risk of Alzheimer's disease. Of course, the big pharmaceutical companies are not rushing to pour millions into a twenty-year study of women on HRT or placebo, because hormones are products of nature, from our own bodies, and neither patentable nor profitable in their simple forms. Hence there is still a medical orthodoxy in some corners that says HRT does not help with dementia, since we don't have a giant randomised controlled trial, the gold standard for research. Even if there was one, I'm certainly not waiting for twenty years, forgetting my car keys every day, to see the results when I know that HRT is good for my body in so many other ways.

Neuroscientists are on the case in the US, less so in the UK. While the Women's Alzheimer's Movement in America funds gender-specific research like Dr Mosconi's, Alzheimer's Research in the UK fails to mention hormones or menopause in the headlines for their latest projects. Why? It's great that wider research is being done, but surely, *surely*, prevention by looking after brain health earlier is better than cure, especially when 'cures' like the amyloid immunotherapy drugs donanemab and lecanemab were largely dismissed in a Cambridge University report because the effect was so small, the side effects were so serious and the drugs were so expensive. Some of the approved drugs suffer from old-fashioned sexism too: the new leqembi drug 'slowed cognitive decline' by 43 per cent in men but only 12 per cent in women. That's not a cure. That's an inadequate braking mechanism – and a drug with an unpronounceable name.

Dr Richard Isaacson, director of research at the Institute for Neurodegenerative Diseases in Florida, told CNN: 'While there is not a clear one-size-fits-all approach, in the right woman, at the right dose, and for the right duration of time, I believe that hormone replacement therapy can be one of our most powerful tools to reduce a woman's risk for cognitive decline and to slow down Alzheimer's pathology. I believe this may be especially true for women with one or more copies of the APOE4 genetic variant, which is present in about 25 per cent of people. It's essential for neurologists and primary care physicians to work closely with gynaecologists and monitor treatment outcomes over time.'

Encouragingly, it looks as though hormone therapy may be particularly helpful for carriers of the APOE4 variant. A small study of 244 healthy women in the journal *Alzheimer's and Dementia* in 2022 showed that starting HRT lowered the bad biomarkers in the brain – amyloid plaques and tau tangles – and they reported that: 'Women at genetic risk for Alzheimer's Disease (carrying at least one APOE e4 allele) seem to be particularly benefiting from Menopausal Hormone Therapy.' The longer the exposure to HRT, the more neuroprotective it was. I can't tell you how much that cheered me up.

Having the APOE4 genetic variant means you are at higher risk of late-onset Alzheimer's disease like Ella's, and only around 1 per cent of people inherit another mutation in genes which causes early-onset Alzheimer's. This is not to say that carriers of either gene will necessarily get Alzheimer's. Lifestyle and habits can outweigh genetics. The Lancet Commission published a 'landmark' report in 2024 on all kinds of dementia including Alzheimer's, naming nine factors that could increase dementia risk – and completely failed to discuss the important role of hormones and HRT in prevention. The lead authors were mostly psychiatrists. The other factors are obviously worth looking at, especially if you cannot take HRT, and everyone should be adding lifestyle changes to their brain protection plan. The nine risk factors were: low education, smoking, depression, lack of physical activity, social isolation, high blood pressure, hearing loss, obesity and diabetes. Lifestyle improvements matter like sleeping well and lowering stress, and looking at 450,000 people in the UK Biobank database, researchers found that higher lean muscle mass was linked with a 12 per cent lower risk of Alzheimer's. That could be due to a healthier lifestyle, but exciting new research in 2024 shows that resistance training (weight lifting) specifically causes structural brain changes in older adults that could reduce the risk of Alzheimer's or mitigate its progression.

On nutrition, Dr Mosconi has also written a book worth checking out, *Brain Food: How to Eat Smart and Sharpen Your Mind,* which advocates a Mediterranean diet. That diet of seafood, wholegrains, nuts, fruit and vegetables could lower the risk of dementia by almost a quarter, according to a recent study from Queen's University Belfast. The Alzheimer's Society analysed sixteen studies and found that regular exercise reduces the risk of developing dementia by 28 per cent and, specifically, Alzheimer's by 45 per cent. So grab your fish oil, your weights and your running shoes and take action.

How to avoid vascular dementia

When it comes to avoiding most cases of vascular dementia, things are simpler: caring for your heart and circulation means you are caring for your brain, and there's lots on cardiovascular health in the Ageproof Yourself with HRT chapter. Vascular dementia is usually caused by mini-strokes and strokes, when there's a sudden blockage of blood supply to the brain, usually due to a blood clot, and also by a narrowing of blood vessels deep inside the brain over time. High blood pressure, which can be lowered by lifestyle changes or statin drugs or sometimes HRT, and physical blockages like malfunctioning heart valves, all contribute to an increased risk. Basically, you want free flow, and no blockages. I had a real-life vision of the disease when I was at the Museum of London some years ago and saw a section of the giant beige Fatberg, a hardened mass of congealed cooking fat (plus the occasional condom and wet wipe) which had completely blocked a 250-metre section of the massive sewage pipes underneath the city, causing back-up and flooding. It was fascinatingly disgusting, and a social media sensation. I realised exactly the same process is happening to our human pipes as we fill ourselves up with trans fats in fried takeaways, in biscuits, in pies, all those ultra-processed foods that cause high cholesterol, leaving fatty deposits that stop or slow the flow in your blood vessels, leaving you short of fuel. In our arteries, the inner lining is called the epithelium, and this is damaged by cholesterol, high blood pressure or smoking, allowing plaque to build up and causing arteries to narrow. When the flow slows in your brain, even by 5 per cent, your mental processes become sluggardly.

In many ways, this is an easy one to tackle, for example by swapping a bucket of fried chicken for something featuring vegetables, lean protein and a dousing of good fat, like olive oil. We all know the foods that are good and bad for the gut–brain axis, but there are other variables. Exercise is also terrific for the brain, because when you do cardio of any sort, you secrete a nerve growth factor that helps brain cells to grow, survive and stay healthy. It helps fix damaged brain cells and grow new connections. Running keeps your brain running, and occasional sprints are even better. A study of over 150 patients over six months showed that those who did high-intensity interval training (HIIT), rather than just daily exercise like walking, had quantifiable improvements in memory – the HIIT helped preserve brain volume, particularly in the memory bank of the hippocampus.

Then there are the benefits of kicking bad habits, like smoking and drinking heavily. My dad, Douglas Muir, appeared in really good health at first glance: he ate well, was slim, and rode a bike for miles into the Campsie Hills in his early sixties, but he had an epic smoking habit. He had managed to go down from 40 Players Untipped a day, to 20 Benson & Hedges, to 20 'low tar' Silk Cut on the day he had a stroke at the blackboard while teaching engineering at Coatbridge Technical College near Glasgow. Douglas was 63, and though the stroke left him disorientated, he had no long-term physical damage that we could see on the outside. He retired, grumpily quit smoking, and began walking and biking again. For over a decade he did really well, but smoking speeds up the narrowing and clogging of coronary arteries, and the damage was previously done. In his late seventies he had a series of mini-strokes, transient ischemic attacks (TIAs), which could strike at any moment; sometimes they'd happen terrifyingly at night when he was sleeping beside my mum. TIAs cause tiny but widespread damage to the brain over time, and he started to have trouble walking and remembering things, as mild vascular dementia set in. Unlike my mum with her later-onset Alzheimer's, my dad always recognised me when I visited, although one time when I visited him at his nursing home, he looked up puzzled and said: 'Who are you?' – but I'd cut my hair and mistakenly dyed it purply brown at the time, so the question was fair enough. We agreed it was still me. Douglas died aged 86, and a week or so before, he'd had enough of it all. 'I'd like a bus to come along so I can just get on it and get out of here,' he said, from his wheelchair. 'You know what I mean.'

It was unbearably sad, but the better news is that vascular problems are, to some extent, reversible unless there's permanent physical damage. You can flush out the Fatberg and often lower cholesterol with lifestyle choices. Again,

HRT through the skin can help keep the endothelium or the artery lining smooth, and one study showed it improved blood flow in postmenopausal women, both those in good health and for those with coronary artery disease. In an observational study of nearly half a million Finnish women over 15 years to 2009 (so mostly on the older HRT), the risk of death from vascular dementia was reduced by 39 per cent for those using HRT. But there are plenty of other studies that show that the older forms of HRT, particularly those containing synthetic progestins, have a higher risk of clots and strokes. Transdermal and body-identical HRT is the safer way to go, and the NHS confirms it does not increase any risk of clots. And low testosterone is a biomarker for dementia in men, so let's hope we get more research into what testosterone top-ups might do for women too.

Talking of men, there's very encouraging news around the use of erectile dysfunction drugs like Viagra and Cialis (generic versions are sildenafil and tadalafil) on vascular dementia and Alzheimer's. Basically, the drugs dilate the blood vessels in the penis, allowing it to fill up and get hard, and they also dilate blood vessels everywhere else too. Viagra was originally developed to treat heart problems and chest pain, and researchers didn't realise the drug's all-over powers until the male patients refused to give their samples back, so happy were they with its erectile effect. Cialis or tadalafil can be taken daily and not just on special occasions, so men can have the long-term health benefits. Would these drugs be good for women's circulation too? We await any research, but the NHS says tadalafil can be used in women with high blood pressure in the pulmonary arteries – under medical supervision – so maybe this is a useful option for those who cannot take HRT.

To some extent, vascular dementia can be slightly reversed by changes in diet. Dr William Li, expert in cardiovascular and metabolic health, and author of *Eat to Beat Disease*, recently said on the Zoe health podcast: 'We know you can reverse heart disease now. We can't do it every single time, but we know it's reversible, and I think dementia is the same way. I think that it's not a runaway train. I think that the more we understand, the more we're beginning to realise we can not only slow it down, but we can even reverse it in some cases.' After all, we know that many people recover from strokes and regenerate parts of their brains.

Dr Li explained that there are 400 miles of blood vessels in our brains, a detail I liked, and that things like clots blocked those roads. When a blood vessel gets inflamed, or has a tear, a scar is formed, then there's more coagulation, and that little lump can block the flow. Plus we also need to drain out the toxins from the brain every night, and let the dangerous amyloid plaques get flushed from our mind's sewers. Good sleep really helps that work better – we don't do plaque recycling so well during the day.

So what's for a dementia-free dinner? 'Plant-based foods, the polyphenols that come in our colourful vegetables, eat the rainbow,' said Dr Li. 'That rainbow helps to heal the blood vessels and keep that lining nice and smooth so blood can flow as well as possible.' Polyphenols enhance the function of the inner lining of blood vessels by increasing the release of nitric oxide, which promotes blood vessel relaxation and improves blood flow. They also help protect blood vessels from damage caused by chronic inflammation, as well as lowering bad cholesterol. More foods on the A-list: oily fish, shellfish, omega-3s and flavonols, which are found in foods like cacao and dark chocolate. Coffee and tea are good too, but alcohol is a toxin for the brain in large amounts. Chronic i.e. long-term, inflammation effectively 'pickles your brain', while a happy gut microbiome lowers inflammation. Food is medicine.

A last trip with Ella

Hindsight is not helpful here when you know there are many things all of us could have done to help our parents' brains stay healthy, but at least we now have the tools to make a difference. I know many of you reading this will have been family carers, and God it's hard and downright miserable looking after parents with dementia – all the more reason that you don't want to give your kids or partner that future burden if possible. As a long-haul carer, it's that frustrating fact that you can't help or change anything, other than be affectionate, play music, and make their lives as easy and comfortable as possible. My mum, even when she wasn't quite sure who I was, liked it when I brought my dog Cara and my kids to visit her in the nursing home.

I was devastated, but disturbingly relieved, after Ella died. I felt I'd slithered out from under a stone slab pressing on my chest and suffocating me. I didn't want to think about it at all afterwards for about a year, and I never dealt with my grief until much later. As an only child, I didn't have anyone to talk to who knew my mum really well, except for a couple of neighbours and her lovely carer Helen, as most of her friends had already gone. I couldn't discuss what she was like, or retell stories to a sibling. That's the Alzheimer's conundrum – you can't make peace with your parent at the end because they're not there, and perhaps haven't been there for years.

My mum died aged 89, a couple of days after I'd visited her in the nursing home, listening to music in the lounge after lunch. After Ella's small funeral at the Clydebank Crematorium, I went back home to London and got on with living life to the full, and put the Alzheimer's experience to the back of my mind, where occasionally it would start a drip-feed of sadness, which I avoided. But I had to confront it all properly twelve months later when I got an email, then another, and then a call from the concerned manager at the funeral home in Glasgow. Ella's ashes were still on the shelf, in a basic urn. When was I picking her up?

I was on my way to the Edinburgh Festival with some friends and two of my children, so I thought I'd go to Glasgow on the way to pick up The Remains (horrible phrase). I couldn't quite think of where to scatter Ella's ashes – we didn't have a house or a garden anymore or a churchyard or a particular mountain that had memories. I arrived gloomily in an Uber at the funeral home, and then things took a turn for the better. The manager gave me Ella's urn in a smart cardboard box, I think it was pale pink, in an elegant bag which might usually have contained a fancy cake or a hat for a wedding. I wanted to giggle. I got back in the Uber, and headed for the West End, where I was meeting a bunch of friends in a bar called the Hillhead Bookclub. I sat Ella on a bench in her pink box, and we all toasted her. I wondered if men came in blue boxes.

I was staying over at a friend's rather grand flat up near

Park Circus, where Ella and I spent a final night together. I thought she would've liked the flat with its high ceilings, plaster mouldings and huge windows overlooking the city. In the sunny early morning, I went for a run through nearby Kelvingrove Park, and realised as I passed the carved stone balustrades of the bridge over the River Kelvin that I could scatter her ashes there. The Kelvin is iconic – a vast, brown torrent that flows from Maryhill, where my mum was born in a tenement, and it runs past the old shipyards into the River Clyde, and out towards the island of Arran (where we went on lots of family holidays on the Caledonian MacBrayne ferry) and the Atlantic. It seemed perfect.

I went back to the flat and collected the fancy bag, but by now there were schoolkids in the park and throngs of people crossing over the bridge to go to work. It wouldn't do to scatter the ashes now. There might be backdraft in the wind. So I took Ella's box down to the banks of the river, beneath overhanging trees, and opened the urn. Inside there was a heavy-duty plastic bag that was impossible to tear open. I had to use my teeth. It was dusty. Inappropriate, but I was getting hysterical with silent laughter by now. I scattered the ashes in the river, and they swirled and drifted into the dappled sun under the branches, in glowing light, and I sat there crying and saying goodbye.

When you've seen Alzheimer's up close, you don't want anyone else to go through that, ever – patient or carer. Yet there's huge hope for us in midlife. We have the latest knowledge now, and choices to make that will alter our path, unlike Ella's generation. Take them.

CHAPTER 6

The Power of Wild Swimming

The musician-philosopher Nick Cave has an 'ask me anything' section on his website, where fans send in questions. Someone asked him, 'What makes you happy?' and he wrote: 'Some years ago, the winter after Arthur [his son] died, I was walking along an empty beach in Brighton and had the sudden impulse to jump into the sea. I was shocked to find that, upon entering the freezing water, I experienced a sudden, violent, radical rearrangement of my relationship with *almost everything*. I discovered that it was simply impossible to grieve in icy water. This revelation began my love affair with cold-water swimming.'

The idea that an icy plunge could stop even grief in its tracks is extraordinary, but I believe him, and there are promising new studies on the positive effect of cold-water swimming on depression. There is nothing more intense or *here and now* than a winter swim, when your body just screams, like Gloria Gaynor on speed, 'I will survive!'

Cave, who is 66, explained further: 'When I am in London, I wake up early, walk through the woods with some other wild swimmers, and jump into the lake. During winter, with water temperatures dropping to freezing, this is nothing less than a catastrophic outrage to the nervous system and an excruciatingly intimate engagement with one's mortality.'

The version of cold swimming or wild swimming that I speak of is not the extreme, exhibitionist, ice-cube-tsunami sport of Wim Hof, but more contemplative and conversational. Sometimes it's spiritual; sometimes singularly hilarious, but never miserable. The iciness brings a laser focus like nothing else. I swim year-round in two places – from the white sandy beaches on the tiny Scottish island of Gigha, and at the public, unheated, 1930s Parliament Hill Lido on Hampstead Heath. It has changed my life. For the last four years, me and my submersible best friend Deborah Ross and my partner Cameron have tried to go three early mornings a week to the Lido. Deborah taught me to swim the crawl in Richmond baths over three decades ago when we were journalism trainees on a crappy free local newspaper. She is now a national television and film critic, so provides the latest reviews and other pertinent advice as we swim in the 'chatty lane', which is the slowest lane. Cameron swims lengths efficiently in the faster lane, wearing a neon orange hat and mirror goggles, while we ignore him and paddle on chatting sometimes alongside the Lido's two mallard ducks (Laney and Drake), who often take to the turquoise waters. I do think you sometimes need a friend to provide a tug of guilt or volley of abuse if you don't turn up in the morning. If you live on the coast, joining a group of local sea swimmers like the Bluetits on Facebook is encouraging, and useful for safety too.

Mere weather is irrelevant to us winter swimmers. I was in New York recently and I read the old motto of the US Postal Service engraved on their grand building: 'Neither snow nor rain nor heat nor gloom of night stays these couriers from the swift completion of their appointed rounds', and nothing stays us from the swift completion of our swim. When the rain is torrential, we swimmers obviously don't mind getting wet, and the raindrops bounce like surreal giant marbles on the surface of the water in front of your nose. We laugh off the 'lobster effect', when our legs turn bright red in the cold. We always swim in the morning on Christmas Day too. When it's (rarely) down to 1 or 2°C, there's ice-crispy frost on the paving round the pool, and the water feels thicker, like blue jelly. I've never done more than a length at those temperatures, but a length alone is quite an achievement.

Every winter day that you manage to get up in the dark, waddle in your duvet coat to the outdoor pool, get naked in the concrete Gulag of a changing room, and plunge in swearing at 4°C, feeling the glacial water slice your legs like a thousand tiny razor blades, you have properly proven yourself. You have trounced the worst the world can throw at you, you're done, and it's only 7.45am. 'We shall overcome' is your mantra for the rest of the day. An hour or so after the ice plunge, you're at your desk still coasting on a massive serotonin high that few recreational drugs can compete with, which is eventually followed by a deep calm.

Cold swimming also comes with superpowers beyond mere euphoria. A regular icy plunge boosts energy, increases your stress threshold, improves your metabolism and glucose balance, lowers nagging physical pain, decreases blood pressure, is neuroprotective and increases immunity. I can vouch for that last one – I've had one cold in the four years since I started swimming, and when I do feel that itching in my throat that augurs a coming infection, it usually disappears within a couple of hours. You don't even have to swim to improve immunity – a Dutch study found that people who showered in cold water from 30 to 90 seconds a day were a third less likely to call in sick at work, compared to a control group. In menopause, swimming can be a huge mental and physical health boost; I've a friend who's had breast cancer and cannot use HRT and she says the icy dips have made a positive difference to her mood and symptoms.

The mental and physical benefits are addictive. You know how people get addicted to horror films because of the 'jump scares' when something evil pops up? Well, I think ice swimming is a bit like that too. It provides a neanderthal frisson of fright in our risk-free modern lives, and we fight back. We were built for this. In time of struggle, and particularly in midlife as we face our own and each other's mortality, and our health gets out of kilter as our hormones become sluggish, cold swimming provides both a massive kick in the arse and a chance to be part of a community of like-minded mad people.

The Scandinavians, of course, have known all this for centuries, but wild swimming is not new to Britain either. I recently spotted a diary entry by English writer Fanny

Burney, on 20 November 1782, four years after *Evelina* – her novel of manners written when she was 26 – took London by storm. This missive is from a winter trip to Brighton: 'Mrs and the three Miss Thrales and myself all arose at six o'clock in the morning, and "by the pale blink of the moon" we went to the sea-side, where we had bespoke the bathing-women to be ready for us. And into the ocean we plunged. It was cold, but pleasant. I have bathed so often as to lose my dread of the operation, which now gives me nothing but animation and vigour. We then returned home and dressed by candle-light.'

When starting cold swimming, the best technique is to begin slowly and swear copiously, and perhaps consult with your doctor first if you have any health issues. Cold water shock is real, and it takes a while to get acclimatised to it; new swimmers can go under, swallowing water as they gasp in panic. Dr Heather Massey of the Extreme Environments Laboratory at the University of Portsmouth explained in a podcast about how best to cope. 'That inspiratory gasp is where you take a big, deep breath in and then rapidly breathe after that: a hyper-ventilatory response. It causes an increase in your blood pressure and heart rate. We can habituate that response with repeated immersions in cold water.' At first, I used to find I felt dizzy sometimes as I climbed out, but now I've acclimatised and that never happens. I've also learned to read the limits of my own body; I know I've been in too long if I can't speak properly. Look out for when you 'stumble, fumble, grumble and mumble' is the cold-swimmer's saying – that means you're out of your safe zone. It's worth knowing that everyone has a different tolerance of time in the water, and it's best not to show off. I wear my wetsuit gloves and socks well into summer, because I have rubbish circulation in my fingers and toes due to Raynaud's Syndrome, and I feel no shame. In fact, my circulation recovers from cold faster now that I torture it regularly.

Getting quickly and warmly dressed afterwards is an essential part of your survival skills. The afterdrop, when body cooling continues after swimming, needs to be taken seriously. When you jump into cold water, all the blood leaves your extremities, like your toes, nose and fingers, and goes to the core of your body to keep your heart pumping and organs functioning. Even when you've left the water, this conductive cooling still continues, so it may take half an hour to really warm up again, and you don't want to tip over into hypothermia, when your temperature drops below 35°C. 'It takes twenty to thirty minutes to cool the deep body to an extent that you reach clinical hypothermia,' explained Dr Massey. 'Loss of awareness and changes in vision are signs that someone is becoming hypothermic.' Delaying dressing warmly 'will only exacerbate any continued cooling as the water starts to evaporate from your skin – a very effective way of losing heat. We have to rewarm from the outside in. The cooling will continue until the warmth finally reaches the deep body. Only then will the body temperature start to rise.' Shivering is a good thing, as it aids that deep-body warming, although I find a hot shower and a flask of hot coffee also helps. The Outdoor Swimming Society has good advice on all this.

Uncool clothing is key, literally. The midlife lady swimmer in her camouflaged, pink-fleece-lined dryrobe is a social media meme, a cliché, and probably one of my friends. (I have a black robe with turquoise lining myself.) We move in herds and people hate us. But what matters is not fashion but the speed at which you can shift your body from near-hypothermia to happiness when wearing one. There have been times when I've not had my dryrobe when the cold has taken me down so low I've had to go back to bed for an hour to defrost. Similarly, even though I consider sheepskin-lined Uggs to be a fashion atrocity, I got a pair in the sales, and the speed at which I can put them on with a Scottish wool sock means I have not yet lost a toe to frostbite.

My friend Deb has strong opinions on dryrobe shaming: 'If you wear the divisive dryrobe, an ankle-length, waterproof dressing gown designed as an outdoor changing robe, with a £160 price tag, then you've probably already been mocked for it. Initially, the coat was made to give surfers privacy and warmth while changing outdoors. But recently, it's been stripped of its original purpose and is worn by middle-class city dwellers on the school run. In my opinion, whatever your class, it looks like you're wearing a tent. These coats should be left to those who *are* doing cold water swimming activities, not those roaming around London Fields with a matcha latte in hand,' she said in her column in *The Times*. Deb was annoyed when a stranger photographed her in her dryrobe and laughed. 'A woman out and about in her dryrobe and she's fair game? Let me give you a sense of how fair game she is. The Facebook group that is dedicated to spotting this grievous crime, and goes by the name "dryrobe wankers", has 73,000 members. That's the population of Hartlepool, say, or Derry. Imagine leaving your house and knowing the whole of Hartlepool (or Derry) is out to get you. Although I don't have to imagine. I know.' Although dryrobewankers blocks faces out when it snaps unfortunate dryrobers, as Deb points out, 'When it's me, I'll know it's me.'

Aside from overcoming dryrobe shame, since starting swimming I've felt truly comfortable with my body for the first time. Obviously, I'm a late developer on this, but hanging out in the Lido's doorless breezeblock changing rooms and naked communal showers with women of all ages puts everything into perspective. There are Caesarean scars, dragon tattoos, breasts without nipples after surgery, bodies that pour lavishly out of bathing suits, others that seem flat and two-dimensional, goddesses of gorgeousness, pregnant bellies, and stomachs like mine that have proudly had three babies and have the stretch marks to prove it. Most people seem 'bien dans sa peau' as the French say, happy in their skin. We're not here for an Instagram-filtered shot – we're here because we're the new Spartans.

And like the Spartans, the tough regime brings strength and healthiness. A hit of cold takes you into flight-or-flight mode, with adrenalin and cortisol pumping up, but regular immersion improves your ability to recover more quickly from stress, and get the body back into parasympathetic rest and restore mode faster. It also gets the lymphatic system pumping, which removes waste and can reduce swelling – even puffy morning-after eye bags. Plus there's promising research on how cold swimming builds up good brown fat, as opposed to unhealthy white fat, and leads to better glucose balance and insulin sensitivity.

Danish researcher Dr Susanna Søberg, author of *Winter Swimming: The Nordic Way Towards a Healthier and Happier Life*, has been studying this effect for over a decade, and explained: 'White fat stores energy in the body, while brown fat is quite the opposite: it uses energy in the body. When you go into the cold, brown fat is activated by noradrenaline, which increases up to 250 per cent within minutes. Once activated, brown fat uses sugar and fat from the bloodstream as fuel to increase heat in your body. So the purpose of brown fat is to keep you warm and not die from hypothermia. It is really clever of nature to give us this little radiator in your body. And this brown fat tissue will also keep you healthy because it uses suspended calories in your body and increases your insulin sensitivity.' Dr Søberg's studies show two minutes of cold exposure is enough to activate the brown fat response. 'The increase in dopamine and serotonin, also very important for mental balance, also happens within these two minutes.' So you could just finish your hot shower with a cold blast, or have a sauna finished off with a cold dip to get the brown fat burning.

For those like me with Alzheimer's in the family, it's worth considering anything that decreases your chances of neurodegeneration, which can lead to dementia, and cold exposure seems to help. Brain scans show that even short-term head-out immersion in cold water increases connectivity between large-scale brain networks, and early research in mice from Cambridge University suggests that cold water swimming could be a preventative for dementia. When the body cools, it increases its levels of the cold shock protein molecule, which is found in hibernating animals.

When a polar bear or a tortoise hibernates, the protein helps protect the brain from damage and allows it to continue to form new connections. Professor Giovanna Mallucci, who led the work at the UK Dementia Research Institute at the University of Cambridge, said: 'Essentially, the cold shock protein enables the brain to protect itself – in this case, against the damage to nerve cells in the brain.' I'm with the polar bears on this, but obviously we're not hibernators. In promising research, however, trials on Alzheimer's-prone mice have shown that the cold shock protein prevents synapse loss and reduces memory problems.

We've discussed the major physical health changes wild or cold swimming can bring, but its effects on mental health are equally if not more astonishing. And they're properly addictive – more so if you can find a secret shore and run in naked. As the late wild-swimming guru and author of *Waterlog* Roger Deakin wrote: 'I can dive in with a long face, and what feels like a terminal case of depression, and come out a whistling idiot. There is a feeling of absolute freedom and wildness that comes with the sheer liberation of nakedness as well as weightlessness in natural water, and it leads to a deep bond with the bathing-place.'

Literally going with the flow becomes a way of life, he explained. 'When you swim, you feel your body for what it mostly is – water – and it begins to move with the water around it. No wonder we feel such sympathy for beached whales; we are beached ourselves at birth. To swim is to experience how it was before we were born.' Deakin's delightful book charts his swimming journey around the UK, diving into Cornish harbours, the rapids of pot-holers' ravines, Cambridge's meandering don-filled river, London's lidos, Bath's baths, Scottish lochs, murky canals, tarns in the Welsh hills, frog-filled moats, mill ponds and disused quarries. The waterscape of the whole country opens up in a way it never has before; it forever changes the way you think about travelling and the seasons. Passing Loch Lomond in early November, Cameron and I park the car and nip in for a quick, glacial hit; in Walberswick on New Year's Day, we run screaming into the waves, as Sizewell B power station glints further down the coast in the low winter sun. We are free to swim anywhere, anytime.

The cheering effect of wild swimming is now being properly investigated by scientists. We know the cold induces short bursts of short-term 'good' stress that helps you manage any chronic, long-term 'bad' stress when it arrives, as well as learning to be calm and comfortable when you are uncomfortable – the 'this too shall pass' skill. A team from NHS Sussex and the University of Portsmouth carried out a trial last year involving eighty-seven people with mental health difficulties, starting some with progressive sea swimming sessions, and a control group who just sat on the beach. 'In the outdoor swimming group compared with the control group, there was a lower number of them seeking depression-specific therapy post-treatment and at follow-up. The use of antidepressants and sleeping tablets, on average, also reduced more,' said Dr Heather Massey, who worked on the project. It turns out she is also a cross-Channel swimmer herself. Next up will be her even bigger study called OUTSIDE, which will investigate the health effects of eight weeks of swimming on almost 500 adults with depression, tracking effects in the short term, and over months afterwards.

I never thought I'd be consulting the *International Journal of Circumpolar Health*, but it turns out scientists in Finland were across this research twenty years ago, and their 2004 study of landlubbers versus swimmers after a winter of cold dips showed that: 'Tension, fatigue, memory and mood negative state points in the swimmers significantly decreased with the duration of the swimming period. After four months, the swimmers felt themselves to be more energetic, active and brisk than the controls. Vigour-activity scores were significantly greater. All swimmers who suffered from rheumatism, fibromyalgia, or asthma, reported that winter swimming had relieved pains.'

Another study involving Dr Massey looked at magnetic resonance imaging (MRI) scans of brains of thirty-three adults before and after a five-minute, whole-body bath at 20°C, and asked them about mood changes too. They measured brain connectivity and self-reported emotional state, and found the bathers felt more active, alert, attentive, proud, inspired and less distressed and nervous after having a cold-water bath. They concluded that the swimmers had better brain connectivity: 'The changes in positive emotions were associated with the coupling between brain areas involved in attention control, emotion, and self-regulation. The results indicate that short-term whole-body cold-water immersion may have integrative effects on brain functioning, contributing to the reported improvement in mood.'

I could have told them that. Sometimes wild swimming is not merely mood-lifting, but a near transcendental experience. On the island of Gigha in Argyll where I go on holiday several times a year, there's a path down to the water that smells of warm marzipan when the yellow gorse is out. It winds enticingly across the field from the road, slipping you glimpses of the sea. Among the gorse bushes there is always a wild bird rave: bluetits and finches and lesser red polls just arsing about, singing, fat with berries for most of the year. Suddenly the gorse walls open up to a small bay, a half-moon of white sand, with the water and sky in whatever state of turmoil they fancy that day. Sometimes in the early morning or evening, the water is glassy turquoise and you can swim into the glittering sunpath, out towards passing yachts and the Mull of Kintyre.

There are other stunning white sands on the island: the twin beaches that join the island to Garbh Eilean (rough rock) and have views out to the paps of Jura, or the shore on the west side looking out to Islay, or on the south to the hills of Antrim in Ireland on a clear day. We swim from them all. Around 170 people live on Gigha, which is seven miles long and just over a mile wide, but there are at least a dozen other year-round wild swimmers, and the oldest is 82. They seem to be completely weatherproof, and sometimes swim in the dark by the lights of the jetty by the ferry terminal on early winter mornings. The regulars include Hannah Storie, who runs the island shop and The Nook seafood takeaway with her partner Joe, as well as doing part-time work teaching new mums on the mainland to breastfeed. (Everyone here tends to have more than one job.) Then there's Morven Beagan, who runs Gigha's Natural Skincare, making her own organic products, and also offers Reiki healing and other treatments. Her sister, Heather Gorman, is a community carer and school assistant, and also has a cake stall (with honesty box) in a blue cabinet outside her house. Heather brought a very good lemon drizzle cake round when I talked with the two sisters about their cold-water obsession, and their extraordinary feat of swimming the channel back from the mainland one summer. I wanted to find out why these three women started swimming, and how a daily plunge in the sea has changed their lives.

Let's start with Hannah, who is 40, and along with having three jobs, has two children, Maisie and Martha, now both at primary school. Hannah began swimming regularly in the winter before the Covid lockdown in 2020, when her daughter Maisie was about nine months old and still breastfeeding, but she'd stopped the early morning feed. 'Morven and Heather had been swimming a lot, and I thought I'd quite like to join them. I wanted to get a little bit of my life back, just a half hour to be me.' By way of swimwear, Hannah threw on leggings and a long-sleeved top and plunged into the winter sea. 'And after my first swim I felt great; taking that time where my world is not going at a hundred miles an hour, and I don't have to think about the kids or anything else. I haven't suffered from post-natal depression or anything like that. But I find that taking time helps, along with the breathing. I used to practise a lot of yoga, and I use my yoga breathing, and you feel you can get through any kind of situation. I think it's the power of peace in that which is phenomenal.'

After a few weeks, Hannah graduated to wetsuit gloves and socks to keep her circulation going, and a rash vest for warmth – and to fend off the occasional jellyfish. Dryrobes also became island wear. She bought one for her partner Joe for Christmas – and he wore it every day to walk the dog. Hannah happily gets up as early as six in the morning to swim. 'I'd be down in the sea and the rest of the house is silent, still asleep. I would have my swim, enjoy it, come home, have my shower, have a cup of tea, and then take the dog out, all before the house moved. It was really nice to have that. And some of the mornings are absolutely incredible. We'd have a seal come across some mornings and swim really close. And then flocks of geese flying over your head.'

During Covid, the islanders enjoyed socially distanced swims and formed groups, for safety as well as friendship. 'When it's really choppy we tend to go in together and it's the best laugh. You come out and your sides are sore from laughing so much because you can't help but get smacked in the face and it's horrible, but it's really funny at the same time.' The only downside, it seems, are the jellyfish that appear in summer at some of the beaches. They're mostly non-stinging Moon jellyfish, but the nemesis is the occasional Lion's Mane, an orangey-brown creature the size of a plate, with a gazillion tentacles. One morning Hannah swam into one, and by the time she got to the school gate to drop off her older daughter, Martha, she was in a bad way. 'You could see it all up my arm, burning everywhere.' She applied antihistamine cream, but was in pain for two days. Vinegar also helps, and my book editor swears by rum – on the skin. But avoidance is the best technique, and occasionally Martha paddles out ahead of her mother in her kayak to check the sea in summer. 'She's on jellyfish watch.'

The Power of Wild Swimming

Morven, who is 56, started swimming five years ago when her other sister, who lives on the mainland in the coastal village of Tarbert, invited her to take to the water with a bunch of local women she swam with regularly. Morven thought they were mad, but joined in one day to see what they were all raving about , thinking, 'This will probably kill me. But immediately it was amazing. All I was thinking about was the water, breathing and nothing else.' The cold felt tingly. 'I thought, whew, that was good. Then I got on the ferry home and was still on a high and could feel every fibre of my being. I felt such clarity, and I started planning my next dip in the water. It was clear pretty immediately that I needed to do that again.' Cold swimming is a bit like religious baptism – get someone in the water once and they're hooked.

Heather, who is 59, was intrigued by Morven's new habit. 'I would never, ever have thought of doing that. But looking back, that would have been roughly the time that I couldn't run anymore. I used to run all the time, but I had joint pain and I'm arthritic in both my knees.' She began swimming, and was soon going most days. When I'm not on Gigha, I always check Heather's Facebook for her regular posts of her early morning view of the little beach – sunrise, crispy frost, lashing rain. 'I don't feel the knee pain in the water and that relief is relaxing, and now I crave the cold feeling,' she said. 'It clears my mind, rejuvenates me,' Morven nodded. 'I think it does literally wash away stuff that doesn't really matter. And I come out feeling like I was a slow computer that's suddenly had a defrag or something. I can conquer my day.' Although this book is not sponsored by dryrobes, we're mentioning them again because in extreme island conditions, they are even more important. Heather bought a second-hand one online. 'I can't imagine my life without a dryrobe. I wouldn't do it. My zip broke, and I didn't have a dryrobe for a whole week, and I couldn't I do what I usually did.'

Sometimes the sea is between 3 and 5°C in winter, and you need to be sensible. Morven had advice: 'It depends how you feel every day, what your body's doing next. It's really important to listen to your body if you've had alcohol, if you haven't had a great sleep, if you've got a bug – that all makes it very different how you experience the cold. It's your guide as to how long you stay in the water – there's no ego in the cold.' Heather agreed: 'In the beginning I got awful shivering if I waited too long to get back home and get warm, and I couldn't heat up all day.' Now, however, Morven and Heather have, over the years, developed what seem to be swimming superpowers, and a couple of summers ago, they decided (along with the primary school's headmistress) to swim across the sea from Tayinloan on the mainland, where the car ferry departs, to Gigha. This journey takes the ferry twenty minutes, and it's about three kilometres. The sisters began training, and local wild swimming instructor Dan the Merman (very entertaining to follow on Instagram @swim_danthemerman_argyll) came to give them a lesson on front crawl technique, and they got thin wetsuits. 'He said, "I'll show you the basics, and you'll be fine",' said Morven. And they were.

On the big day, a friend guided them in a fishing boat, and they set off from the beach near Tayinloan. 'The tide caught us, and we did more than four kilometres, when it should have been three,' said Heather. 'So it took us over two hours in the water.' They did have to stop for a while when Morven got cramp, they drifted off course, and took a break in the boat. I asked her if she swam the crawl the whole way. 'We swam every stroke you could imagine. And we actually invented some more, to help stop us cramping up. Sometimes you just kind of need to let your legs go and float on your back.' Not surprisingly, there were some jellyfish to be negotiated in the murky middle of the channel, but a huge welcome was waiting for them at the Gigha jetty – and a huge cooked breakfast with a dram. 'Oh God, I was just so emotional,' said Morven. 'It felt so good,' said Heather. The sisters had also set up a charity sponsorship on a JustGiving page, as their father had been taken into care due to dementia. So from the small start of winter dip, there was a lot of healing of different kinds, and a massive sense of achievement. 'I had never swum any distance before,' said Morven. 'You never know you can do something until you do it. So you just keep going. We just kept going.'

Since the population took the icy plunge into rivers, lakes and the sea during Covid lockdowns when public swimming pools were shut, Facebook groups for the damp and mildly deluded have mushroomed around the country: Wild Swimming – Scotland has over 157,000 members and recommends secret spots and group events, while The Bluetits Chill Swimmers encourage people to give cold water swimming a go, and join a free community run by volunteers, which also helps you find swim buddies. The resilience and health benefits – mental and physical – are almost miraculous, but there's something about the wild and cold swimming movement that perfectly plays into the need for midlife eccentricity and rubberwear – odd costumes worn at odd hours by odd people. I'm proud to be part of it.

BODY

CHAPTER 7

Ageproof Yourself with HRT

What if I told you there is a natural potion, made from soy, that will miraculously increase your healthspan, sexspan and lifespan and help protect you from many of the creeping diseases of old age? That this potion is scientifically proven to lower most women's future chances of getting heart disease, brittle bones, dementia, Alzheimer's, colon cancer, joint pain, depression, Type 2 diabetes, urinary tract infections, and it might even stop you from going blind in later life? Better still, this potion is cheap as chips and easily available right now. Sign me up for that, you'd say. What's not to like?

That potion is body-identical hormone replacement therapy – HRT – and it's had the worst PR campaign in the history of the universe.

Along with my colleagues in the new menopause movement, I am here to alter that negative public narrative for a positive one. It could change millions of women's lives for the better. I'll explain in more detail later, but what's happening is people (and some doctors whose education is not up to date) are still confusing the old oral combined HRT made from *synthetic* progestins and estrogen, which had a very small increased risk of breast cancer, with the new version: *natural* body-identical HRT, which is much safer. Body-identical HRT simply contains molecular copies of your own hormones, estrogen, progesterone and sometimes testosterone, all made from soy derivatives. Numerous clinical trials have proved body-identical HRT has a completely different, healthier effect on your body and mind because you're topping up your natural hormones, rather than swallowing some drug that's alien to your body. The old synthetic HRT is still available, but it's being prescribed less and less by menopause experts and the NHS in the twenty-first century, because there's a better choice now.

Obviously, each woman's path is different, and you need to consult a doctor or menopause specialist on whether HRT is right for you. For the majority, starting HRT in perimenopause, around menopause, or even a few years later will not only vanquish the smorgasbord of symptoms, but it will also increase longevity and quality of life, and women need to be told that's an option as soon as possible. Why have we been informed otherwise? Why are we still being fed inaccurate, scaremongering headlines about older, riskier forms of HRT? As American urologist, podcaster and menopause campaigner Dr Kelly Casperson said: 'The most dangerous thing we did to women was tell them that something their body naturally makes will kill them.'

She was referring to what I consider a crime against female humanity which was committed over twenty years ago, in 2002, when a massive research project on 26,000 patients, the American Women's Health Initiative (WHI), put out a shaky set of results and a terrifying press release which claimed that HRT increased your risk of breast cancer, clots and strokes – but they exaggerated the risks. Millions stopped taking HRT and suffered the miserable consequences of being plunged back into menopause. Those screaming headlines were seared onto midlife women's retinas forever – until now. Years later, the scientific truth has come out: the study eventually showed a 23 per cent *lower* risk of breast cancer among women who took estrogen-only HRT, which is given post-hysterectomy, and even the women who took the old combined HRT – made from a synthetic progestin named medroxyprogesterone acetate and estrogen extracted from horse urine – had a tiny increased risk of breast cancer, and the lead author of that study admitted that it did not show a 'statistically significant' difference in rates of cancer among women who were on HRT versus placebo. We also know now that the new body-identical HRT now available is much safer and better tolerated.

What's more disturbing is that the WHI study is still being cited today in advice for women starting HRT in perimenopause or around menopause, but the average age in the study was 63, some were as old as 79, and 40 per cent had been smokers and the majority were overweight – two major cancer risks right there. We know that HRT is far more effective if started a good decade earlier, around menopause. Two of the original WHI authors have published an apology for the misinterpretation of the study, admitting it caused many women to miss out on the benefits of HRT and another, Professor Robert Langer, said: 'Good science became distorted and ultimately caused substantial and ongoing harm to women for whom appropriate and beneficial treatment was either stopped or never started.' The leading thinker in America on the menopause, obstetrician and gynaecologist Dr Mary Claire Haver, who is also author of *The New Menopause*, explained in the *Guardian* that the WHI study's legacy has to be challenged by a new generation. 'This is what I call the old menopause, versus the new menopause. With the old menopause, it's the same old researchers who are just trotting out their tired data. They are all PhDs and they sit in labs and they never see patients and they just crunch data. I'm like: I'm not going to let you hurt women. I'm done. I'm going to use my power to tell you guys no, and we're not going to stand for this. We're going to keep giving women hormones.'

We have better data now to show that the newer body-identical transdermal HRT does not increase the risk of clots or stroke, according to the NHS, and guidance from the leading NHS Chelsea and Westminster menopause clinic is that the risks come mostly from the old synthetic combined HRT, and transdermal estrogen in a spray, patch or gel works well with 'natural body-identical progesterone which has a non-significant breast cancer risk'. A number of large observational studies have shown natural progesterone has low-to-no breast cancer risk, and the old synthetic progestins like the medroxyprogesterone acetate are what caused cancer cells to proliferate. Thus for most women, the massive benefits of HRT outweigh tiny risks. For women with a history of breast cancer, HRT is still mostly not advised, but it also depends on which form of breast cancer, from estrogen-receptor positive to triple-negative (which has no estrogen receptors), and that requires a conversation with an oncologist and/or a menopause specialist.

The health benefits of body-identical HRT, as well as its quashing of most menopause symptoms, are acknowledged by thought leaders in the international menopause movement, including those who wrote the British Menopause Society's consensus statement on HRT. And yet ... everywhere I go, women are still saying things like, 'I don't want to go on that stuff. I want to take the natural route through menopause.' Let's be clear. There's no solution more natural than topping up your natural hormones, and it's unnatural to pump your body full of ashwagandha or black cohosh or red clover supplements. Everyone needs to assess benefits and risks depending on their individual medical history, but I hear from women that their doctors, who were trained decades ago, are still adhering to the old information they were taught at medical school, when the old HRT was considered risky and you had to stop it after five years. Professional menopause education is growing at last, but as Dr Haver says in her book, 'Medicine is a slow-moving ship – it takes a very long time to course-correct.' Turning that supertanker of fear is not about truth – the science is all stacked up and footnoted – but emotion. It's about a *feeling*.

How do you change those feelings? By providing information that's as powerfully emotional as it is factual, which is what we did when Linda Sands directed, and I produced, the first of two documentaries, *Sex, Myths and the Menopause*, which were presented by Davina McCall. When viewers watched women just like them crying as they suffered the misery of depression and brain fog, and not just hot flushes, and witnessed their joy at getting their lives and hormones back, that changed opinion. As did the visual moments where we demonstrated breast cancer risk with Davina holding up pink and white plastic balls in a giant ball pit. She showed them that drinking a couple of glasses of wine every day or being overweight are far greater risks for cancer than any kind of HRT. When she put a body-identical HRT patch on her arm on camera, people went to their GP afterwards and said: 'I'll have what Davina's having.' There was a shortage of those estrogen patches for months.

We've seen not just a sea change but a tsunami of better-informed women rushing out to get the safer HRT since the menopause movement kicked off, and many other radical doctors and campaigners like Menopause Mandate and Carolyn Harris MP brought it to tipping point. A million more women in the UK have started HRT since 2021, making 2.6 million in total out of around 13 million menopausal women, the largest percentage in the world, and part of that is what academics and newspapers hilariously now call 'The Davina Effect'. But the serious side of the Davina Effect is this more widespread dissemination of information. Menopause has become a digital health revolution, mostly through social media, through peer to peer sharing such as Facebook support groups for women, but also through access to professional advice, particularly with doctors taking to

Instagram and reaching thousands of women. Armed with information, patients are taking their future health into their own hands.

The first point of call in taking ownership of your midlife health is knowing your own body. One of the questions I get asked by women every week is, 'How do I know I'm in perimenopause?' Perimenopause can last for up to ten years before the menopause, when, on average, periods stop at 51 for white women. It's often a year or so earlier for Black women, and a study of women in India found the average age of menopause was 46. Plus, 1 in 100 women under 40 go into early menopause. So there's no typical perimenopause or menopause, and pinpointing its start is more or less up to you. Blood tests can read your hormone levels, but the problem with these is that your hormones are like the weather, different every day, and NHS guidelines recommend that in women aged 45 and over, perimenopause and menopause should be diagnosed on symptoms and menstrual changes, rather than relying on blood tests. So the most useful answer is that your symptoms will tell you the truth. These may include: hot flushes, night sweats, brain fog, memory lapses, difficulty concentrating, fatigue, joint pain, hair loss, mood swings, vaginal dryness, sleeplessness, weight gain, itchy skin, reduced sex drive, headaches and migraines, anxiety, depression, heart palpitations, urinary tract infections and muscle aches. I had eleven of those twenty symptoms. Now, on HRT, I have none. Keep a journal of your symptoms for a few weeks. Download one of the many menopause-symptom lists available online, like the one from The

Menopause Charity, or just use the top twenty symptoms listed above, and tick the ones you have regularly.

If you think you are in perimenopause or menopause and decide HRT is something you might be interested in, the next challenge is going about asking for it. When I'm talking in workplaces, people always say, 'But I don't know what to ask my doctor for.' Or 'Do I need to have my hormone levels tested?' or 'My doctor says I'm too young.' You may have a doctor who is well informed, but menopause coverage only increased in the Royal College of General Practitioners' training curriculum recently, so I wouldn't bet on it. Even if they've opted in, I've studied their non-compulsory e-learning menopause module and it's rather limited. The best way forward is to walk into your doctor's surgery armed with your health data – and this is why it is worth tracking your symptoms. Take the symptom list into your GP, and say you'd like to see if HRT will help – remember, you can try HRT for a few months and decide if you get on with it, or whether you need a different prescription. You do not have to commit to a lifetime on the stuff.

It is important to also be informed as to what you're asking for. The safest and best-tolerated HRT is body-identical – specifically transdermal estrogen (estradiol), which you take through the skin in a gel, patch or spray, and micronised progesterone, which comes as a capsule you take before bed, as it also helps you sleep. I use the estrogen gel, which I rub on my arms morning and evening, so I have a steady flow of hormones over 24 hours. The progesterone helps with mood and calm, but it also keeps the lining of your womb thin, as estrogen causes it to build up. So you need the two hormones to stay in balance, and for many women, adding testosterone gel is the final of the triumvirate, and there's a whole chapter coming up on that fabulous female hormone. Women who have had a hysterectomy and/or their ovaries removed are usually offered estrogen-only HRT.

There are other hormone choices available for women who find the gel or patch a hassle, or live with disabilities that make this impractical, and there is also a new pill which combines body-identical estrogen and progesterone called Bijuve. It's a convenient choice, but it means you can't alter the dose of estrogen to suit you. We may need different amounts, as everyone's skin absorbs estrogen differently. For instance, it turns out if I have the average two pumps of estrogen a day, I feel the occasional hot flush coming through, but if I have three pumps, I don't get any. So that's the correct dose for me, discovered by trial and error and signed off by my NHS GP. It all takes a while to settle, and minor vaginal bleeding can be common in the first three months of starting HRT, but if it lasts for six months or more, you need to get it checked.

Getting into the gritty detail here, I also have fibroids in my womb, like millions of women, and I found that the estrogen sometimes gave me breakthrough bleeding and spotting, so I now have a five-year Mirena coil that prevents the bleeding, and I still take micronised progesterone for my brain and the chill-out factor at night. Even though my Mirena coil has a low local dose, it contains a synthetic progestin with a small risk of breast cancer, similar to the contraceptive pill, so I've made the informed decision to take that risk because HRT is essential to my quality of life.

Next time round, I'm planning to get one of the smaller coils if I still need it, the Jaydess or the Kyleena, which has a much lower dose of progestin and is safer, but only lasts for three years. If you can avoid synthetic progestins in later life, it's a good idea. One of the combined patches contains estrogen and a progestin together (which may be an option if you don't tolerate natural progesterone well) but using an estrogen-only patch with a micronised progesterone capsule is safer. That's in the GPs' e-learning module: 'Oral micronised progesterone has likely less risk of breast cancer and VTE [clot risk] than older progestogens [progestins].' A small percentage of women are progesterone-intolerant, and sometimes taking the hormone vaginally as a pessary rather than as a pill works better for them.

Getting the right dose may take a few prescription adjustments with your doctor, as every woman's hormones are different. It took me a while to get my hormones balanced, and if you want more detail on menopause and HRT, check out my previous book *Everything You Need to Know About the Menopause (but were too afraid to ask)*. Now I'm sorted, my hormones are steady and predictable every day, and it's delightful not dealing with a moody menstrual cycle anymore. I asked my @menoscandal Instagram feed what HRT had done for them, and here are a few of the hundreds of replies, many of which emphasised mental health: 'White jeans every day, emotional stability, on HRT lost weight, fighting for HRT made me fight for myself generally, ability to speak up, far better sex life, ability to put myself first,' said one. 'With proper HRT, actually feeling less volatile than in the forty years previously,' said another. And finally, 'My life was fantastic until menopause. It all came crashing down. Mental and physical health. The best thing was taking HRT and going back to my perfectly normal beautiful life. Otherwise, I don't think I would be here. I hated everything about menopause.'

HRT is usually prescribed to banish menopause symptoms, but while researching it, I became increasingly fascinated by the protective effects of estrogen and progesterone if you continue taking them long term, something that is beginning to emerge as more medical papers on the subject are published. It turns out that we have a fantastic gift for women on our hands when it comes to longevity. HRT can be a literal lifesaver; we know that women who lose their hormones earlier in life due to hysterectomies and the removal of ovaries in surgical menopause are far more likely to die prematurely of cardiovascular disease and get dementia, due to long-term hormonal deficiency. Hormones can extend our lifespan, but they can also extend our healthspan. Presently life expectancy in the UK for women is 83, compared to 79 for men, and in the US, it is 79 for women and 73 for men. But women spend 16 per cent of their lives in poor health, compared to 13 per for men. Women live longest, but they don't live in wellness. This is where replacing hormones can make a huge difference. We are beginning to understand that for the first-time ever, the majority of women no longer need to face the sudden accelerated ageing process that follows midlife hormonal loss. Topping up these natural hormones can extend the time we spend in good health, rather than just miserably surviving.

There are hormone receptors all over our bodies, like keyholes waiting for the hormone key to come along and turn them on. They're in our brains, our bones, our organs, our muscles and our vulvas, and unexpected places, like our eyes. Almost two-thirds of cataract patients are women (including my mum Ella), and the problem starts when estrogen begins to disappear in perimenopause, but it turns out that HRT significantly decreases the risk of cataracts. Estrogen stops eyes getting dry, helps with tear production, which may protect the lens in the eye. HRT also lowers the risk of glaucoma, the chronic eye disease that can cause vision loss and blindness by damaging the optic nerve. The longer you stay on hormones, the better for your eyesight.

That's just one example – and it almost seems like a miracle, until you begin to realise that so many of the problems we put down to 'just getting old' are not just due to age, but to preventable hormone loss. In an earlier chapter, I covered HRT's protective effect against Alzheimer's – latest UK studies show it can half the risk – and in two upcoming chapters, I explain how hormones and other measures can help prevent osteoporosis and urinary tract infections. I worked as the lay writer (for free, obviously) on The Menopause Charity's *Transforming Women's Long-Term Health* report along with menopause specialists Dr Radhika Vohra and Dr Sarah Glynne. Over months, they crunched the numbers and read hundreds of scientific papers, and this is what we learned when we put the jigsaw together: combined HRT reduced colorectal cancer by over 25 per cent, halved the incidence of coronary heart disease when started within ten years of menopause, lowered blood pressure and cholesterol, reduced the risk of Type 2 diabetes by 30 per cent, reduced the risk of dementia by over 30 per cent, halved the risk of fractures due to osteoporosis and improved osteoarthritis. As Dr Glynne explained: 'Plus those benefits are likely to have been underestimated because most women in those older studies received synthetic hormones.' Of course, all the hormones in the world will not protect you if you have a seriously unhealthy lifestyle in terms of exercise and nutrition. One study showed eating ultra-processed foods, compared to a Mediterranean diet rich in fish, vegetables and fibre, could make your biological age over five years older.

Everything I'm saying here about HRT has solid science to back it up, and you can read a simple summary of all the evidence on disease protection in the endnoted document *Transforming Women's Long-Term Health* on The Menopause Charity's website. It's not rocket science, but gender bias in medicine means that it's not part of common knowledge or doctors' education right now. The message that ought to be going out to the majority of women is that they should take HRT if they can and if they want to, because it's a smart way to protect your body from the vicissitudes of old age which start when hormones bail out. As Dr Haver says: 'A generation of women has been disadvantaged by not being offered HRT.' Only 4 per cent of American women in menopause use HRT, compared to 19 per cent in the UK, the world leader. 'It should be 90 per cent.' I know some women who have had breast cancer can't or don't want to take hormones, and I've written a chapter on help for that in my previous menopause book. But for now, I'm talking about the majority of women who can massively benefit.

Take the example of the doyenne of television's *Bake Off*, Prue Leith, who is 85 and has been on HRT since she had a hysterectomy and her ovaries removed in her forties due to fibroids. Could there be any greater advertisement for the long-term health benefits of hormones? 'Every day, confronting my wall of necklaces and earrings, I think I should be getting rid of some of them, not adding to them. (But "not needing" is not the same as "not wanting" is it?) Every time I slap a hormone patch on my bum, I think of my doc telling me (not because she believes it, but she needs to cover her back) that continuing with HRT in my eighties could be the death of me. I've been on it since my forties and thank it for my energy and generally upbeat attitude. If I die, I die, but it's been a good life,' she wrote in *The Spectator*, and she told *The Times*: 'Doctors like to say "change your diet" or "do more exercise" or that HRT is a cancer threat, but that's nonsense – all the latest research shows that the risk is minimal. They don't like to prescribe HRT because of the cost of the drugs, but the benefits are incredible.'

The popular hormonal revolution – the shouty older women, the radical doctors questioning the status quo, the extra millions in HRT expenses to the NHS, and the growing positivity around HRT in the US – has been met with mild horror by some parts of the medical establishment. Even the International Menopause Society – which frankly should know better and would do if it listened to the speakers at its own conferences – put out an Instagram post in 2024 which announced: 'It is important to counsel women from the outset that menopause symptoms such as hot flushes and sleep disturbances, mood swings and brain fog will usually improve with time and may not require treatment. The difficulty is in knowing when these symptoms will improve, and it is important to *not let women suffer indefinitely* if a conservative approach is adopted.' (My italics.)

In what world do doctors decide how long they're going to 'let women suffer'? Why don't they give women the medically correct information at the outset and allow them to make their own decisions? Are women's lives so worthless that losing five or ten years to nasty symptoms around menopause is considered acceptable? Do we not deserve to sleep, to be happy, to have our memories in good shape? Do we not deserve long-term health rather than sickness?

So what do we do? We educate ourselves, and we share what we know and learn with others. Dr Vohra said that getting the message about HRT's long-term health protections out to economically deprived and underserved communities is key to inclusivity, but racial inequalities and lack of education often stand in the way, with only 5 per cent of Black and 6 per cent of Asian women using HRT compared to 23 per cent of white women. 'South Asian women have a higher risk of osteoporosis, and many don't know about the bone-building benefits of HRT,' she said. 'Diabetes is also higher in Black ethnic and South Asian groups. There could be huge benefits for women, and improved health outcomes could save the NHS billions.'

Most people have not heard about the long-term restorative power of hormones, and we are sometimes given the impression in the media that only weak and feeble women give in to the siren call of HRT; that we must power through the menopause transition and everything will be fine at the other side. It won't. We have to take action one way or another, as menopause itself is a health risk, so over 50 we need to live healthier lives to compensate. Menopause is a permanent hormonal deficiency, and until now we have had to tell ourselves positive stories about 'The Change' to keep our courage up. We need to counter that belief and misinformation: menopause is a health risk; hot flushes are not power surges, but outages. In fact, the more hot flushes you have, the higher your future risk of Alzheimer's disease. I recently chaired a myth and menopause event in a beautiful deconsecrated church in Bristol with the author of *Hagitude* and *Wise Women*, Sharon Blackie. Her work unearthing old myths and stories of powerful women in ancient times is wonderful. She negotiated menopause without HRT and said: 'I burned and I burned, burned myself alive in some great conflagration of long-suppressed emotion but instead of being consumed, I was transformed ... I feel utterly incandescent. Menopause systematically strips away trappings of womanhood and sexuality we've clung to or had foisted on us throughout our lives.' She added, 'Sometimes we refuse it, postponing the inevitable with hormone therapy and hair dye.' Sharon still has some hot flushes now, but has chosen not to take HRT because of another existing medical condition, and the choice of approach to menopause depends on every individual's wants and needs. We should remember, however, that as empowering as feminist stories of witches and hags are as models as we start to age, the cultural aspects should not be confused with medical facts.

We need to listen to the stories of older women who

have been on HRT for decades, who can tell us about the decisions they made. Now that breast cancer risks have disappeared or diminished, the NHS says, 'There's no fixed limit on how long you can take HRT, but talk to a GP for advice. You'll usually have a review of your treatment every year.' I intend to get into my coffin clutching my HRT, as do many more women and doctors who have read the science and want to stay on hormones for life. I talked to the elegant Paula Keats, who at 77 is a splendid example to us all. She has been on HRT for thirty-three years, and intends to keep enjoying the benefits.

Paula worked in HR in international banking in London for over thirty years. 'I know what it's like to work long hours in a position of responsibility, in a demanding, largely male-oriented environment,' she said. She also was unable to have children, after an ectopic pregnancy revealed she had problems with the shape of her uterus, so she decided to get sterilised. All was fine gynaecologically until she started to have heavy, painful periods. She booked in with her company doctor, gynaecologist Dr Gavin Webb-Wilson, who discovered a large ovarian cyst, so she had a hysterectomy and her ovaries removed at the age of 44. They also found Paula had fibroids and extensive endometriosis. At that point in the 1990s, women were often sent home after operations without hormones, but she happened to have Mr Anthony Silverstone at the Portland Hospital as a consultant. 'He told me I must have been feeling pretty awful for quite a while, and that he really wanted me to feel well again and not have to deal with the effects of a surgically induced menopause, hampering my recovery. So he'd given me an

HRT implant that would last for six months, and I could continue that if I wanted.' Paula had lucked out with these two consultants: Dr Webb-Wilson was an early member of the British Menopause Society, and Mr Silverstone was a menopause specialist.

'As the weeks passed, I felt so much better than I had for years,' said Paula. 'In particular, I no longer still felt exhausted when I woke, which had been the case throughout my thirties, and I'd thought it was due to working long hours. My abdomen felt lighter, my energy levels had greatly improved, and my eyes were brighter. I felt like a new person!' She stayed on HRT with the guidance of Dr Webb-Wilson, and after a couple of years changed from implants to using estrogen gel, and has stuck with it ever since. When the WHI report and breast cancer headlines came out in 2002, Paula and her doctor made the decision to stay on her HRT because she was thriving, and she is now in her retirement in her late seventies. 'I intend to continue to avail myself of HRT indefinitely, for its undoubted benefits beyond the menopause. I believe that HRT, together with exercise, a healthy diet and mental stimulation, will help me to retain my independence, quality of life and keep me out of the doctor's surgery for as long as possible.' She finds she has not lost much muscle, and still 'totters around' in high heels on special occasions. 'I'm somewhat amazed that I still feel better than I did in my thirties. I take Zumba classes twice weekly, sing in a choir and recently passed my Grade 8 singing exam. I take no medication, my blood pressure and weight are normal (I'm a size 10) and I visit my GP just once per year for a flu jab and have an obligatory annual online HRT review.'

Every time someone suggests Paula should stop HRT at her age, they are put firmly in their place. 'It's puzzling that menopause seems to be the only hormone-related condition that's not routinely treated in the same way as replacing hormones for diabetes or a thyroid deficiency. After "The Change" has taken place, female hormones do not miraculously reappear, so why stop using them? I ask myself why this is, and whether men would be treated in the same way?'

I was sitting next to Paula in the theatre the other day, and looking at her gorgeous smooth skin, not the usual skin of a 77-year-old, and here we come to one of the little bonuses of taking HRT long term – estrogen fights wrinkles. Women lose up to 30 per cent of the collagen in their skin over five years in perimenopause and menopause due to loss of estrogen, and decreased collagen and elastin synthesis lead to thinner skin and wrinkles. Whole body HRT keeps estrogen levels up, and that worked well for Paula, but if there are specific areas – crow's feet, laughter lines, eye bags, evil scowls – that need help, it's worth considering a regular dose of one of the estrogens – estradiol or estriol – that you get in special face creams or (much more cheaply!) in using the gentle cream or gel for your vulva and vaginal dryness on your face. That cream is available over-the-counter as well as on prescription in the UK. Facial estrogen increased collagen production by 6.5 per cent over six months in one study. The trials have been small but promising, with one showing 15 women already on general HRT had a 'significant increase in dermal collagen' after 16 weeks of using 0.01 per cent local estrogen cream on their faces. Another double-blind placebo-controlled trial on ninety women of a topical face cream containing estriol, as well as glycerin, Vitamin E and oleic acid, showed an 88 per cent improvement in skin elasticity, and a 70 per cent improvement in hydration after three months.

The cosmetic use is off-licence medically in the UK, and sadly your GP won't prescribe gentle estrogen for your face, but this is not a medical textbook, so I'll just pass on my own experience. A couple of years ago, I started putting a tiny dab of my Blissel estriol vaginal gel on the thin skin under my eyes every day, and my one-woman experiment has diminished my eye bags. I am not alone. New York dermatologist Dr Ellen Gendler confessed to *The Cut* that she had been successfully using the low-dose vaginal estrogen cream Premarin as an eye cream for the last *twenty years*, and she also suggests it is good for the back of the hands. 'I have no problem using estrogen on the face,' she said. 'It's my staple!' That's my skin longevity tip. Don't all rush at once.

While we have scientific evidence that estrogen is good for your skin, it appears that you can stick the word 'menopause' on any old pile of ingredients in an 'age-defying' cream and sell them at an added premium in a pink pot. Does Boots' No7 Menopause Skincare Nourishing Overnight Cream have any hormones in it? No. Does No7 Menopause Skincare Instant Radiance Serum have anything different from other serums which tend to include hyaluronic acid, collagen and ceramides? No. Dermatologist Dr Sajjad Rajpar, an expert on menopausal skin, told me he had looked at five 'menopause'-labelled face creams. 'They all claim to put back what the skin is missing because of the menopause – but we know the only thing that does that is estrogen. I looked at the active ingredients in these products, which were mostly antioxidants, chemicals that reduce free radical damage. They're used in anti-ageing products anyway. Some creams contained peptides, which are collagen-stimulating chemicals, and all of them had a moisturising effect.' But was there anything unique about these active ingredients which would make them special for menopause, I asked? 'No,' said Dr Rajpar. 'These products would work just as well for a man or a premenopausal woman.'

There are far worse rip-offs out there, but I'm citing Boots because these products have the 'Gen-M Menopause-Friendly' accreditation tick, which is supposed to reassure shoppers that the item 'can help relieve, ease or support one or more of the 48 menopause symptoms'. I don't think we want our menopause symptoms supported, we want them crushed, but that's what it says on the Gen-M 'Menopause Partner for Brands' website. Supermarkets like Morrisons, Tesco and Sainsbury's have whole shelves of M-Tick approved products, including – ridiculously – ordinary Colgate toothpaste, multivitamins and Dove deodorant. 'We call it the *MenoChain*, where every business, regardless of sector, has a role to play,' said Gen-M, and they charge big companies like Boots £25,000 to be a 'Global Influential Heavyweight' and small businesses pay £5,000 to be an 'Independant Trail Blazer' (their bad spelling).

I talked to Emma Heathcote-James, the soap manufacturer who appeared in the chapter on neurodivergence, and she mentioned she had been approached by Gen-M, who suggested she add the word 'menopause' to her soap packet. 'But it's already moisturising,' she answered. 'Why would I do that?' Emma decided not to pay the £5,000 for the official tick, or change her product. Gen-M also put their M-Tick on Tena incontinence pads, and like many of these meno-products, the less women know about their own hormones and HRT, the better for menopause capitalism. I'd like every pack of Tena to have a box on it which says, 'Ask your doctor for vaginal estrogen. It is safe even for women who have had breast cancer, and reduces urinary incontinence. Also do some pelvic floor exercises if you can.'

The global menopause market is estimated to be worth $24 billion by 2030, and sales depend on women *not* being given their own hormones back cheaply. Scaremongering around HRT and keeping women debilitated by their symptoms is good for business. The less women know, the more likely they will be to buy the VolcanicX bracelet to 'relieve "meno-bloat" in 48 hours', or menopause knicker magnets to stop hot flushes, or menopause chocolate for mood swings. How daft do manufacturers think we are?

I also wonder if there are other reasons why female hormones are demonised, when the scientific data is there, proving that replacing them is hugely beneficial to women's short- and long-term health. Is it deeply ingrained ageism, the idea that once fertility has gone, we should be quietly shelved as worthless? Or it is fear that older women, freed from motherhood, will use their reinvigorated sexual, political and hormonal power for themselves?

CHAPTER 8

Reclaiming Testosterone

For me, discovering almost a decade ago that testosterone was a female hormone was like discovering a new planet. Female testosterone seemed wildly speculative, an unlikely idea from a male galaxy far, far away. Frankly, I thought the London menopause specialist offering me it was a bit weird. But then I started taking testosterone, in a tiny quantity, as part of my hormone replacement therapy, and the rest is history – or rather herstory. Quite simply, a daily pea-sized blob of testosterone gel gave me my intellectual and libidinal oomph back in midlife. I started investigating why, listened to other women's experiences, spoke to pioneering doctors, read the latest science papers, and wondered how profoundly female health and longevity might be affected in the future by 'The Big T'. Ongoing research is already pointing to the amazing effects of reclaiming this hormone and topping it up in later life.

However, there's been a bit of a balls-up along the way to us understanding and reclaiming our own hormone.

We now know that the chemical messenger testosterone is made in men's testicles, adrenal glands and brains, and in women's ovaries, adrenal glands and brains. So we could just as easily have named women's testosterone 'ovasterone'. Dr Casperson, a board-certified urologist, notes: 'The androgen receptor is encoded by a gene on the long arm of the [female] X chromosome. Tell me again why we call this a male hormone? Men literally get the receptor from women. Stop gendering hormones. They are in all bodies.'

Why has there been such a gender divide, awarding estrogen solely to women and testosterone solely to men, even after we knew that both genders have both hormones? We also know that testosterone can change or 'aromatise' into estrogen too, in men and women. Why has testosterone been tagged as a hormone of aggression when at natural levels in women it is subtle and complex in its effects? Why has there been this medical silence? Perhaps it's because until now, medical research focused on women as breeders, and therefore on the procreating hormones estrogen and progesterone. Our fertility was more important to society than our virility – which, by the way, means strength and energy as well as libido. The focus on female reproductive health has resulted in long-term neglect of our post-reproductive health, despite the fact that we spend almost forty years on average in that age band. Labelling testosterone as a 'sex hormone' hasn't helped either, when its effects are far more wide-reaching than simply libidinous. This bias will eventually be swept away, by women themselves, radical doctors, and the more recent destabilisation of hormonal binaries in the trans and non-binary movement.

Understanding that testosterone is not a gendered hormone – not a male hormone but a people's hormone – throws a Rosie the Riveter spanner into decades of cultural and medical assumptions. It's a radical shift in mindset because testosterone isn't 'his' hormone after all. Despite what we were all wrongly taught at school, testosterone is produced in significant quantities in the female body. Neuroscience has opened a window into women's brain scans – we can now see all the testosterone receptors there, and we have discovered there are more receptors all over our bodies, including our breasts, eyes, vulvas and, of course, muscles. Those receptors are ready and waiting for the hormone to dock and the lights to go on. We are all testosterone-fuelled Gladiators now; we know that men, women, trans and non-binary people all have the hormones testosterone, estrogen and progesterone, just in a different variety pack of quantities.

While the NHS only officially prescribes testosterone to women for Hypoactive Sexual Desire Disorder (HSDD) – a negative-sounding label from last century that basically means low libido – further research indicates that trans-dermal testosterone might help with more than sex drive and better orgasms, including improving women's memory, mood, poor concentration, sleep, stamina and motivation. It's a powerful female hormone which may be key to pre-venting some of the damage caused by natural ageing. While estrogen and progesterone levels crash when we enter menopause, our testosterone supplies deplete steadily down-wards throughout our lives; at menopause, they're at about half the levels we had in our early twenties, or less. It varies with each woman. For those of us in midlife with testosterone running on empty, as my own blood tests showed, the top-up is a godsend, the third leg of the three-legged stool of estrogen, progesterone and testosterone.

Lorraine Laneres, a 56-year-old staff nurse from my hometown of Glasgow, is full of enthusiasm about testosterone after her own experience. She was already using basic estrogen and progesterone hormone replacement therapy after an early menopause in her forties, but discovered testosterone was the missing link: 'If I didn't get testosterone, I'd have to give up my job as a nurse, because it has been a game changer for my brain fog. Without it I'm slurring my speech, can't string sentences together, can't focus. It's like switching the lights down to dimmer level without it, then when I take it, it's like switching the lights on to full.' Lorraine often works on acute medical elderly wards, and added, 'I really need my brain working to make up intravenous infusions, as well as being on the ball to administer their meds and notice medical concerns. I noticed the huge difference when I did without testosterone for a week once – I couldn't get through to get my repeat prescription, and I was looking after my mum with Alzheimer's, so couldn't leave the house. Once I got the testosterone back, I could function again, even on difficult days.' For midlife multi-taskers like Lorraine, with huge responsibilities at home and at work, testosterone really matters.

The 'Time for T' conversation is already playing out beyond the walls of academia, and testosterone supplementation for men's health is all over the bio-hacking and bro-longevity podcast network, along with the science to prove its efficacy. I ran a surprisingly popular ten-day 'Ten Things You Need to Know About Testosterone' series on my @menoscandal Instagram and wrote a feature in *The Times*, making the science around testosterone easy to understand. Around the world there are forward-thinking clinicians, the Futurists of the menopause world, making the latest science around testosterone easy to understand, like @kellycaspersonmd and @drmaryclaire in America, @menopause_doctor in the UK, and in Australia, @drcericashell, all worth following for their wisdom.

There's an animated conversation around testosterone among women on social and traditional media, and I always find when I'm giving workplace talks on hormones and the menopause that the atmosphere in the room gets electric as we discuss it. It's a sexy topic. Columnist Bryony Gordon wrote a spread in the *Daily Mail*, extolling her experience of taking the hormone along with her HRT. She reported, 'A much higher sex drive, more motivation for exercise, yes, but more importantly to me, a *joie de vivre* that has been largely absent since I began going through quite early menopause two and a half years ago.' As Gordon lifted weights in the gym and had impromptu sexual fantasies on the London Underground, she wondered, 'Is this what it feels like to be a man?' She was less anxious too, her obsessive-compulsive disorder disappeared, and she was just more relaxed about not sweating the small stuff. Patients report these positives in spades using female-appropriate doses, but are often met by pooh-poohing from the traditional medical elite, whose education happened when the two sexes were segregated in separate silos – the breeders and the leaders. The Royal College of GPs guidance suggests GPs ask for 'specialist help' if they don't feel 'competent' prescribing testosterone to women in menopause. But they can prescribe it directly for men when blood tests show low levels. One woman who wrote to me about her struggles to get her own hormone back said, 'It's like getting unobtainium' (which was the name of the powerful mineral in the film *Avatar*).

Testosterone for older women often receives negative press, with headlines complaining 'prescriptions soar'. You can feel the fear of destabilisation. But in fact, only a tiny number – around 8,000 out of the 13 million UK women of menopausal age – are prescribed testosterone as part of NHS hormone replacement therapy. Should it be more? Professor Isaac Manyonda, an obstetrician and gynaecologist at St George's NHS Hospital London, has been prescribing testosterone to women for over three decades. He's learned his craft of titrating hormones to each woman's needs along the way, because there's not much in the textbooks. He's inspiring. In particular, Professor Manyonda prescribes testosterone to younger women who have a surgical menopause due to hysterectomy or removal of their ovaries. Although the adrenal glands can make testosterone too, there's usually a huge hormonal crash added to recovery from major surgery. Often these women are sent home without HRT, and most are not offered testosterone, only estrogen. 'I think it's absolutely irresponsible to remove the ovaries of a premenopausal woman and just wash your hands of her,' he said. 'Every medical professional has a duty to have a conversation about what to do about the menopausal symptoms she is still going to get.' Often, he puts a long-lasting testosterone pellet in as he closes the wound, so that the patient's hormones don't plummet following surgery, and they then come back six months later and work out what HRT they need long term. 'The idea of just castrating women and offering them nothing at the time of surgery? That's irresponsible, barbaric.' But it happens all the time. Professor Manyonda's patients are part of a lucky minority. If a man had his testicles removed, would they send him home without testosterone?

Testosterone doesn't always work for everyone, however. A minority of people find it makes them irritable or angry, or gives them acne or a bit more body or facial hair, but the Menopause Research and Education group estimate that it has a positive effect on libido for around 60 per cent of women. It's also not going to magically rescue your libido and relationship if other things, like exhaustion, boredom or an impending divorce, are standing in the way. However, a survey of over 900 UK women showed that in almost half, the addition of testosterone to HRT 'significantly improves mood-related symptoms such as anxiety and irritability, as well as concentration and memory'. This is such a fertile area, but it's still being sidelined, perhaps due to ageism too. There were millions of angry hits on TikTok for the 2024 song by Farideh, which shouted out about this lack of scientific research: 'No we've never really studied the female body'. She emphasised the dismissal of women's reports of their own health, rhyming 'psychosomatic' and 'dramatic, hormonal and erratic'. Farideh's list of mystery matters included: 'Morning sickness, endometriosis, menopause, migraines, PCOS . . . ', and you could add testosterone to that list of neglected issues.

A deeper look into cutting-edge research indicates that testosterone might help protect us against dementia, cardiovascular disease, osteoporosis and possibly even breast cancer. You heard the good news here first. In 2019, a panel of experts from international menopause societies called for more clinical trials on testosterone's effect on osteoporosis, muscle and brain health in older women. In 2024, Cardiff University and Dr Louise Newson announced the upcoming ESTEEM randomised controlled trial of over 400 women who will either be given testosterone gel or a placebo gel, and asked to complete a menopausal quality-of-life survey over a year. There's already some pioneering work out there – often started decades ago and ignored – so here are ten fascinating pieces of scientific evidence which show why this neglected hormone might play an amazing role in wellness and longevity. Preventative medicine at its best.

Ten Things You Need to Know About Testosterone for Women

Testosterone is women's biggest hormone

Testosterone is the hormone women make in the largest quantity, except during pregnancy. The NHS says, 'women produce three times more testosterone than estrogen before menopause'. Levels peak in our early twenties, halve in our forties, and slump in our sixties. Estrogen and progesterone fall off a cliff at menopause, around 51, but testosterone just dwindles slowly away. For many women, topping up testosterone to natural female levels after surgical or natural menopause can be a game-changer. Yet in a humdinger of gender bias, there's no testosterone gel or cream available for women on the NHS, so patients have to measure out a messy tenth of the male daily dose of gel. (Men with low testosterone are liberally prescribed top-ups for fatigue, depression, anxiety, low libido, muscle and bone health, poor memory, erectile dysfunction, and even night sweats – many of which mirror menopausal symptoms.) In America, the Food and Drug Administration (FDA) has not approved testosterone for women, so female patients have to get it compounded privately or use the male version. Only the Australians have approved female testosterone, Androfeme, a cream specially measured for menopausal women – in pink packaging. A testosterone patch for women called Intrinsa was approved in Europe until 2012, but the manufacturers dropped it due to lack of sales. Now demand for testosterone is growing, and a new patch is in trials at the University of Warwick.

It can improve sex drive

With half of women aged 45 to 55 saying they had 'low to no interest in sex' in a Fawcett Society poll, the role of testosterone (as well as estrogen) may be key to libido. The UK National Institute for Health and Care Excellence (NICE) guidelines say: 'Consider testosterone supplementation for menopausal women with low sexual desire if HRT alone is not effective.' The official diagnostic term for this, Hypoactive Sexual Desire Disorder (HSDD), has heterosexist and patriarchal undertones – hypoactive means inactive, desire probably means 'Ooh doctor, I can't satisfy my husband in bed anymore', and disorder implies chaos and failure. The idea that you might want to just perk up and enjoy masturbating again is not on the cards. GPs or menopause clinics also carefully look into other health, relationship and psychological factors before prescribing, which is not the case for erectile dysfunction drugs, of which 4.5 million were prescribed to men in the UK in 2023, many over the counter. Double standards? Yes indeed. Particularly when a meta-analysis has confirmed the sexual benefits and low-to-no-risks of testosterone at female levels. Professor Susan Davis of Monash University in Australia published a major study in 2019 that stated: 'Testosterone acts directly in the brain and influences sexual functioning at a central level (sexual desire, fantasy, thoughts, etc) and it also increases blood flow to the genitalia so women are more likely to feel sensation of arousal and orgasm.' As your test case here, I can confirm that testosterone optimises orgasms, perhaps even better than before . . .

It can help with vaginal dryness and protect against UTIs

We don't think of testosterone when we're talking about the common symptoms of vaginal dryness and increased urinary tract infections in menopause, but it's a major part of the picture. Usually, vaginal estrogen is prescribed for what's called Genitourinary Syndrome of Menopause

(GSM), or when low lubrication is caused for some people by the synthetic progestins in the contraceptive pill. Yet one of the most effective new preparations is prasterone, with the brand name Intrarosa, which contains dehydroepiandros-terone (DHEA), which converts to estrogen and testosterone in the body. Our vulvas and clitorises are full of testosterone receptors. You might have guessed that. The prasterone pessary stops dryness, improves intimacy and feeds the vaginal microbiome that helps protect against urinary tract infections. It plumps up the tissue – it's like a Chanel anti-ageing serum for your vagina. Studies show prasterone, like local estrogen, is also safe to use for breast cancer survivors. Intrarosa is approved by the NHS – but guess what? It's hard to get prescribed as it costs the NHS £15 for 28 pessaries, and vaginal estrogen is cheaper, but you can buy Intrarosa privately for about £22. In the US, Intrarosa retails between $128 and $274. A huge mark-up.

Testosterone may help prevent osteoporosis

When testosterone is combined with estrogen HRT, it results in better bone density than with estrogen alone after meno-pause. This is particularly important for women who are at higher risk of osteoporosis either in early menopause or after the removal of the ovaries in surgical menopause. Similarly, testosterone can also be used to improve dwindling bone density in women living with anorexia. Testosterone in-creases bone-building cells called osteoblasts, making them last longer and work better, which helps prevent osteoporosis. Interestingly, there have been small studies of this going on since the early 1990s, all of which show positive results – which have largely been ignored in mainstream osteoporosis treatment. In a small trial in 1995 of thirty-two postmenopausal women over two years, they found that treatment with combined estrogen and testosterone was more effective in increasing bone mineral density in the hip and spine than estrogen alone: 'Bone mineral density increased more rapidly in the testosterone treated group at all sites.' Add to this that we already have proof that low testosterone puts men at increased risk of fractures, and extending the research to apply to women seems a no-brainer. But the promising studies mentioned above are decades old, so why has more investigation not been done when two-thirds of osteoporosis sufferers are women?

Low testosterone levels double the risk of heart disease

A 2022 investigation in *The Lancet* discovered that women over 70 who had low blood testosterone – but not low estrogen – had twice the risk of a cardiovascular event than women with higher testosterone. One of the investigators said this year that 'testosterone has been overlooked as a hormone with favourable cardiovascular effects in women' and called for 'robust randomised controlled trials to determine the effects of testosterone in women with heart failure'. There's also a tiny but cheering study of women with chronic heart failure being given testosterone patches for six months – and afterwards their walking speed and oxygen use improved compared to a placebo group. Testosterone can help dilate arteries and lower the build-up of amyloid plaques. This is such a simple way to lift up women at a time of their lives when they are really struggling – so why is this being neglected as a potential treatment?

Testosterone may lower the risk of breast cancer

Transdermal testosterone has not been shown to increase the risk of breast cancer, but the latest news is even better: women aged 55 and over who were using supplementary testosterone had a 50 per cent *lower* risk of breast cancer, according to an observational 2024 study of the American TriNetX healthcare database. The study looked at 20,000 women with and without testosterone over three years, and users had a 'significantly lower' risk of an adverse cardiac event, deep vein thrombosis or breast tumours. Obviously, there's a caveat that HRT use entails a healthy bias – users tend to be better off, more engaged in their health and more likely to take exercise – but this is a hopeful direction for future breast cancer research in randomised controlled trials. Dr Rebecca Glaser, a pioneering physician in Ohio, has experimented with combining testosterone with aromatase inhibitors (a post-operative breast cancer drug which prevents androgens like testosterone converting to estrogens) in menopausal breast cancer survivors for almost two decades, and said: 'Testosterone therapy has proven invaluable, dramatically improving the health, sexuality, and quality of life of thousands of women. Testosterone combined with an aromatase inhibitor should be considered in patients with symptoms of estrogen excess or a history of estrogen-receptor-positive breast cancer.' Dr Glaser found in an observational trial that patients using testosterone-only HRT, without estrogen, were less likely to have a recurrence of breast cancer than those not using it. That's positive news, but a one-off trial is not enough – we need large-scale studies. We see so many women taking to the streets in pink-ribbon charity runs, raising money for breast cancer charities. But perhaps we need to also be suggesting where this cash might go when it comes to new research.

Memory and cognition may be boosted

A small 2013 study by Professor Davis shows that testosterone alone improves memory. This is also what many women report anecdotally when using testosterone as part of HRT, as brain fog disappears and intellectual clarity returns. Davis worked with ninety-two healthy postmenopausal women, who were not receiving estrogen therapy, and assigned them to either testosterone gel or a placebo for twenty-six weeks. Before treatment, subjects underwent comprehensive testing of their cognitive function. After treatment, the testosterone group 'had a statistically significant and clinically meaningful improvement in verbal learning and memory'. Testosterone also improves most people's spatial abilities, although in my case, I still struggle to parallel park the car. Rachael, who appeared in the chapter on mental health, said that after testosterone was added to her HRT, 'my cognition improved in a real and measurable way. As a young woman, I was able to do cryptic crosswords and other puzzles very easily. During perimenopause and postmenopause I lost that ability, as well as no longer being able to follow new recipes.

Within a month of taking testosterone, I was completing the crosswords and baking complicated French pastries and breads like ciabatta and baguettes like I'd been making them all my life. The testosterone not only gave me back my cognition to do it but the motivation to try.' Let's call it the Bake-Off hormone.

Testosterone may increase resistance to Alzheimer's disease

The female brain is full of testosterone receptors, and we already know that men with low testosterone can have a higher risk of Alzheimer's. Dr Lisa Mosconi, director of the Alzheimer's Prevention Program at Weill Cornell Medicine in New York, has already established the significance of estrogen in protecting the brain against amyloid plaques, which can be a precursor to Alzheimer's, and she is now looking into testosterone. A 2024 study of over 500 women, comparing normal brains to those with cognitive impairment, showed that lower testosterone levels in those carrying the APOE4 gene (which can increase Alzheimer's risk) were associated with worse cognition, processing speed and verbal memory. If you're an APOE4 carrier, hormone levels are worth paying attention to early for protection, along with nutrition and exercise. Again, we should be asking whether hormones are being studied in research funded by the international Alzheimer's charities.

In middle age, muscle declines –
testosterone helps maintain it

We know from Olympic doping scandals that illegally high doses of testosterone help improve strength when it comes to sport, but at normal physiological levels it is also great for maintaining regular muscle health, as it stimulates the growth of muscle fibres and builds lean muscle mass. When testosterone levels lower in middle age, and estrogen disappears, women are more prone to muscle-wasting or sarcopenia. Along with an appropriate exercise routine, testosterone can help make a difference. One study in the journal *Menopause*, following women whose testosterone was topped up after having a hysterectomy, showed improvements in muscle mass over twenty-four weeks. Yet again, testosterone pumps up the volume, and muscle health is so important to our general health as we age, lowering the risk of chronic disease and high blood pressure, while helping to burn calories and increase cognitive function.

Does testosterone at normal female levels make you hairier?

Large doses of testosterone like those trans men choose to take can result in a beard growth, baldness and voice deepening. But a panel of international menopause experts concluded that testosterone therapy in doses providing the natural level of a premenopausal woman might cause 'mild increases in acne or body/facial hair growth in some women', but nothing more. 'I've never seen a woman whose voice changed, in years of prescribing testosterone,' said Professor Manyonda. 'I have seen one or two women with a slight increase in the size of their clitoris.' Not entirely worrying, and we know many women find their clitoris shrinks in perimenopause and menopause due to vulval atrophy, so that could be a positive turnaround.

In practice, any menopausal women who suffer acne or hair growth can simply reduce their dose by trial and error – everyone's hormone tolerance is different, and I think we're smart enough to titrate that a tiny bit ourselves. One woman messaged me on Instagram: 'I have noticed a significant increase in my cognitive function. It feels like debilitating brain fog has lifted. The increase of hair on my legs is not ideal but that's a swap I'd take any day of the week!' Of course, some women love their body hair, and for others, what's a little strip-waxing compared to the multiple benefits testosterone may bring?

Looking back over this body of research, I wondered if there was any other medicine that had such amazing potential – for men and for women in midlife – that had been so mysteriously ignored? The exaggerated breast cancer risk headlines for HRT I mentioned in the last chapter is part of it, but the other stumbling block is that hormones are a product of nature and cannot be patented, and so Big Pharma is in no rush to fund the research. Always follow the money. Maybe research funds will have to come from governments, academia or charities instead.

*

There is plenty of anecdotal evidence regarding testosterone supplementation, but even though women are reporting positive effects far beyond libido, these reports are mostly ignored. 'There is this kind of gaslighting that happens in which women's lived experiences in health are just completely denied,' said Dr Lauren Redfern, executive director of the non-profit women's information site Hormonally, and author of a PhD on women and testosterone. Dr Redfern worked on her thesis for seven years, researching the history and also sitting in on menopause clinics where women were being prescribed testosterone as part of their HRT, reporting many powerfully positive experiences. 'Women are talking about testosterone on social media, talking about it in these spaces because they are struggling to be heard elsewhere.' Dr Google, Dr Tiktok and Instagram are often where information is gleaned about menopause, hormones and even discussions of the risks of the older synthetic hormones in the contraceptive pill. Menstrual apps like Clue and Flo – which is used by one in four women in the USA – are moving into the menopause and hormone space, and will soon be massive purveyors of information, opening a new avenue for women's health. 'I think the distribution of information on apps and social media may be unwelcome because it's a destabilising of the hierarchy and medical systems that are about control,' says Dr Redfern. But if the medical establishment won't create that space for women to discuss their need safely, information is going to find alternative routes.

There is an old-fashioned negativity about this positive news on wellness and longevity, particularly from traditional institutions like the British Menopause Society, who should be leading the calls for new, rock-solid testosterone research. They put out a press release in 2024 after I wrote 'Ten Things You Need to Know About Testosterone' in *The Times*, saying 'Testosterone is not an "essential" hormone for women' – which is just bonkers. What on earth have all those testosterone receptors all over our brains and bodies been doing all this time? They added: 'There is no evidence to support claims that testosterone will help with other symptoms associated with menopause or prevent bone loss or dementia.' To the contrary – there is plenty of evidence above, and many menopause specialists have spoken about it at recent medical conferences. There may not be randomised controlled trials of hundreds of thousands of women yet, but the nascent research I have detailed and endnoted above has thrilling potential. Why live in fear when you could live in hope? Why not look into the future?

'I think the reluctance and fear is because we haven't conducted enough clinical trials,' said Dr Redfern. 'This was the big thing that came up in my research that was incredibly frustrating. As an anthropologist, your research is always dismissed as colloquial evidence. So it doesn't matter, right? Doesn't matter if you've collected 40, 50, 500 accounts of women that say, "my memory improves" because that doesn't count.' The NHS in the UK is cautious too, both medically and economically. If we all rush at once for prescriptions, it could cost the NHS around £40 per menopausal woman each year – and it costs £372 for men who need a larger quantity. The NHS cost of testosterone for women is probably around £320,000 a year in total, using 2023 figures. The NHS cost of erectile dysfunction drugs is £15.5 million. The disparity is astounding, and the disparity it reveals in the bedroom is equally worrying for relationships.

'Medical sexism is real,' said Dr Maria Uloko, who works in California. 'I'm a board-certified urologist who specializes in sexual health for ALL sexes. Men and women are not getting the same level of care, access to care or even scientific integrity in their care. It is so deeply ingrained in our system that we don't even notice it. So let's give some very obvious examples: hormones are celebrated for men's health, and fear-mongered in women despite both potentially causing cancer and side effects.' She pointed to many other areas where gender bias occurs, in particular when 'vasectomies are done under local anesthesia or sedatives as standard practice. An IUD [coil] placement however is done without medication despite the immense pain that can be associated with it.' Dr Uloko has written a superb meta-analysis of testosterone and libido in women, along with fellow, or should I say sister urologist, Dr Rachel Rubin, and their conclusions are very encouraging.

Product availability is similarly unbalanced between men and women. In 2004, the US Food and Drug Administration (FDA) rejected the Intrinsa testosterone patch only for women who had undergone surgical menopause, saying it was clinically effective, but lacked long-term safety data. But the European Medicines Agency (EMA) went ahead and approved the patch for the same use. When the manufacturers went back and asked permission to use the patch on a larger group of women in natural menopause, the EMA said the safety data wasn't good enough, and eventually the patch was withdrawn in 2012. Meanwhile, testosterone treatments for men were being handed out like sweeties – by 2020, 31 products had been approved by the FDA for men.

Fear of its very 'maleness' has made us tremble before testosterone, when in fact it is an integral part of women's lives and in particular their health in later years. Natural testosterone reaches a nadir at about 62 years on average – and then, surprisingly, takes a turn for the better for some women as they head towards 70, sometimes even heading towards premenopausal levels, according to one report. No one seems to know why, and the science is spotty and sporadic so far. The later-life testosterone turnaround was news to me, but it perhaps explains why we have more hairs on our witchy chins as we age. Or why Ruth Bader Ginsburg remained a radical feminist judge on the US Supreme Court until she died aged 87. Or why actor Judi Dench became the first female member of London's heretofore all-male Garrick Club aged 89. And harking back, how about Queen Elizabeth I, who died on the throne aged 69? As she said: 'I know I have the body of a weak and feeble woman, but I have the heart and stomach of a king.' And perhaps the testosterone levels too.

What's shocking is that extreme gender bias in medical research is still prevalent in received opinion and the media. *The Times* ran a story in 2024 saying 'Testosterone Prescriptions Soar for Women', with negative comments from doctors, but many of these prescriptions turned out to be gender-affirming hormones for younger women, and not for menopausal ones. Yet despite the limited use, the disapprobation was forceful. Dr Heather Currie, a gynae-cologist who is the former head of the British Menopause Society, said in the article: 'Many of us who work in this field are baffled, and quite concerned, by the massive increase in the use of testosterone.' Is it because we might have bigger, better orgasms in later life?

Also in 2024, the *Guardian* ran an article under the headline '"Frightening" How Easily Women Are Able to Get Testosterone, Say Doctors'. There was something deeply shaming and disempowering about that headline, with a whiff of patriarchal control. It was as though we women were furtively creeping around, getting a hormone which would allow us to have sinful sex. The article did acknowl-edge that we know testosterone works on far more than libido, but the story focused on a journalist's ease at getting a private prescription from the Superdrug online chemist, and how in the absence of the correct information, women might use the wrong quantities, and get too liberal with the T. The article warns of dire consequences in this case, referring repeatedly to risks and side effects while failing to at any point specify what these might be. The real story here is not the ease of getting testosterone expensively and pri-vately, but the stonewalling and dismissal of women whose health would benefit, but are not given access to bloodwork, care and prescriptions on the NHS unless they manage to get on the waiting list for a menopause clinic.

Dr Redfern is in her thirties, and she and I often spend time trying to understand the deep resistance to a hormone which is full of potential. We think it is partly generational: a few of the old-fashioned, middle-aged menopause specialists worry about 'inappropriate use' of the hormone, particularly if everyone rushes at once. It's good feeling strong and confident, but how far do we testosterone users want that to go? It's an interesting choice, and trans and non-binary rights are in the air in the menopause and midlife space, but mostly unmentioned by traditional medical professionals. Dr Redfern said: 'The issue is about gender destabilisation. Women growing beards and men losing erections disrupts the binary and throws the structural categories that help us maintain the fabric of society into question. It's a big spectrum, and people are using different hormones for different reasons at different doses. But I think a part of the desire for the status quo here is maintaining stability about what the organic component or biology of men is, what women are, and who trans people are. The category of non-binary of course pushes all that to the boundaries.'

One of the most fascinating moments in Darcey Steinke's book *Flash Count Diary* is when she considers how much more gender fluid she feels after menopause, while still being in a good relationship with her husband. She decided to not take HRT (unfortunately her understanding of it is outdated) and suffered brutal hot flushes and a dry, painful vagina. Steinke has shortish hair, and when a young man packing her bag in the supermarket called her 'Sir', she decided she rather liked it: 'Defeminization is not on the list of menopausal symptoms. Even if ungendering were listed, it would be framed as negative rather than as the rare opportunity it is to finally slip outside the brutal binary system,' she told BuzzFeed. Dr Redfern commented, 'What Steinke does really well is pull out the similarities between menopausal and gender-diverse people, explaining that both groups occupy a sort of liminal space, and are often actually persecuted by social and cultural systems.' Hormonally, of course, there are similarities too. Midlife women are topping up their hormones to earlier levels so they don't suffer, and trans and non-binary people are also using hormones to achieve a natural equilibrium for themselves. 'Both camps want to experiment with their hormones for good reasons, often for mental health,' said Dr Redfern. (It is worth noting that there are risks: large doses of testosterone, used in gender-affirming therapy for trans men, can increase the risk of metabolic syndrome including conditions like high blood pressure, and Type 2 diabetes.) But why is using a small amount of the hormone to replace your deficit and prevent some of the vicissitudes of ageing seen as somehow self-indulgent? While I'm all for wisdom, maturity and ageing disgracefully, I'm less keen on creaky joints, lost memories and replacement hips.

The testosterone uprising is part of the wider menopause movement among women and clinicians. Aside from the growth of period power among younger women, and the recent pro-abortion movement in the US, there have been few challenges to the healthcare status quo when it comes to women. 'What the menopause campaign represents is one of the few times in women's health – other than like the women's lib movement in the 1970s when we were pushing for access to birth control – that we have seen a political movement, pushing back in the same way,' said Dr Redfern. Is there also something pleasurably transgressive about reclaiming a 'male' hormone? It's empowering. So many studies have linked it in the past to power and aggressive behaviour, which is perhaps why it was so readily gendered as male, these being considered more masculine traits. But like gender, testosterone has its own complex and nuanced identity that is neither 'male' nor 'female' but works with and on aspects of both. 'Testosterone has an identity and that's what we forget,' she said. 'But it's far more complicated than that. The endocrine system is super clever and it has these modulating effects where the different hormones will interact to help stop certain reactions. The endocrine system is like an orchestra, and the pituitary is the conductor, and all the different hormones of the different sections in the orchestra. And when you have a different section that's not quite playing in tune, it throws it all off balance.' Professor Manyonda agrees: 'Using estrogen and testosterone together is key. My belief is that we should not be giving one without the other: they are complementary. Both hormones together probably have a synergistic impact we don't understand as well as we could do.'

Access to testosterone still belongs to an elite – those rich enough to get it privately; those educated enough to even know it exists; and, in the UK, those able to fight long and hard for their own health within the NHS system. I asked two different London NHS GPs for testosterone as part of the estrogen and progesterone HRT I was already getting on the NHS, and they both refused me, saying this was a 'specialist decision'. The second one referred me on to an NHS menopause clinic. (At that point I'd made a documentary in which we'd interviewed medical experts and three women who made video diaries over three months on the positive effects of starting testosterone, so the GPs' negativity didn't put me off.) Eventually, after seven months on the waiting list, my menopause clinic appointment arrived. Within five minutes, the gynaecologist gave me testosterone 'for libido' and I've been on it ever since for sharpness, energy and resilience too. What a waste of a desperately needed gynaecological appointment, when a GP could easily prescribe it. But such are the barriers still in this patriarchal space.

We also need to think about the consequences of *not* topping up testosterone, for those who want it. So many wider health issues like low bone density, cognitive decline, obesity and cardiovascular disease are signs that preventive healthcare is needed, and testosterone and estrogen insufficiency may be the underlying cause. There's a plague of 'poly-pharmacy' out there where doctors are prescribing women antidepressants, statins, sleeping pills and even semaglutide weight-loss drugs like Ozempic, when fixing hormonal imbalance might be the answer. Dr Redfern describes the way women's rights to testosterone have been stolen as 'gland larceny', which would be hilarious if it wasn't such a profound loss in terms of understanding our health.

Medical institutions and clinicians should be leading the way on changing this perception and embracing the health-protecting possibilities of testosterone. Instead, they are stuck in the patriarchal mud, and, just as it has in the menopause movement, the impetus will come from women themselves, readers of this book like you, and

forward-thinking, maverick doctors. Here's a natural product which can potentially protect against bone and muscle
loss, cardiovascular disease and dementia, lengthening your
lifespan and your sexspan. Let's celebrate it. Yet the fear
from medically and socially conservative forces around the
Reclaim Testosterone movement is almost as panicked as
the reaction to the Reclaim the Night feminist movement
for safer streets back in 1977. That will change. We have the
knowledge, and eventually we'll take the power.

CHAPTER 9

The Importance of Being Cliterate

'Everyone talks about needs and anxiety and everything like that in midlife, but no one talks about the elephant in the room, which is the sex and the libido part and the vaginal dryness and the changing personalities,' said Emma Sayle, founder of Killing Kittens, a hedonistic, sex-positive community where women take the lead. 'Sex just gets ignored and it's huge. You're not talking about it. You know you don't want the sex your partner wants. Or maybe you're not having it at all and it's just like right, fuck you, you know what, I'll get it somewhere else. What if men and women and partners actually had conversations about sex with each other? Spoke about it, went through it together?'

The lack of mutual communication around our desires and expectations stands in the way of pleasure, especially among Boomers and Gen Xers who grew up in a different era. There are double taboos for some around talking about menopause and sex without shame, with the added squirm of navigating the rich vocabulary of genitalia. So it's rather refreshing to get a relaxed take on it all from Emma, who is 46 and married with three children. Her community Killing Kittens is both a giant chatroom where you can talk safely about sex, and a portal to real-life parties every month, which can be a postmodern version of swinging, leading to casual sex in a safe, contained way, or just some kissing, touching, talking or flirting. I noticed one is called The Clitoratti, held at a secret location in a spa with hot tubs and plunge pools in London's Covent Garden, and there are extravagant balls, cocktail soirees and dress-up parties with themes like 'Hedonism' and 'Kreatures of the Night'. Only women can join the parties, but they can bring a man as a partner or a guest, and everyone needs official ID. The name comes from an old-fashioned warning about the dire consequences of self-pleasuring: 'Every time you masturbate ... God kills a kitten', and thereafter 'killing kittens' became a codename for women masturbating. Emma decided to reclaim the phrase and simultaneously reclaim the night. Two-thirds of the partygoers are female and everyone wears masks until the 'playspaces' open later in the evening. There's no pressure to use them, Emma told me. 'You can just have a drink and hang out.' There's also a strict policy of 'hugs not drugs'; consent is mandatory 'meaning no creeps and consent to communication'; and there are trained staff with red LED armbands if anyone needs help.

Obviously Killing Kittens is not for everyone, but it opens the door to a deeply liberating way of thinking and talking about sex. We may not all need adventures and affairs, but even the happiest of relationships probably needs a midlife MOT in bed. Sexy parties are the lighter side of some fairly dark times around intimate relationships in midlife, when affairs, break-ups, and perhaps just a constant low hum of dissatisfaction bring painful confrontation within ourselves and with others. The peak decade for divorce for men and women is in their forties – smack in the middle of perimenopause chaos for the couple.

Many of the women attending these Killing Kitten events are in their late thirties through to their fifties, and this is just one example of how women might choose to revamp their midlife sexlife. As we enter midlife, sex changes – and that's fine. But how can we make that a positive change? Relationships become more vintage than fresh, affairs blossom, and single women, non-binary and trans people want to explore new possibilities and sexual fluidity. Then there are physical changes, for both men and women, which have a profound impact on both our desire for sex and the practicalities. While some people are perfectly content to say sex is no longer for them, and long-term relationships morph into comfy companionship, for those who want to stay in the game (half a century in, with perhaps another half-century of pleasure ahead!), sex may need a radical rethink – physically, hormonally and psychologically.

We also need the language to discuss these issues. Often by the time we get to midlife, both men and women are chronically underinformed about the female body and genitalia, let alone how it's going to change over this period. It wasn't until my friend Portia gave me a Christmas tree ornament, a 3D printed fuchsia pink plastic anatomically correct model clitoris, that I realised quite how large they were. The only organ on earth solely dedicated to pleasure is shaped like a wishbone curving round either side of the vagina: long-legged, voluptuously bulbous, with a perky head, the only part you can actually see. I think men and women need to hold one of these models in their hands to become fully clitorate, and as Portia pointed out, grinning, 'We realised there was much more to explore.' As the clitoris dangled from the tree, I understood how much of it was hidden from view, and how vast the invisible play area of 10,000 nerve endings is around the vulva.

'We learned about sex behind the bike sheds, from *Jackie* magazine, from Alison at school, who was the first to get a bra and her period and was the font of all knowledge. Very little of what we learned was even true or useful,' said Dr Claire Macaulay, creator of The Pleasure Possibility coaching programme, and Catholic-educated herself. 'As a consequence, we may have been living our whole sexual lives with some wonky beliefs and ideas and not really getting what we want – or knowing how to ask for it.' Dr Macaulay is a brilliant combination of sex-positive and medically informed, which helps around menopause and midlife. She set up The Pleasure Possibility – virtual or in-person coaching for people who 'want deeper intimacy, body confidence, and great sex'. But she started her career as an NHS oncologist in Glasgow.

Many of Dr Macaulay's patients with breast cancer were facing early chemical menopause due to treatment. As a result, they often found their sex lives were hugely impacted. One patient, a breast cancer survivor, came in and said: 'I don't know what's worse. The fact I might die of cancer one day, or the fact that I can't have sex with my husband.' Aside from feeling awful after chemotherapy or radiation, with the resulting hair loss, it's often afterwards in recovery that menopausal symptoms like dry vaginas erupt in patients, caused by the anti-estrogenic cancer drugs. And while many cannot or decide not to take hormone replacement therapy, there are changes to nutrition, lifestyle and exercise that can help, all detailed in other chapters here. Dr Macaulay suggests her post-cancer patients in menopause can still safely use incredibly low-dose vaginal estrogen, available from GPs, to help with sex and a healthy vulva. The local estrogen builds up over a few weeks and then needs to be taken regularly to maintain the collagen in the vulva and vagina, and prevent dryness and many urinary tract infections. In terms of safety, a study of almost 50,000 women in the *Journal of the American Medical Association* showed that vaginal estrogen did not increase the risk of death after breast cancer; in fact, topical estrogen users were healthier, but only 5 per cent were using it. So many women are being left to suffer unnecessarily.

But it's not just cancer patients that need vaginal estrogen for comfort – pretty much every single menopausal woman does eventually, but we're not told that. Problems can begin in perimenopause, even when women are still having periods. It's very unpredictable and everyone is different. So many midlife women stop having penetrative sex – or grin and grimly bear it – because their vaginas are painful. They may also give up riding a bike, or wearing tight jeans, due to itching and discomfort. The thinner, papery skin results in pain, 'a sharp, crisp-packety dryness', as one of my friends said, or even tearing of tissue, which can make penetrative sex impossible, and can also cause the clitoris and labia to shrivel up. Moisturiser or lube may help temporarily, but they are not going to change the core problem of hormone loss. Fortunately, the tissue in the vulva can be lubricated and get its plumping collagen back by using topical vaginal estrogen regularly, in a cream like Ovestin or pessaries like Vagifem or Vagirux, available from GPs on the NHS. Blissel gel is also mild and soothing. In the UK you can buy Gina (short for Va-Gina?) pessaries over the counter in pharmacies. In America, the cream is one of the cheapest drugs available, at around $20. The Rolls-Royce of vaginal preparations is Intrarosa (prasterone) pessaries, which bring up estrogen and testosterone levels in the vulva, where there are receptors for both hormones.

Dr Rachel Rubin is one of America's top urologists and sexual health specialists in her practice in Maryland, and she explained what's happening. 'This is not just vaginal dryness. This is Genitourinary Syndrome of Menopause, a very serious condition caused by lack of hormones. So, yes, it's about pain with sex, decreased orgasm, decreased arousal. As a sex doctor, those are important to me, but so is the bladder, and you're susceptible to both genital and urinary symptoms.' It's somewhat scary talking to Dr Rubin about what happens in your fifties or sixties or later if you don't use vaginal estrogen. She's seen a lot of vulvas in her time, and says the changes are not properly explained in medical textbooks – so far. 'Did you know as you go through menopause your labia minora shrivel up and disappear?

Those pink inner wings shrivel up. I don't like to call them lips, I think it sounds gross, but nobody taught your doctor how to look at a vulva. We use speculums for pap smears maybe once in medical school, but we need to understand more: that when hormones change, there are consequences.' Your clitoris shrinks too without top-up estrogen. She estimates that around 7 per cent of women use vaginal estrogen, and at least 80 per cent could do with it.

Hormone replacement therapy helps improve vaginal dryness, but many women (like me) need a top-up of vaginal estrogen too. The estrogen in full-body or systemic HRT also helps perk up libido. The 'use it or lose it' theory about regular sex preventing vaginal dryness is not true. While you may still lubricate on arousal, that's not going to maintain collagen or bring your missing hormones back. Aside from Dr Rubin's scientific explanation of that, I also have confirmation from my friend, Stephanie Theobald, author of *Sex Drive – On the Road to a Pleasure Revolution*, which charts her 3,497-mile midlife trip across America in search of orgasms and deeper understanding of desire and sensuality. Stephanie's had more sex than perhaps anyone I know. She's reached menopause and is a big fan of vaginal estrogen cream.

Topping up our hot female hormone testosterone helps libido too, as we discussed in the previous chapter. Testosterone makes women feel sexier, and improves orgasms for most of us. Gender bias in medicine has buried that good news for far too long. As a woman in the UK, you can ask your GP for body-identical testosterone gel for 'low sexual desire', but as discussed in the previous chapter on this hormone, there are huge barriers in place to women accessing this. You have to be diagnosed with what's officially and perhaps sexistly known as Hypoactive Sexual Desire Disorder, and usually have to be settled on estrogen and progesterone HRT first, plus getting an appointment at an NHS menopause clinic for a testosterone prescription can take months or even years.

There's a spectacular disconnect here in the treatment of men and women sharing the same bed. Men can get testosterone from their GPs after a blood test, and prescriptions for erectile dysfunction drugs are given immediately, or they can take 'little blue pills' like Viagra (sildenafil) over the counter in a few minutes, and they don't have to answer lots of probing questions to prove that they, too, have Hypoactive Sexual Desire Disorder. In the UK in 2023, over 4.5 million drugs for erectile dysfunction were prescribed, costing the NHS £15.5 million, and over half of men say they experience erectile dysfunction at some point. They also get testosterone topped up for general health if levels are extremely low, while women have to prove that we're on our knees and failing our partners when it comes to having sex. It's grossly unfair, and there are no female testosterone products available on the NHS, so we have to make do with a tricky tenth of a squirt of the male gel. You'd think they could find a female-friendly dispenser bottle. It's not much to ask.

As the campaigning and podcasting American author and urologist Dr Kelly Casperson told me: 'Urologists here are already very comfortable with testosterone because we safely give ten times the dose to men every day. So we already have this comfort with hormones improving men's quality of life – why is it not the same for women? It's really a gender equality thing for me. When a man comes in with low libido and erectile dysfunction, we don't tell him that "this is just how it is now", the way doctors dismiss women in menopause. We don't ask him if he'd like an antidepressant. It is so foreign that we would ever treat a man like that.'

Aside from topping up hormones, in America there is a 'little pink pill' for women: the drug Addyi (flibanserin), which was initially developed as an antidepressant and has been approved by the Food and Drug Administration for women who have Hypoactive Sexual Desire Disorder. Addyi targets neurotransmitters in the brain that increase arousal and decrease inhibition, but it's not available in the UK so far because of the reported side effects, which can include dizziness, fainting and low blood pressure. The drug also shouldn't be taken while drinking alcohol, which puts a lot of people off. Interestingly, 10 per cent of users of Addyi in the US are men. It can work the other way round too: the erectile dysfunction drug Cialis (tadalafil) increases blood flow to the body and the genitals for men – and it can do exactly the same for women, increasing arousal and lubrication, but no one's done a major study. Gender bias again.

We're fixing men, but we're not fixing women, and that brings gender imbalance in the ability to maintain a sexual relationship – or just have fun. Dr Casperson fights for equality by providing science-backed information on her long-running You Are Not Broken podcast, and believes women's sex lives are being neglected because we define menopause as the end of periods and fertility, rather than as a low hormone issue. 'Our definition is wrong and close-minded. Because when a person comes into my office, and they haven't had sex in seven years, and their last periods were ten years ago, they can't fathom that this is a hormone issue.'

Sex is often a point where the physical and the psychological intertwine, medically referred to as 'psychosexual', and it's often hard (and not necessarily helpful) to delineate between the two. Examples include 'chronic vulvovaginal pain', as well as vaginismus, when the vaginal muscles involuntarily tighten when penetration is attempted, making intercourse difficult or impossible. Vaginismus is often described in textbooks as 'a common female psychosexual problem', which may be the case if there's previous trauma or you're not keen on the penis-owner, but Dr Casperson thinks there is a lot of misdiagnosis out there of these long-term conditions. Some are less 'psychosexual' and more physical. 'Most of what I see is very easily corrected conditions, but because the medical community hasn't learned about the vulva, how it works, how to keep it healthy and how to diagnose common conditions, these patients are deemed difficult to treat and never given hope that they will get better. I'm on a mission to change that.'

Of course, some problems do go much deeper. Psychotherapist Dr Kalanit Ben-Ari, who specialises in couples therapy, as well as running courses online, said that previous trauma can re-erupt in the maelstrom of midlife, percolating into the bedroom, making everything more complex. 'Traumatic events, stress and emotional upheaval can influence your sexual well-being and your relationship, and that can affect desire, trust, and connection. I try to help couples find pathways to healing, and there are practical things you can do around communication, mutual understanding, and asking for emotional support.' Women and men on antidepressants, particularly SSRIs (selective serotonin reuptake inhibitors) such as sertraline or escitalopram, can find it harder to reach orgasm. There are so many other layers here too, wrapped up in religion, or a very rigid upbringing, and the past. Serious sexual trauma often needs long-term therapy work, which can be somatic, possibly involving touch therapy. Dr Macaulay has trained in bodywork and somatic therapy and explained: 'Gentle touch might help with some specific issues, say if someone's never had a sexual partner, or wants to recover from significant sexual trauma. We create a therapeutic contract so that they can experience touch and have a different bodily based understanding. They can trust someone, and be in control. And for a lot of people, that is life-changing.'

We need life-changing help for changing lives at this time. And yet Dr Macaulay finds women are often still playing the same roles in relationships and in bed they grew habituated to years ago, when they have grown up into very different people. 'Midlife is throwing up questions, added to the anxiety, irritability, intolerance and even depression caused by hormonal changes. The impact on mental health can be profound, draining and isolating. It's a very vulnerable time.' She also has clients coming in hoping their partner will change, but find it's up to them instead. 'The world is full of "If only they would ... " But what if they don't? What if they never do? If you are waiting for someone else to change in order for you to be happy, you might be waiting a long time. Women are conditioned to be good, be kind, care-take, not cause a fuss or be selfish. We have been primed to people-please, dismiss our own needs and deprioritise ourselves.' Midlife can be a time to step back and look at your own needs and wants – in your wider life but also in the bedroom.

To open up the wider conversation, Dr Macaulay created the free Midlife Sex Festival online last year (2024), featuring her interviews with experts and sexperts. The talks included tantric sex and menopause, kink, better sex through mindfulness, sex after cancer, relationship diversity, awkward conversations, erectile dysfunction, the 'later-in-life lesbian movement' and sex outside of the hetero-normative box. That's increasingly common. Dr Macaulay broke out of the hetero-normative box herself in midlife and is now living happily with her female partner and explained: 'I wasn't sitting pining after women my whole life. You know, I married a man in good faith and loved him. We had good sex together. But that relationship ran its course, which is what I often hear from women. I met him when I was 17. And I think women go through a more reflective moment of personal development. It took me some time before I left, because I had kids, and, you know, people try to carry on. It's not just that perimenopause or menopause happens. I think these things have been coming for a long time. The menopause, the transition, your kids being a wee bit older, that gives you the boldness to get on and do something about it. It was completely inexplicable in some ways until you start to look back and think, yes, my emotional connection with women was always greater than it was with men. So it just happened.'

There is some fantastic inspiration for change out there: classic books like Esther Perel's *Mating in Captivity* about the tension between domesticity and desire in long-term relationships, or Dr Emily Nagoski's *Come as You Are*, which explains accelerators (sensuality, romance etc.) and brakes (stress, distraction etc.) on sexual arousal, and affirms diverse sexual experiences. Orgasms are not the be-all and end-all, wrote Dr Nagoski: 'A more revealing question might be, "What percentage of the sex you have do you like?" Orgasm is not the measure of a sexual encounter. Pleasure is the measure of a sexual encounter.' Obviously, a lot of tantric sex is about the delicious erotic charge of delaying orgasm. I've seen a lot of discarded paperbacks of the *Fifty Shades of Grey* series in second-hand bookshops recently; the mainstream is moving on from breathlessly cheesy S&M to more nuanced fare. Actor Gillian Anderson's liberating collection of anonymous readers' fantasies, *Want*, features a pink cover with a light switch on it, and, she says, 'reveals how women feel about sex when we are totally free to express ourselves'. The book has genderqueer contributions too, and is curated into sections including 'Kink', 'Rough and Ready', 'Gently, Gently', 'The Captive' and 'Power and Submission'. It is a twenty-first-century update of Nancy Friday's groundbreaking *My Secret Garden: Women's Sexual Fantasies* from 1973. As one reader said back then: 'Finding that book made me understand that I was no lascivious freak, destined for a wanton life.' These books may give us not just erotic ideas, but the words to ask for what we want.

'We don't know how to communicate our own needs, repair after a fight, prioritise intimacy and connection, or help each other grow. We are not taught how to create a healthy partnership,' said Dr Macaulay. Her career change came partly out of her own sexual exploration and curiosity. 'It was also about erotic energy and the connection between sex and success and confidence.'

Not communicating properly helps to keep the orgasm gap going strong; studies show that 95 per cent of heterosexual men usually or always orgasm during sexual intimacy, compared to only 65 per cent of heterosexual women. Women think they're broken because they can't orgasm from normal penetrative intercourse, when surveys show less than 25 per cent can. Also, depending on the study, between 53 and 85 per cent of women admit to faking orgasms, mostly during intercourse. We've all done it, although perhaps not as well as Meg Ryan in her classic *When Harry Met Sally* scene. Even the experts in this area admit to faking orgasms. At the Swell Sex Symposium in New York in 2024 (you can still access the talks online), Emily Morse, a doctor of human sexuality and host of the long-running Sex with Emily podcast, said: 'I faked orgasms more than I'd like to admit. In fact, I got good. I would fake multiple. Sometimes I was like, I'm a professional, I could go pro. And I also thought that if you had to talk about sex, then, you know, there was a problem in the relationship.' The conference was packed with glamorous midlife women nodding and laughing. Dr Morse continued: 'What I realise is that a lot of us do not talk about sex. We really just don't. We don't talk to our friends. A lot of us don't even talk to our partners.

That's where I found myself about twenty years ago, when sex was really disappointing. If my partner had a good time, well, it must have been a success. Like he had an orgasm, like we're good. My sex back then was really performative. Trust me, I did all the things, like arching the back and the moans. I did it all.'

Lesbians, incidentally, do much, much better in sharing pleasure, and don't report an orgasm gap, due to understanding a similar body, and being cliterate. Many men really need to work on their cliteracy; so often penetrative heterosexual sex leaves the clitoris high and dry, untouched and unloved, partly due to unrealistic portrayal on screen, be it in movies or (most) pornography. I watched a hell of a lot of erotic scenes in cinemas during my seven years as a film critic, and I am still dumbfounded by the number of times a woman comes ecstatically in approximately one minute while having heterosexual sex up against a wall or on a kitchen counter.

We also need to reduce shame and embarrassment around sex and advocate for what we want; vibrators and other sex toys often help to loosen up conversations and inhibitions. As Dr Morse said at the sex festival: 'I've learned that sex toys are a game changer, and lube is a must-have. My dream is a lube on every nightstand.' (Water-based lubes are best. Glitter or weird colour is a no-no for a healthy vaginal microbiome.) She also wants women to use toys to take a more holistic view of their sexuality and understand the importance of being in the body, being self-aware, and centring a sex life on pleasure rather than penetration. 'Not the old in and out. Right? That's what we need to talk about.'

While it is brilliant to go into a female-friendly sex shop, ask for advice and handle the products – we all have different good vibrations – obviously many people prefer a discreet cardboard box in the post. I still get an annual catalogue from my friend, former nurse Samantha Evans, who runs the online sex toy company Jo Divine. I met her while filming a segment on vibrators for a menopause documentary, and I left with a goody bag containing tubes of lube and a 'Satisfyer' vibrator, which provides increasingly popular air-pulse stimulation for the clitoris, as well as a variety of vibrating speeds. 'A great all-round sex toy,' said Sam. It's killed a lot of kittens. I think there's now a more advanced version which you can control from a phone app too. What's hilarious is how mainstream all this now is: the *New York Times* Wirecutter product review site has detailed analysis of magic wands and whatnot from a regular vibrator expert, Bianca Alba, and I was looking for vacuum cleaner reviews on the *Good Housekeeping* website when I also found 'The best vibrators to buy now, tested by 130 women. From rabbits to bullets, the Good Housekeeping Institute tried a range of sex toys to find our winners.' Housewife's choice takes on a whole new meaning.

There's added pleasure to be had by maintaining muscle strength in the pelvic floor, and there's not enough emphasis on that in the UK and US. After I'd had a baby in Paris, I was sent by the French state to a few weeks of free and uplifting pelvic floor exercises in a class – *La Rééducation Périnéale* – which was very much about putting the mother first. For sexual pleasure, urinary continence and preventing future womb prolapses, playing with your pelvic floor

muscles, doing kegels or other exercises, is really important, particularly as tissue starts to thin in perimenopause.
There are apps, online courses and even books addressing
pelvic floor exercises. One, by Coco Berlin, is described as
a 'bestselling guide to pelvic floor training for radiance,
confidence, and a fulfilling love life'. Its title? *Pussy Yoga.*

The bulk of this chapter has been about finding your
sexual confidence and joy again through understanding
what is happening to your body and what your options are,
but we cannot finish without mentioning those who find
perimenopause turns out to be a wild peak in their sexual
life, like nothing ever before. This is known as the perimenopausal sex surge, and some millennials, the oldest of whom
reach 44 years old in 2025, may well be heading there as
they enter their 'millenopause'. Not every woman gets the
surge – most experience a dimunition of desire – but those
who have very high peaks of estrogen as their body fights
waning fertility towards fifty can find they just want to have
sex all the time. Hinemoana Baker wrote *Perimenopause and
Libido: A Personal Story* on the women's health app Clue, describing 'the nuclear-powered juggernaut my libido seemed
to have turned into ... I'm hornier for much more of my
cycle than ever before.' There are threads on Mumsnet with
confessions about the surge lasting for years, as well as its
effect on vibrator batteries and long-term relationships.
As Mumsnetter BigPussyEnergy noted in 2024: 'Trouble is
the middle-aged men can't keep up! My sex drive is higher
now than when I was married, although it did increase
around 40, after divorce. Now 50, and my boyfriend only
wants it once or twice a month. I'd have it every day, so we

compromise about once a week.' She had also started taking HRT and testosterone, adding to the hormonal hothouse. I must also recommend here the first literary novel to truly tackle the perimenopausal sex surge, *All Fours* by Miranda July, who says of her character's sudden rampant desire: 'Was this the secret to everything? This bodily freedom? It felt intuitive and healthy, as if promiscuity was my birth-right as a woman.'

While other 40, 50 and 60-somethings in sensible shoes are wheeling their travelcases onto all-inclusive cruise liners, with crochet classes, trivia quizzes, bingo and Sinatra singalongs, you could be taking a different kind of trip altogether. I'm not on commission here, but the upcoming Killing Kittens Mediterranean cruise from Barcelona to Mallorca via Florence might be your thing: seven days of sightseeing, seven nights of sheer hedonism. Imagine what you could pack in your wheelie case. Imagine who you might be on returning. We may not all be keen on cruises or cruising, but it's powerful to think of this time of midlife as an odyssey, with menopause at the centre of it, not as a negative, but a lightbulb moment for change.

CHAPTER 10

Viva la Vulva

How exciting is it to discover a thriving, powerful ecosystem in your body that you had no idea existed? I certainly didn't know the phrase 'vaginal microbiome' until a few years ago, and it's been a joy and a relief to discover what it does – and how we can control it. While tons of media attention and fascinating scientific research has welcomed in the gut microbiome, and brought Professor Tim Spector and Zoe international prominence and cookbook and supplement sales, the vaginal microbiome has had less attention, perhaps because everyone has a stomach but only half of us have a vagina, and that's just a bit embarrassing. So let us now bring the vaginal microbiome – or vagibiome as I shall intimately refer to it – out of the darkness of the crotch into the light, and celebrate its wonders.

The vagibiome, first mentioned in science around two decades ago, is literally your 'lady garden', a euphemism I have always hated, but which now makes sense. The vagibiome is basically a constant bacterial party going on in your whole vulva area, and the key is to keep your good, protective bacteria thriving, so they stop pathogenic viruses and fungi in their tracks. It all looks very exciting under a microscope: little smooth bacteria torpedoes fighting off ugly, spiky ones. The good bacteria are mostly strains of lactobacilli (which you also get from food like live yogurt or kefir) that protect the vagina and urinary tract from evil bacteria like E.coli, which can cause urinary tract infections (UTIs), bacterial vaginosis, unusual vaginal discharge, and even kick off kidney infections. If we look after our vagibiome, it looks after us. If we don't, well, we all have an epic UTI disaster story.

Mine was in my twenties, when I was writing a book about female soldiers going into combat, and I was embedded on exercise with some of the first women marines on Parris Island, South Carolina. The girls were tough, had big boots and big water bottles, and knew what they were doing. I had a mini Evian bottle and my gym shoes. I got hot and exhausted and kept on reporting for a few days, until I found I was feverish, needing to pee painfully every half hour and my back was really sore around my kidneys. I thought I could lubricate my way through it by drinking tons of water and cranberry juice, but to no avail. I didn't just have cystitis (a bladder infection) but a full-on kidney infection and I ended up in a creepy doctor's office in a strip mall paying a wodge of dollars for a consultation and super-strength antibiotics. My vagibiome (if only I'd known I had one then) had been badly treated, and I've been overly prone to UTIs since then – until, that is, I learned about my vagibiome and how to take care of it.

There are two peaks for UTIs in women: in their twenties and early thirties, and later when they go into perimenopause onwards. Younger women with flourishing sex lives are often on the progestin-only contraceptive pill or coil, which can reduce natural vaginal estrogen and leave the vulva dry and the bladder, urethra and kidneys more prone to infection. This can also happen to mothers who have lowered estrogen during breastfeeding. UTI rates shoot upwards again when women hit 45 and are perimenopausal. It won't surprise you to hear that this is yet another part of your body affected by falling estrogen (and testosterone too). Lack of estrogen around menopause means the good bacteria in the vagibiome can be more easily replaced by pathogenic ones, particularly if you've been prone to UTIs over the years: after sex, or when you dehydrate, or just inexplicably, again and again (once the nasty bacteria colonise your vagibiome, they often lurk silently there even after the UTI stops, ready to attack again).

Estrogen keeps your vulva area nicely acidic, which suits the lactobacilli, and when it disappears, the environment gets more hostile and alkaline. Aside from encouraging good bacteria, estrogen also helps collagen production, and collagen disappears from the vulva by up to 30 per cent in the five years after menopause. Dry vaginas and urethras with thinner skin are more prone to infection. We invest millions in collagen supplements and anti-ageing serums for our faces, but it never occurs to us that precisely the same process goes on down below. No doubt because we are never told any of this.

*

Women make up the majority of the 1.8 million hospital admissions for UTIs over the last five years in England – not to mention a gazillion more GP appointments. We are an astonishing thirty times more likely to get UTI than a man, and UTIs can cause fevers and pain – that knives in your pelvis, razorblades in your pee feeling – and are occasionally fatal. This is not just a gender health gap – it's a dangerous crevasse. Basic ignorance of the science around female bodies and the vagibiome is causing unnecessary misery, antibiotic resistance, and even sepsis-related deaths. For years, doctors have repeatedly prescribed antibiotics to treat UTIs – a short-term cure that often leads to long-term problems, including killing some of the good bacteria in your stomach microbiome and reducing its diversity. Then there is the issue of antibiotic resistance. This is no small matter. The NHS death rate for hospital UTIs is 4 in 100, rising to 1 in 10 in those aged 95 and over. Sometimes, antibiotics no longer work – a quarter of women have a UTI strain resistant to certain common antibiotics. Pharmacies have been able to give out antibiotics over-the-counter for UTIs without tests since 2024, but there is no data yet on any growth of antimicrobial resistance.

We know that antibiotics are sometimes necessary, but we also now know that there are other options – preventative ones. According to the *American Journal of Obstetrics and Gynecology*, we can halve the risk of UTIs by giving women in perimenopause and menopause a safe, incredibly low dose of vaginal estrogen, which plumps the tissue back up again and feeds the vagibiome. Large studies show it is safe for most breast cancer patients too, it's a win-win on the sex front, and you can take it alongside normal HRT. It also tends to reduce the too-frequent need for urination. Professor Chris Harding, a consultant urologist at Newcastle upon Tyne Hospitals NHS Foundation, told me: 'Vaginal estrogen replacement works and it's great to have a non-antibiotic alternative to increase prevention. I sometimes use it in premenopausal women, too, to change the microbiological environment of the vagina.' Another hormonal solution, perhaps the best, is the Intrarosa (prasterone) pessaries mentioned in the Testosterone chapter, containing DHEA (dehydroepiandrosterone), which converts to estrogen and testosterone, and binds, with restorative powers, to the estrogen and many testosterone receptors in the vulva. Vaginal hormones come as a cream, gel or pessary and are cheap, costing the NHS around £5 for the tube of estrogen cream. Meanwhile, hospital admissions in the UK for people with UTIs stand at around £400m a year. Neglect of this simple prevention is another astonishingly stupid omission in our medical system. If the science on vaginal estrogen has been there for thirty years, why has the medical establishment failed to pass it on and give women the best advice?

On the non-hormonal front, oral or vaginal probiotic supplements and a healthy, low-sugar diet with prebiotics from fermented foods like kimchi will help keep your vagibiome flourishing. Four strains of lactobacilli, particularly lactobacillus crispatus and lactobacillus rhamnosus, are showing good results in lowering UTIs, as well as helping with thrush and other problems. I'll talk about the exciting new research on this later, but reporting directly from my own vagibiome, with years of UTIs behind me, I've found that vaginal estrogen plus a lactobacillus rhamnosus oral supplement every day means I don't get infections, and I have to pee less often. It has made a massive improvement to my day – and night.

What about the other alternatives sold over-the-counter to cure UTIs? Do any of them really work? D-Mannose, cranberry capsules, sodium citrate powders for cystitis, cranberry juice? There's lots of snake oil being sold in this space, so I took advice from Professor Harding, who told me about the European Association on Urology guidelines which researched lots of promising non-antibiotic options, including certain probiotics taken orally to improve the vaginal microbiome, and the sugar supplement related to glucose, D-Mannose, which might also prevent certain kinds of bacteria from sticking to the walls of the urinary tract and causing infection, and which helped in a few small trials. D-Mannose didn't work for me, but we're all different. Cranberry products and particularly juice, however, seemed to be marginally effective in scientific trials, but drinking water in large quantities also has a positive effect. Sodium citrate powders can help provide symptom relief, but don't seem to have any effect on bacterial infections, and can interact badly with some antibiotics.

So it looks like probiotics are the big winner here, and a major round-up in the *New Scientist* in 2024 said probiotics definitely help treat urinary tract infections. Taking a vaginal probiotic, either on its own or with an oral probiotic for four months, reduced the incidence of urinary tract infections in women with a history of recurring UTIs. Probiotics are living micro-organisms, live bacteria, and ones like lactobacillus crispatus, rhamnosus and reuteri, or bifidobacterium lactis and longum, are able to suppress the growth of urinary pathogens like E.coli. Studies seem to show that the most effective lactobacilli for controlling UTIs are lactobacillus rhamnosus and lactobacillus reuteri. My oral probiotics – you can get a mixed dose or a specific one which particularly works for you – cost me £19.99 for sixty capsules, and I just order them from a reliable mainstream supplier on Amazon. I thought vaginal pessaries would be best, but mysteriously, the oral and vaginal versions both seem to work – it all ends up in the same microenvironment down below. I asked a doctor about it, who put it simply: 'There's a lot of bacteria travelling back and forth in your pants and it gets everywhere.' Keeping your gut microbiome flourishing with a varied, vegetable-centric diet and consuming the probiotic foods like kefir, kimchi and kombucha will also help your vagibiome. And using bubbly bath bombs, or glitter lubes, or vaginal deodorant sprays is an incredibly bad idea – your vagina is self-cleaning. Water alone is good.

Of course, we may all need different lactobacilli and probiotics depending on the needs of our individual vagibiomes, which are unique to each of us, and to some extent finding the right combination is a bit of trial and error.

As I discussed in the previous chapter on sex, when vaginal estrogen falls in menopausal women, it can result in Genitourinary Syndrome of Menopause (GSM) and this only becomes a bigger issue as we get older. I got the lowdown on the urinary aspect when I visited the campaigning urologist

Dr Rachel Rubin in her office in Maryland, replete with pink anatomically correct vulvas and cute clitoris models. 'The serious issues are discomfort, pain when sitting, irritation, burning and itching of the vulva, urinary frequency and urgency. And the thing that kills elderly people all the time is urinary tract infections, which can lead to sepsis, worsened dementia, and death.'

Understanding the vaginal microbiome in older women could be life-changing for millions, and there is encouraging research. In one California study of over 5,000 women with the average age of 70, more than half had reduced UTIs after a year on vaginal estrogen and a third had none whatsoever. Dr Rubin is a crusading campaigner on this: 'We have millions of people in nursing homes who are dying of UTIs, and we have lots of data since the 1990s to show that vaginal hormones massively decrease urinary tract infections. We have new data. We have old data. We have so much data. The problem is that nobody's talking about it.' What about our mothers, our aunts, our older friends who don't know this? Can a simple intervention with regular vaginal estrogen make a huge change to their comfort and health?

The suffering and the science are often ignored by supposed experts too. A 2023 NHS England press release on UTI prevention advised women to stay hydrated, and wash themselves more. (Do people really think women haven't got the 'wipe front to back' message yet?) But the advice failed to mention vaginal estrogen at all, despite aiming warnings at 'older adults' and their carers. This is probably due, as usual, to gender bias in medicine, as well as embedded disinterest in the post-fertile vagina and possibly a complete misunderstanding of the safety of local estrogen.

To make matters worse, in the US the Food and Drug Administration 'black box' warnings on vaginal estrogen have not been updated and still list risks like blood clots, stroke and even memory loss, which have now been proven incorrect. The patient warning leaflets for vaginal estrogen products in the UK are outdated too. No wonder doctors are cautious. Dr Ashley Winter, a Los Angeles urologist colloquially known as 'The Angel of Estrogen' on X (the vagibiome is spreading on social media), said: 'In the US, vaginal estrogen has been approved by the FDA for vaginal dryness and painful sex – but not for an overactive bladder and UTI prevention, although we know it overwhelmingly works. So there's an education gap. I never learned it in medical school. That's why you have to bootstrap the education through social media.'

Sometimes a simple UTI can be a turning point, especially in our later years. It was for my mum, Ella. She was living at home independently with Alzheimer's disease, helped by her carer Helen who went in twice a day. But when Helen and I were both away for two days one August, the replacement carers failed to turn up and Ella became dehydrated, confused and delirious. She was taken to hospital, diagnosed with a UTI, and given intravenous antibiotics. By the time I flew in that evening, my mother was crashed out asleep. She rallied a bit physically over the next few days, but not mentally. The UTI had taken its toll. For the first time, she didn't recognise me and sometimes thought that I was her mum. That's a heartbreaking moment. Ella wasn't eating properly, so Helen and I took turns to come in and feed her, something she had always managed by herself. She struggled to stand or go to the hospital bathroom. Although the delirium went and she recognised us again, something had shifted mentally. Ella never came home to her flat. She started using a wheelchair and moved to a nursing home where she died less than a year later.

Now I know that dehydration was the cause of the UTI, and even if Ella had had decades of vaginal estrogen, it might have made no difference. But I had no sense until then that UTIs could have greater consequences and permanent physical and mental losses. There is already emerging evidence that infections, including UTIs, are themselves associated with an increased risk for dementia, according to a *Lancet* study. Professor Harding explained: 'UTIs can cause delirium, specifically in elderly patients, and that can make them disoriented and affect their cognition. A severe infection might just be sufficiently debilitating to cause it and then getting back to your baseline is quite difficult.'

How many UTIs like that could be avoided? Back in 2015 when Ella died, I had never heard of vaginal estrogen or atrophy, but now when I think of the truckloads of incontinence pads arriving every week at care homes like hers and the other women sitting in constant genitourinary discomfort on those plastic-covered armchairs with the television blaring, I wonder if we couldn't do more. So I talked to Dr Charlotte Gooding, a British Menopause Society specialist and GP in the north-east of England. 'UTIs are a large chunk of GP workload in primary care and it's mostly women of menopausal age. The majority of my home visits are to older women, particularly in care homes. Carers often ring up to say a patient is unwell and delirious with urinary symptoms and I've got to assess whether to try to keep her in the community or send her to hospital – and look out for sepsis. Mortality from urosepsis is huge, and UTIs can lead to further problems, for example when people get delirious and need to go to the bathroom, they might climb over the bed rails and fall and break their hip. I've seen that many times and it makes me incredibly sad walking round care homes, knowing we could do more to prevent UTIs in the first place.' Over half of hospital UTI admissions are for people over 65 and a quarter of all sepsis cases are related to UTIs – that's more than 50,000 a year in the UK.

Dr Gooding believes that no one is looking at the bigger picture and takes direct action when she can. 'Twice weekly estrogen pessaries, such as Vagifem, are very effective, but can be tricky for older women who might have dexterity issues and their carers don't always have time to help. But an Estring hormonal vaginal ring is great, like a floppy hairband with a jelly consistency and you can bend it to slip it in and leave it there for three months to estrogenise the tissues.' She sees improvement 'even for women in their eighties. In patients that have cognitive impairment such as dementia it's even more important, a UTI can cause serious worsening of their mental state. Some people find the idea of consent to vaginal rings difficult, and I understand that, but sometimes there is a medical "best interest" argument for that kind of care. So much better than ending up catheterised or using incontinence pads or with urosepsis.'

But while Dr Gooding is doing good, many medical

professionals are not up to speed on the efficacy of vaginal estrogen. She explained: 'I wasn't taught about menopause in my medical training. I wasn't taught about the role of estrogen in bladder functioning. We were just taught to treat UTIs with antibiotics, and it can make your heart sink, watching people go round in circles, in and out of hospital and care homes with embedded UTIs that we can't seem to help.'

Men suffer UTIs, too, making up about a fifth of cases. I remember my dad, Douglas, had a UTI a couple of times after he had a catheter following a stroke, but there was no mental change or delirium, although that can happen. For men, a UTI can often mean something more serious, and Dr Gooding says they tend to get seven days of antibiotics compared to the three offered to most women. 'Men are just designed much better – everything is more spread out and they've got a longer urethra meaning its harder for bacteria to reach the bladder. When they get a UTI, it is often a sign of something else going on in the immune system – their prostate affecting the emptying, or cancer, or being catheterised.'

The time to get to know your vagibiome is now in order to protect it in the immediate future and for the years to come. If you're unsure where to even start, there is a growing market in vagibiome testing, which might be useful for you to work out which bacterial strains are low level or non-existent in your body. Daye in the UK has a simple £99 test using a 'diagnostic tampon' which you put in for twenty minutes to gather a sample of your vaginal fluid, and then send off to their labs for testing. The results show your levels of lactobacilli, which might show which particular strain is missing, and help you 'understand your risk of vaginal infections like thrush or bacterial vaginosis'. Similar work is being done by the female founders of Evvy in America, which also does research: 'Our mission is to close the gender health gap by discovering and leveraging overlooked female biomarkers – starting with the vaginal microbiome. With a simple swab, you're not only taking control of your own health but improving research and treatment options for women and people with vaginas everywhere.'

There's a massive female health gap around the need to urinate all the time as you head into menopause, and that moment when you refuse to go with kids on a trampoline because of potential leakage, or literally pee yourself laughing or coughing. In medical terms, this is known as stress incontinence, and there's also urge incontinence, 'when you feel a sudden, overriding urge to urinate, and urine will leak either at this time or shortly afterwards', and also overflow incontinence when 'you are unable to fully empty your bladder and may leak urine frequently'. I looked these definitions up on the NHS Guy's and St Thomas's Hospital website – and they did *not* mention vaginal estrogen in their list of treatments, an extraordinary lapse of communication and knowledge. There is, in fact, a large body of research on this, and looking at thirty-four studies on 19,000 women in total, estrogen massively improved incontinence. Indeed, one study showed just twelve weeks of estrogen cream meant that almost half of women could now cough without a surprise pee. Daily pelvic floor exercises will help to keep muscles strong, but estrogen will make the skin in the bladder and urethra less thin and more elastic.

So peeing a lot is not an inevitable part of ageing. The news is spreading fast – there's even been a literary foray into the urinary tract. My neighbour, novelist Nina Stibbe, recently published *Went to London, Took the Dog*, a diary of leaving her family home in Truro at the age of 60 and running away to London for a year. 'I've always been prone to laughing and weeing myself a little bit,' she told me, 'but I was out with my dog, Peggy, in the city, and we got into a tussle over a chicken bone in the street and I weed myself and had to walk back with wet trousers. I realised I'd just been ignoring it for years.' In the book, Nina wees herself laughing while having spaghetti with the writer Nick Hornby. She began to use Tena Lady pads for safety and tried pelvic floor exercises, which didn't make much difference.

It was at that leaky point I first met Nina and her land-lady, author Deborah Moggach (also featured in the online dating chapter), at the launch of my 89-year-old neighbour's painting exhibition. As we walked home afterwards, we discussed the joys of general hormone replacement therapy and vaginal estrogen, and Debby said: 'Will that stop Nina peeing herself?' I suggested there was hope, posted my book through their door with the relevant page marked, and Nina went on HRT and vaginal estrogen. The HRT took a while to settle down, but the Vagifem was instantly popular. 'It made a difference within a week. I'm almost completely cured now, dry as a bone,' she said. Nina got her mum on vaginal hormones, too. 'She'd been on and off antibiotics for UTIs for ten years, and now she's doing much better.' Nina had been worried about including the 'UTI narrative arc' in her book, but it turned out to be an incredibly popular topic on her book tour. 'The audience is loving it.'

So now we know about the vagibiome, this glorious eco-system that lives within us and has only recently been investigated. The lack of interest until now reeks of medical misogyny. We're not just talking about UTIs here; we're talking about a whole generation of women who have felt shame around this, kept their miserable urinary symptoms secret, and just carried on necking Nurofen and antibiotics. What matters now is education, education, education – telling women that prevention is key, and that local estrogen and probiotics will help.

CHAPTER 11

Pumping up Your Muscle and Bone

We know that until recently, the healthcare system was deep-designed to keep men, rather than women, alive. Men are the default, and when it comes to our bones, the reality of this neglect is stark. Imagine a roomful of women. Imagine half of them breaking a bone. What will it be? Hip? Spine? Wrist? Neck? Imagine the plaster casts, the metal screws, the pain, the immobility, the loss, the grief – a third of those who break a hip will die within a year. You probably know one of them: an aunt, a mother, a neighbour down the street. This is our Zimmer-framed reality today: one in two women over 50 in the UK and the US experience a fracture due to osteoporosis. Men don't reach those sort of statistics until they are much older. And the same *could* be true for us – if we take action, now, to maintain hormones and muscles. The recurring theme throughout this chapter is that when it comes to osteoporosis, prevention is key.

Osteoporosis is insidious because it's invisible, and not on the radar for most women in midlife. I met a new osteoporosis patient, working mother Narelle Chidwick, when I was giving a book talk in Henley. Narelle was only 49 when she was sent for a DEXA bone scan by the NHS after injuring her ribs during a family skiing holiday. 'They told me I had the bone density of an 80- or 90-year-old woman, and a high fracture risk. I was properly shocked. I cried. I got really depressed. I didn't see it coming. I had early menopause at 46, but I'd been exercising, doing Pilates, eating well.' Now, ironically, Narelle and her 80-year-old father both have osteoporosis, but she is on a mission to try to rebuild her bones, more of which later.

Thanks to massive gender bias in medicine, and perhaps a lackadaisical disinterest in post-fertile bodies, midlife women like Narelle are not being told early enough about the simple preventative action they can take to maintain healthy bones – and this looks different for women from men. Two-thirds of osteoporosis sufferers are female for a reason: when hormones start running out around menopause, bone strength declines by 10–20 per cent. Men's hormones don't crash to the same level until they're in their seventies or eighties. Fragility fractures – the inexplicable sort that happen when you just trip over, or casually bang into something – rise exponentially in women from their late forties onwards. Low bone mineral density means your bones are brittle and look like a Crunchie bar inside, honeycombed with big holes. Most women don't know that. 'Your bones are silent until they break. And then they scream,' said Dr Vonda Wright, an American orthopaedic surgeon who is evangelical about getting the message out to women, not just in midlife but to younger women who may have low bone density due to missing periods when training for sport, dieting or being on certain contraceptives. Women aren't aware of the damage that has been done until far too late. 'It's crazy that women here usually only get DEXA scans once they are 65, when much earlier screening would mean we could halt the damage,' says Dr Wright. It's a very exasperating case of shutting the stable door after the horse has bolted – and broken a bone.

Instead of protecting bone health, we're dealing with the aftermath – extremely gruelling and invasive operations that bear a huge cost for both the NHS and the patient's health. Dr Wright talked about the tragedy of seeing frail women in hospital gowns after massive operations asking her, 'What's happened to me? I'm not who I used to be.' I spoke to another orthopaedic specialist, Dr Bill Robertson-Smith, an NHS senior surgical care practitioner at Northampton General Hospital. Bill is a brilliant woman, with wild curly hair, surprising earrings, and an iconoclastic and questioning attitude to women's healthcare, perhaps because she came to bone surgery after retraining later in life. I caught her one day as she emerged from theatre: 'We've been operating for nearly three hours, and I've just finished suturing a wound the length of the upper thigh of a woman in her eighties who had a peri-prosthetic fracture – that's when they've had a metal hip replacement, for example, and have now fractured the bone around it.' A big operation takes two pairs of hands, and Dr Robertson-Smith works alongside a senior consultant orthopaedic surgeon. I asked her to explain what happens in theatre in laywomen's terms.

'First, we cut through the skin, fat, fascia and muscle of the upper thigh before we get to the bone itself, and there's a lot of blood loss, so we have to cauterise blood vessels as we go along.' There's spurting? I ask, uneasily. 'The larger bleeding vessels will need to be tied off. Sometimes we remove the hip replacement and put a much longer implant into the femur, and sometimes we need to put a plate against the whole bone with long screws up to 50mm.' With a power drill? 'Yes, the tools are a bit like the ones in B&Q. We put metal cables around the plate. Then we wash the wound with saline, put local anaesthetic into the soft tissues and sew up each layer: muscle, fascia, fat, and finally put clips on the skin like a staple gun. We cover the wound with a special dressing that draws up the blood, so they don't get an infection.' Reading it back, the description has echoes of a body-horror movie like *Saw* but Dr Robertson-Smith is deadly serious. 'That operation and rehab costs the NHS about £30,000' – and could be preventable.

Dr Robertson-Smith has been on the front line for the last eleven years, and has grown increasingly frustrated by the lack of preventative care. It hangs heavily on her like the lead apron she has to wear when operating, so surgeons can X-ray as they go along, attaching screws to bone. 'The use of HRT wasn't part of my education in orthopaedics, and medical colleagues have said the same. What a difference it would make if we could discuss the benefits of HRT on bone health, and signpost patients to primary care for further treatment if appropriate.' But medicine works in silos, and menopause experts, surgeons, endocrinologists and rheu-matologists rarely confer. Progress is glacial. What might happen if they all looked at the world together through hormonal glasses?

There are two effective ways to protect women (and some non-binary and trans people) from fractures: the first is life-style, incorporating serious muscle-building, weight-bearing exercise, along with Vitamin D, magnesium and calcium-rich foods; the second is using hormone replacement therapy to slow bone loss and promote new growth. Using the two options simultaneously is an even better strategy. While it has proved almost impossible for the NHS to get the sedentary midlife population interested in jumping rope or lifting weights, it is cheap and easy to offer HRT to those for whom it is suitable, and it is approved by the NHS and the US Food and Drug Administration for strengthening bones and reducing breaks in menopausal women. Because HRT impacts on other menopause symptoms such as energy levels and mood stability, this often encourages a healthier lifestyle too.

The good news is that HRT can increase bone density by 7 per cent on average over two years, and reduce spinal fractures by a third. A meta-analysis concluded: 'HRT has a consistent, favorable and large effect on bone density at all sites.' Someone recently emailed me their DEXA bone scans, two years apart after starting HRT, and density had gone up 10 per cent – but I suspect some of that is the effect of weight-bearing exercise too. In one study, HRT increased spinal density by 13 per cent over a decade, while the untreated comparison group had 5 per cent bone loss. So bring on better bones. Throw away your Zimmer frames!

Not so fast. While we now know that HRT = Stronger Bones, healthcare professionals on the front line in the US and UK rarely consider that option. I wanted to change that once I knew the science, and with a research grant from Henpicked – Menopause in the Workplace, I worked on an investigation for months in 2024 with Dr Robertson-Smith. As part of the investigation she sent Freedom of Information requests asking for treatment data on nearly seventy NHS Fracture Liaison Services (FLS) in England, Wales and Northern Ireland. The FLS is 'the gold standard for fracture care' in treating osteoporosis in people over 50 who have broken a bone, according to the Royal Osteoporosis Society (ROS).

Our data revealed that in the last seven years, a massive 356,229 women had been treated by FLS clinics. Guess how many were offered HRT afterwards? Just 169. 'I was astonished it was so low,' said Dr Robertson-Smith. 'Around three-quarters of those women would be over 65 and un-likely to typically be offered HRT, but thousands of younger women in their fifties and early sixties who could benefit from bone-protective HRT were never offered that option either.' That's despite the fact HRT can work well alongside osteoporosis drugs, and the NHS website says: 'HRT helps to prevent osteoporosis by increasing your level of estrogen. It's particularly important to take HRT to help prevent osteoporosis if your periods stop before the age of 45.' It's also worth noting that women lose up to 6 per cent of their bone mass in perimenopause, so the earlier the better with starting hormones, and more so if you have low Vitamin D. One study of over 700 women in Iran, where covering up means women don't get much Vitamin D from sunlight, showed 10 per cent of perimenopausal women had osteoporosis but had no symptoms – yet.

It's not simply estrogen that makes a difference to bone health, but the orchestra of hormones, in particular natural testosterone in men, which is converted into estrogen in the body. Testosterone protects bone strength in women too. Dr Robertson-Smith explained: 'The main role of estrogen in bone health is to prevent bone loss, but we also know that progesterone also has an important part to play in stimulating bone growth. There is also a positive association between testosterone and bone mineral density, so all of these hormones are important.' Men with low testosterone levels earlier on in life are more likely to get osteoporosis as they age.

There is a lot of promising research out there, but the resources used by women to access information, such as the Royal Osteoporosis Society website, are not exactly HRT-friendly. An 'HRT' word search in 2024 brought up an old headline about breast cancer risk, and the HRT section is outdated compared to British Menopause Society guidelines, failing to make clear the safest choices, and starts unhelpfully: 'There are more than 50 different HRT products ...' leaving women flummoxed. I told the ROS about the sub-optimal experience for female users, but they replied: 'We make every effort to ensure our information is up-to-date and accurate ... we will review your feedback when we next update our HRT information.'

And if you're not aware of the benefits of HRT on your bone health, you're unlikely to be given that information by your GP. Although Narelle went through an early menopause, she was not offered HRT by her GP. Instead she was prescribed bisphosphonate drugs after her bone scan aged 49, as well as calcium carbonate and Vitamin D. Bisphosphonates inhibit bone resorption, which is the breaking down of bone tissue – bones are a bit like tree branches, growing, shedding and renewing all the time. Bisphosphonates cost £50 to £100 a year, and are the first-line NHS treatment for both men and women. But patients often complain of gastrointestinal, joint and flu-like symptoms. Due to that, and the fact no one can actually see whether they are working, around 40 per cent of patients come off bisphosphonates within a year, and 85 per cent with three. That's not very effective.

Narelle found the calcium carbonate and bisphosphonates caused weeks of painful constipation: 'You could feel it, like ropes in your stomach.' She called the ROS helpline to understand her scans and get advice, and then waited months for an appointment with an NHS rheumatologist. In the meantime, she started HRT for separate menopause symptoms with her GP, and felt a lot better. She is using what NHS menopause experts consider the safest option: estrogen gel or patch through the skin, and Utrogestan pills containing body-identical progesterone.

The rheumatologist said Narelle could stop the bisphosphonates and calcium carbonate pills if she wanted, and that HRT, calcium from food and Vitamin D supplements were acceptable for the moment. Treatment was about 'age and stage' and worth revisiting regularly. 'That gave me some confidence. Also, I knew my mother, who's in her late seventies, has been on HRT for years and is only just going into osteopenia.' Osteopenia means slightly lowered bone density, and is not as grave as osteoporosis. We should all look at what's happened to our mothers and sisters and aunts, and consider whether it's worth taking protective action early.

Some of the most effective preventative action can be lifestyle changes, and again we need to educate ourselves as to what this should look like. Narelle looked exasperated when she showed me her hospital letter suggesting she walked for thirty minutes, three times a week. 'I knew that wasn't anywhere enough for bone density – I was already walking 10,000 steps a day and exercising when I got the diagnosis,' she said. She's slim, fit and energetic, and runs a business called Live More With Less, helping people to simplify and transform their lives and homes, but more rather than less was what Narelle needed in terms of weight-bearing exercise. She did her own research online and learned more about the importance of muscles in her health. Among other experts, she discovered Dr Gabrielle Lyon, the American author of the bestseller *Forever Strong*. When I interviewed Dr Lyon, she said: 'Muscles are key to osteoporosis prevention, to holding up our skeletons.' She has almost a million followers on her @drgabriellelyon Instagram, and a mission to make muscles big, in both senses. 'People think of bones as the end point of this silent disease, but low muscle mass is the first sign of low bone density.' Dr Vohra agrees and says muscle mass is a useful early indicator of skeletal health, informing women of the need to take preventative action before they have to resort to expensive hard-to-get scans. The NHS exercise guidelines recommend aerobic exercise for over two hours a week, including cycling and walking along with weight-bearing or resistance exercise twice a week – but most people don't follow those instructions. 'We'd be better doing more social prescribing, sending people on the NHS for six weeks' free training at a gym – but sadly that's still a postcode lottery.'

Loss of muscle mass is called sarcopenia, and women can see a drop of up to 10 per cent from early perimenopause to postmenopause. This is what we need to guard against. high-intensity interval training (often referred to as HIIT) – short, sharp shocks with heavy weights – is the way forward, according to Dr Lyon: 'The best way to safeguard your independence is to protect your skeletal muscle mass. Muscle is the only organ system we can directly control, and you can't build it without resistance training and eating plenty of protein.' Narelle was lucky and worked with a private trainer who created a programme of strength and impact exercise three times a week (but you can find similar programmes free online). In the American LIFTMOR trial, 101 women over 58 years old with osteoporosis or osteopenia were split into two groups and monitored over eight months. Those in the group that did conventional exercise twice a week had a 1 per cent loss of bone density in this time, and those doing supervised high-intensity interval training – squats, deadlifts and jumping chin-ups twice a week for thirty minutes – gained almost 3 per cent. It worked – fast. Why aren't we getting that message out to women?

'Because we're the Special K generation,' said Narelle. Gen Xers grew up with messages favouring skinny over strong. Remember the 'Special K' TV challenge from two decades ago, which told women they could 'drop a jean's size in two weeks' by replacing two meals per day with bowls of sugary cereal? Or adverts for Nimble, white bread so light at fifty calories a slice that women floated off in hot air balloons. More than thirty years since Madonna flexed her biceps on the Blonde Ambition tour, prompting shocked headlines, there's still a sense for older generations that muscles are masculine. Dr Lyon concurs: 'There's still a cultural perception that muscle is not attractive; it's been very fringe for so long. Muscle is the organ of longevity.'

Also out there on the battlements changing public opinion alongside Dr Lyon is Dr Wright, an orthopaedic sports surgeon and longevity expert with a million followers on her Instagram. She is an evangelical believer in muscling up. I spoke to Dr Wright, who is 57, and you will either see her in hospital scrubs with her specs on, or in a short leather dress with her magnificent muscled legs. She explained: 'I lift *heavy*! You need deadlifts, squats, bench-presses, chin-ups. Four reps, four sets. Lots of reps with namby-pamby pink weights are garbage. You can also stomp up and down the stairs and that helps too.' She added: 'Building muscle is the one thing you can do to save your life, save your metabolism, save your bones, prevent you from falling down, and build brain resilience.'

Dr Wright also authored a groundbreaking 2024 medical paper in the journal *Climacteric,* which officially named the problem: the Musculoskeletal Syndrome of Menopause.

'This means the collection of symptoms caused by estrogen loss from perimenopause onwards, including joint pain, muscle weakness, decreased bone density and increased risk of arthritis and fractures. Estrogen doesn't just increase bone density – it reduces inflammation in our joints. So many women come into my clinic with frozen shoulder at this age – not due to injury, but because of inflammation.' Frozen shoulder affects 10 per cent of women in the UK at some point in their lives. This very naming of Musculoskeletal Syndrome of Menopause is a major step forward in helping women and doctors join the dots between hormones and bone and joint health, as is Dr Wright's insistence on sharing her knowledge on public platforms, despite backlash from traditional colleagues. 'How dare an academic surgeon like myself want to educate women and come out of my ivory tower to talk to people on Instagram?' Her muscloskeletal paper has had over a quarter of a million downloads – that's Taylor Swift-level popularity for academia.

In the paper, Dr Wright advocates holistically for exercise, vitamins and nutrition. One of her catch phrases is 'Sugar bakes you from the inside', as it's inflammatory. Her own joint pain really improved when she gave up sugar. She is also a massive advocate for protein, and suggests consuming one gram of protein per ideal pound of body weight every day – lean chicken breasts, lots of eggs, tofu, nuts and oily fish. Protein is crucial because it makes up about half of bone volume, and calcium-rich foods like yogurt and kefir are also a win. Fresh vegetables, legumes and fruit are essential (she grabs handfuls of raw spinach and just eats them in passing) and the fibre in those and wholegrains really matters; Dr Wright describes fibre as a 'new BFF' and you should aim for 25g daily, like a cup of beans, two or three fruits, or a tablespoon of flaxseeds, as it helps decrease inflammation and maintain lean muscle mass, which in turn supports bone density.

There is so much we can do to protect our bones in later life. But there are also barriers. As well as being a gender issue, this is a socioeconomic issue: the worse the economic deprivation, the worse the bone health. Dr Radhika Vohra, a GP with a special interest in women's health and medical advisor to The Menopause Charity, has done groundbreaking research over the years on menopause and ethnicity in the UK. Some Asian women are at higher risk of osteoporosis – smaller bone size can lead to lower area bone mineral density, and genome-wide studies have identified a genetic link to osteoporosis in East Asian populations. As I mentioned above, some Muslim women who cover up or spend less time outdoors in the sun are often short of Vitamin D. Many Asians are also lactose intolerant so can miss out on calcium from dairy products. Better and more specific advice is needed. 'Menopause care is lacking for people from economically deprived and ethnic backgrounds: there's more early menopause too. Disparities in lifestyle, nutrition, education and poverty mean women are losing bone mineral density earlier, and less likely to get help.'

Absurdly, there are barriers to prevention at GP level too. Dr Vohra astonished me when she explained that the 40-plus health checklist for all women doesn't mention osteoporosis or menopause, instead concentrating on high blood pressure, cholesterol, diabetes, body mass index, exercise and alcohol. 'General practice gets paid to keep a register of patients already diagnosed with osteoporosis, but they don't get paid for preventing it. The first-line treatment advised is a bisphosphonate, and the DEXA report with recommendations does not mention HRT. Yet osteopenia is that lovely window when you can change things for women, and we miss it.'

As ever, it's worth following the money. Improving prevention would be bad news for the osteoporosis Big Pharma business, which makes $16 billion worldwide annually (that's the equivalent to the GDP of a small country). Pharmaceutical capitalism thrives on sickness-care rather than preventative-care, and many pharma companies lavishly sponsor conferences and osteoporosis charities in order to promote their wares. Of course, there is a real need for bone-strengthening medicine to protect people once osteoporosis sets in, and the Royal Osteoporosis Society website has a useful guide to the various drugs. They include Denosumab, which prevents bone resorption and costs the NHS £732 a year; Abaloparatide, approved for treating osteoporosis after menopause for women at high risk of fractures at £3,534 a year; and Romosozumab, which stimulates bone formation and reduces loss, but may increase the risk of a heart attack, and costs up to £5,133 a year. By contrast, estrogen and progesterone HRT costs £140 a year. Many of these drugs, such as bisphosphonates and denosumab, can also potentially make the bones too hard, causing rare problems with jaw growths and atypical fractures, so patients are advised to take a 'drug holiday' of at least a year every three to five years to mitigate these risks. HRT, on the other hand, keeps bones in their naturally rubbery, flexible state because it maintains collagen. We want to bend when we hit the ground, not crack.

This is a humongous public health issue, costing the NHS £4.6 billion a year for women and men. Positive change could come in three ways: by paying GPs for osteoporosis prevention, by educating healthcare professionals, and by giving women choice and knowledge. The ROS says a quarter of people don't even know what 'osteoporosis' means, so we need a public and social media campaign, as there has been for menopause. The research grant from Henpicked went towards creating professional resources for doctors, and an information pack for women, as well as a downloadable poster. Its slogan? Give Your Bones a Break.

I learned so much researching this chapter, and obviously I sit at my desk typing, plotting and going on Zooms for most of the day, except when I am swimming, occasionally running, or walking the dog. None of it, except the lackadaisical running, is seriously weight bearing, so I began to obsess about my potentially flaccid muscle and the need to rip my muscles and jolt my bones into regrowth. On a deadline, I didn't have time to travel back and forth to a gym, and I'd rather be outside anyway, but I began to add little 'exercise snacks' to my day. These are much advocated by my friend Lavina Mehta, who has written a book called *The Feel Good Fix*, which advocates exercise snacking: a plank here, a bunch of sit-ups there, some weight lifting here, some squats on a coffee break, nothing taking much more than five minutes, stuff easily sneaked in at work. Lavina started her snacking business on YouTube in Covid lockdown, when she persuaded her 76-year-old mother-in-law, Nisha, to do chair workouts alongside her athletic leaps. They went viral.

Inspired, I devised a system of doing blocks of twenty-one sit-ups while drying my hair, giving it a curious windblown look, and I started using the kitchen counters for arm exercises, taking my full 9st bodyweight, until the counter started to crack. I then began taking the dog for its evening sniffari to children's play areas, where I swung from monkey-bar to monkey-bar. I do dead-drop hanging – basically hanging like a gibbon for a minute from a pole or tree – which increases shoulder mobility, improves upper body muscles, and helps with posture if you sit at a desk all day. You feel taller afterwards. I have also started climbing trees, which I hadn't really done since I was 12, and I'd forgotten how much I enjoy it – challenging, a tad dangerous, and entertaining when you drop suddenly down into the park, a mad 60-year-old woman in running gear with twigs in her hair. May you find your own path to muscle power.

CHAPTER 12

Avoiding the Midlife Muffin Top

'Muffin top' is a horrible term, but I wanted to get your attention and dig specifically into how we change shape in midlife, and the health risks that brings. Why do we mysteriously grow a roll of fat above the waist of our jeans, and gain weight around our stomachs? Why do our arms suddenly sprout 'bingo wings' when we are eating exactly the same foods as we used to and taking the same amount of exercise as before? Let's approach these questions through the lens of science and research. Like so much in midlife, understanding the latest science and investigating the changing machine of your body makes a positive difference to the way you feel and act.

Having researched this chapter, my consideration when I'm choosing what to eat now is: 'Will it make me strong?' not 'Will it make me fat?', a question which hung guiltily around my neck for years like a nutritional albatross. We all know so much more now about the role and importance of food – eating the rainbow, pumping up protein and filling up on fibre are about health and not just calorific content. And yet calories have long ruled this conversation for so many of us, particularly women. I'm average-sized and like many women you'd never know I'd had a problem with food. Yet I spent a couple of my teen years with intermittent, secret and undiagnosed bulimia, desperate between bingeing on Mars Bars and throwing up to get into size 10 drainpipe jeans, lying on the floor to pull the zip up. Even when I felt better about myself and the bulimia ended, that self-critical gremlin stayed with me for years. The reason I mention my early disordered eating here is because midlife's stresses and hormonal changes can bring back anxiety around food that we thought we'd overcome, and return women to the disordered eating of their teens or twenties. 'The hormone changes and psychological changes in midlife can be very similar to those of teenagers,' psychotherapist Dr Kalanit Ben-Ari explained. 'So if you had a vulnerability as a teenager, and it wasn't processed, and you have emotional baggage that wasn't processed, it might show up again. We revisit the things that are unresolved.'

Midlife body image is reflected in a hall of distorting mirrors, and that's partly because in perimenopause and menopause, your body composition changes – much like during puberty. It's good to know that we can once again blame our hormones and not our habits for what's happening, and use this moment to take action rather than panic. Perimenopausal and menopausal women naturally stop making the strongest and most prolific form of estrogen (estradiol, the one we put back with HRT) and instead start making a weaker estrogen called estrone in fatty tissue, often round their waist and tummy. It's a vicious, tubby circle: as estradiol falls, so does your insulin resistance and your ability to burn fat, and there is an increase in visceral adipose tissue – the fat that surrounds your organs in your abdominal cavity. Menopause leads to a shift of fat build-up from subcutaneous to visceral tissue, where estrone is produced to compensate for lack of estradiol.

That particular estrone-producing fat also increases breast cancer risk by 20 per cent or more: 'Estrone activates pro-inflammatory genes associated with poor estrogen-receptor positive breast cancer outcomes', according to a recent study. While estradiol is healthy and anti-inflammatory, the second-rate estrone causes inflammation. The combination of this, and a steady decline in female testosterone, which helps maintain muscle and metabolism, means we're in trouble. So if you can avoid building up that kind of fat, through replacing your hormones and/or making lifestyle changes, it's really worth it for your future health.

There's a duvet of estrone-producing fat wrapped round most middle-aged women in the US and UK, and while we shouldn't fat-shame, we should fat-explain. This is not just about dress size, it's about increases in the risk of diabetes, dementia, cardiovascular disease, joint pain – and the miserable effect on mental health. The data is sobering: weight gain rises for everyone with age, but it takes a big leap up for women their mid-forties. In the 45–64 age group, 72 per cent of women are overweight, and of those, 30 per cent are obese. Those figures worsen with deprivation and disability too. The changes are slow and insidious: in the US and UK, women hitting menopause put on around 1.5lbs every year on average, and every pound pumps up their blood pressure. The majority of American women over 45 have high blood pressure or hypertension, which increases the risk of heart disease or strokes.

What should we do? It's clear regular dieting isn't working for the majority. Do we hand out weight-loss drugs like Ozempic, Wegovy or Mounjaro to everyone? Latest figures from America show one in eight people have used one of these drugs, and 6 per cent are presently using them. That's 15 million Americans. Figures are much lower for the UK, around 50,000, but rising rapidly. Semaglutide drugs like Ozempic mimic the hormone GLP-1, which is released from the gut after a meal. The hormone helps insulin work properly and feeds back to the brain to make people feel full. That satiety signal from the gut to the brain stops us from overeating. (It's interesting that doctors give out higher-than-natural doses of expensive patentable hormone-mimicking semaglutides, but they're more reluctant to give out the cheap, natural, unpatentable hormones in HRT.)

In the US, obesity has gone down by 2 per cent since these drugs were widely available, and they also help counter diabetes and improve heart health. In the UK there have been gushing endorsements and many before-and-after photoshoots with journalists and celebrities. The Health Secretary Wes Streeting announced a new partnership between the government and US pharmaceutical company Eli Lilly who make the appetite-reducing drug Zepbound and will invest in trials. He said: 'Our widening waistbands are also placing significant burden on our health service, costing the NHS £11bn a year – even more than smoking. And it's holding back our economy.' Prime Minister Keir Starmer added: 'This drug will be very helpful to people who want to lose weight, need to lose weight, very important for the economy so people can get back into work.' At the moment, a monthly supply from UK supermarket pharmacies is around £169 if you have a prescription from a private doctor, and in the US, the cost is much higher: Wegovy retails at $1,349 per month. Semaglutides are already available on the NHS to tackle obesity, but there are many caveats and long waiting lists. The NHS is, sensibly, combining the use of semaglutides with new lifestyle and nutrition apps, which offer a programme for long-term weight reduction. The criteria for accessing weight management medication means patients have to have at least one weight-related disease such as diabetes or high blood pressure, and a body mass index (BMI) of at least 35.0 kg/m², or at a lower threshold depending on circumstances.

Semaglutides are not a bad idea as a kickstarter for weight control, better health and diabetes management, particularly for people living with obesity, but they do come with some potential health risks. The main side effects are nausea, diarrhoea and constipation, bone and muscle loss, as well as rarer cases of thyroid tumours, pancreatitis and kidney disease. The effects on mental health are relatively uncharted, but the warnings on semaglutide products differ.

Wegovy's label mentions potential risks of anxiety and depression, while Ozempic's does not. Yet the huge positives of losing weight on physical and mental health – the return of joy in life and bodily confidence – probably outweigh most risks. However, in the weight-loss gold rush, we just don't have the necessary long-term research studies. There is some concern that semaglutide can reduce free 'happy hormone' dopamine levels in the brain that may eventually lead to anhedonia, which is a loss of interest in pleasure, and the psychiatric safety of the drug is now being monitored by regulators in the US and Europe. Then there is the question of long-term effectiveness. Will many patients have to stay on these potentially risky drugs forever? One study found that people who stopped taking semaglutides regained two-thirds of their weight within a year, so clearly a complete and courageous re-engineering of eating and exercise is needed when the drug has done its work and permanently leaves the body. And that's hard. Without changes to lifestyle, everything reverts, and staying on semaglutides forever is not only expensive, but has health risks, particular to bone density.

Yet for many the dream seems to come true, and the appetite-suppressant drugs are largely effective. Celebrities from Oprah Winfrey to Stephen Fry to Sharon Osbourne have had a go, and two English newspaper columnists I've met, Sarah Vine and Allison Pearson, have written about their transformations in midlife on diet drugs. '"How do I know the fat jab works? Because I'm on it!" Sarah Vine reveals how it has changed her life,' said the *Daily Mail* headline. Sarah, 58, who at one point weighed 16st, had early menopause, and was on track for Type 2 diabetes. She managed to get down to 13st with diet and exercise, and then plateaued. Her private doctor offered her Saxenda, similar to a semaglutide, and she lost another stone. 'Initially, I had a tiny bit of nausea – a common side effect – but nothing so drastic as to make me want to stop. Gradually, I began to notice that I wasn't all that hungry anymore. And when I did eat, I ate a lot less, as though I had already eaten half a plate of food before even picking up my knife and fork. It was an almost imperceptible shift. And, slowly but surely, the dial on the scales began to go the right way again.' She wrote that she is now maintaining her weight on low-dose Ozempic. 'Food, which once used to be such a source of anxiety and guilt, is no longer my enemy. It's just fuel. I eat when I'm hungry, and I don't have to worry about eating too much because it's simply not possible. I am also much less likely to crave sugary treats ... Physically, I feel so much better. Being lighter means my joints don't hurt, and it's a joy not to be lugging those extra pounds around every day. My blood pressure has come down, my skin is better – and I no longer hate the person in the mirror.'

That's life-changing in terms of physical and mental health. American research has also suggested weight-loss drugs could substantially shrink the opioid crisis by muting addiction and alcoholism, and there are also positive effects on the risk of stroke and heart disease. A survey of over 7,000 people who used semaglutide-type drugs on a Weight Watchers' programme found 45 per cent reported decreased alcohol consumption. On the downside, users can experience loss of bone density in the hip and spine, and muscle wasting appears to be around 15 per cent in just over a year, and as we saw in the previous chapter, maintaining muscle and bone mass is key, especially for women in midlife who are already losing both due to hormones leaving the building during menopause. Here, weight-lifting exercise can help maintain muscle and bone as patients lose fat. Obstetrician and gynaecologist Dr Mary Claire Haver, who wrote *The Galveston Diet* and *The New Menopause*, thinks semaglutides can be incredibly helpful – when taken sensibly. On her podcast she explained: 'What's happening today is a frenzy over GLP-1s [semaglutides]. A lot of people are getting it from people who don't understand how it works and what happens to the body. But you never want to sacrifice muscle mass to get to a number on a scale. That muscle mass is going to keep us out of a nursing home. This relentless pursuit of thinness as a measure of health is the worst thing. We're worried we're going to see the possibility of an epidemic of osteoporosis in women and men who have not been properly counselled in the use of these GLP-1s, because they lose so much muscle.'

With that risk in mind, Allison Pearson, who is 64, has a personal trainer and goes to the gym twice a week in an attempt to keep up her muscle and bone strength while on Mounjaro. In her *Telegraph* story, 'My Miracle Weight-Loss Jab Has Changed My Life', Allison explained: 'There is no shame in doing anything that makes you healthier ... After three weeks, I weighed myself and I'd lost half a stone. Around 4.5 per cent of my body weight. Admittedly, most of that is chins. It's good to see my jawline again. And it's a hell of a lot cheaper than a facelift.' She suffered from constipation and took to prune juice, but that has been the only problem so far. 'I am unshackling myself from the ravening Cookie Monster and retraining my appetite for when I go it alone. I am eating mainly protein, getting most of my carbs from vegetables and, astonishingly, not missing chocolate. Without my regular sugar fix, which I mistook for happiness, I definitely feel calmer too.' In terms of bone and muscle loss, along with weight-bearing exercise, combining semaglutides with HRT seems to be a winner, creating higher weight loss, while the hormones in the HRT help to protect bone density and muscle mass.

The weight-loss jab is a miracle for capitalism too. The Danish pharmaceutical firm Novo Nordisk, who patented the drug Ozempic, have a $418 billion market capitalisation – worth more than the GDP of their own country. I recently met someone who'd taken out her entire pension and invested it in Eli Lilly shares. She'll just have to cross her fingers that these drugs turn out to be largely safe and hope there's no huge class-action lawsuit in years to come. Weight-loss medicines are a part of the predatory economic cycle of Big Farming, Big Food, Big Health Insurance and Big Pharma, particularly in America. In this cycle, high-fructose corn syrup is added to ultra-processed foods delivered to your door, creating a ticking obesity bomb defused by medical insurance paying pharmaceutical companies for weight-loss jabs. But what if the semaglutide rush heralds the end of the fast-food culture, those profitable products high in fat, salt and sugar? What if we no longer want the McDonald's double quarter pounder with cheese at 740 calories, twenty chicken nuggets at 890 calories, or the big breakfast with hotcakes at 1,080 calories? Research by JP

Morgan suggests that people on semaglutides spend up to 17 per cent less on food in the first six months, and in an attempt to milk the trend, Nestlé has launched its Vital Pursuit brand featuring frozen pizza, protein pasta and sandwich melts as 'a companion for GLP-1 weight loss medication users'. It's a brilliant piece of doublethink.

But what if you still want to lose a bit of weight for your health, without going down semaglutide alley? What if calorie counting has never helped you, regular cardio exercise isn't working for you, and cravings lurk evilly, waiting to pounce in the mid-afternoon slump? Let's look at the ways to rebuild a healthy relationship with eating, and find the right types of food that work with a changing midlife body. For a start, there is one food that works like a semaglutide on your metabolism, holding back hunger because it takes such a long time to digest, and that's simply protein, preferably lean, like chicken, fish, tofu, beans and unsalted nuts. I interviewed Dr Gabrielle Lyon, an expert on nutrition, muscle and longevity and author of *Forever Strong,* who explained that we need protein to build muscle, and muscle burns fat. 'The issue isn't body fat, but lack of sufficient healthy muscle tissue. You can't build muscle without dietary protein. Your choice of food is really important.' Dr Lyon herself is an extraordinary lean, mean, protein-fed machine, and she can lift gargantuan weights without chipping her nail varnish. 'It's common for women to put on central adiposity whenever hormonal change is going on, and there are practical ways to combat that. We need to be fitter, stronger, and build more muscle mass by lifting weights three times a week.' She favours 30g of protein twice a day (30g equals a chicken breast, or a cup of nuts, or five eggs) and says we need to change our attitude to pumping iron. 'We think it's not for us, it's not for women to be strong, it's not for women to lift weights, and muscle was seen as very fringe.' Long-term benefits of more muscle, aside from a stronger body and bones, include a faster metabolism, less risk of disease, better mood, as well as lower triglycerides, a type of fat (lipids) found in your blood. Triglycerides store extra calories ready to use as energy, but if there's too much, that can cause hardening of the arteries and risk of stroke. So muscle matters, or as Dr Lyon put it: 'Muscle is the organ of longevity.'

Aside from protein, there are also cheap, old-fashioned (mostly Scottish) foods like barley and porridge which may well be 'Nature's Ozempic', according to a new report which says that more fibre in the diet may boost levels of the hormone GLP-1. Meanwhile, weight-loss programmes and diet books are losing sales as weight-loss drugs replace their words of advice. I have always thought you can guess what's in most of those books by their titles, so there's no need to actually purchase them. For instance, *5-2: The Fast Diet* does precisely what it says on the tin, as does *Intermittent Fasting* and *Glucose Revolution*. *How Not to Eat Ultra-Processed* is also self-explanatory – just don't do it. I remembered the consternation and constipation when my mum went on the *Grapefruit and Boiled Egg Diet* for a week, long ago, and that's how I fell down an internet rabbit hole investigating wacky diet books of yore. Although it's not entirely relevant, I'm just sharing some titles for your delectation in case they help. There's the religious route: *I Prayed Myself Slim*, as well as *Help Lord – The Devil Wants Me Fat!* and *What Would Jesus Eat?* (loaves and fishes, obvs). There's astrological advice in *Diet Signs – Follow Your Horoscope to a Slimmer You.* Husbands are also considered: *How to Take 20 Pounds Off Your Man* tells readers to use 'stealth, subterfuge, trick and treat' because 'he alone cannot save himself'. I was especially attracted to two vintage titles: *The Sexy Pineapple Diet* and *The Viking Method: Your Nordic Fitness and Diet Plan for Warrior Strength.* What we do know is that diet books sell, but diets very rarely work, so diet books sell more. What we have to do instead is grasp the science of how food works in our bodies.

The high priest of food science nowadays is Professor Tim Spector of King's College London, who has brought understanding of the stomach microbiome to the not-starving masses, and on the way created the Zoe nutrition empire, which handily combines research and profit. Professor Spector does sell healthy eating books – his latest is the *Food for Life Cookbook* – but the work his team has done on the gut microbiome is genuinely very useful. I interviewed him a while ago when my partner Cameron and I tested out the Zoe scheme and were each given a free Continuous Glucose Monitor (CGM) for two weeks to track our blood sugar peaks and dips. We also had to agree to Zoe anonymously harvesting our data for future research. (The Zoe monitoring and follow-up assessment package now costs £299. In America you can get a two-week CGM monitor programme over-the-counter for $49.) We would also provide a sample to discover the dark secrets of our microbiomes, the community of trillions of micro-organisms living in our guts.

The diversity of those bacteria and other microbes is really important – a wide range of good bacteria protects you from infections and disease, and a small range (say if you favoured double cheeseburgers every day) puts you at risk. Eating ultra-processed food (UPF) for two weeks increased harmful bacteria and reduced the biodiversity of people's microbiomes by up to 40 per cent. UPF is basically food that often contains high levels of sugar, salt and fats, with added ingredients like artificial flavours, emulsifiers, colouring, sweeteners and preservatives which you wouldn't use in home cooking, and the microbiome isn't keen on them either. Professor Spector added that 'diet and depression are clearly linked; your gut microbiome affects your mental health too'. He described the gut microbiome as an 'incredible pharmacy' within us, with individual microbes helping produce vital chemicals like serotonin, which affects brain function and mood. Studies have just begun on the links, but low diversity in the microbiome seems to be linked with higher levels of depression, and that some specific types of bacteria are more abundant in depressed people. Professor Spector said that 'quite big changes begin in the microbiome around perimenopause; the way that you metabolise food changes as you age. As women get older their post-meal blood sugar levels get larger.' That's why we need to change what and how we eat, for our physical and mental health.

The idea with Zoe is that after two weeks of tests and monitoring, they help you work out a personal nutrition programme, and you can also spot how you react individually to various foods. I found it fascinating at first, as Cameron and I stabbed what seemed to be a pin on a big sticking plaster into our arms, leaving the CGM there for fourteen days. It linked to the Zoe app on our phones, and measured the peaks and troughs in our blood sugar levels day and night. For a while, it was high drama: a mere banana could send my glucose spiking; yet waking up in the morning, I was clearly close to death, comatose on the glucose ratings. I shuffled around steadily eating dry nuts in case the CGM had a hissy fit, but I mostly stayed between the high and low lines. Cameron, perhaps due to being a man, had an even steadier glucose level, even though we are the same age. It didn't seem fair. Professor Sarah Berry, the nutritionist leading research at Zoe, told me why that might be. 'In our study, peri- and postmenopausal women had higher blood pressure. They had worse insulin sensitivity. They had higher cholesterol. They had higher inflammation. They had higher visceral adiposity.' This was a sudden change for the worse, whereas men's risk factors just get steadily higher with age. Menopausal women had an increase in circulating blood sugar, and unfavourable post-meal responses to fat. As usual, diminishing estrogen – estradiol – is the culprit. The whole caboodle also causes bloating, gas and discomfort, and do I remember rolling around with stomach pain at night during perimenopause. But when Professor Berry looked at women on HRT, 'they had significantly lower blood pressure, lower heart rate, less bad cholesterol, and significantly better insulin sensitivity'. They also had less stomach fat and lower inflammation.

So obviously HRT was helping me quite a bit, but it turned out my microbiome and glucose mechanism could do better. I drank a rare glass of Chardonnay on an empty stomach at a medical conference to see what would happen on the app, and my blood sugar went through the roof. Sirens. Wearing the CGM was like having a bossy teacher nagging you all the time: a railway snack shop – all KitKats, apple juice, white bread sandwiches and syrupy cereal bars – suddenly looked like Dante's Inferno in terms of glucose spikes, and there was nothing sensible to eat. You also have to consume a nasty bag of fatty muffins on one day, and sugary muffins another, so Zoe can see how your body processes fat and sugar. A few hours after eating, you have to take a large blood sample (I believe the kits have improved), and unfortunately I was on a train with a friend in that time window, so that was quite messy and scary for the other passengers, although funny for us. There was also the 'collect your poop sample' day (I'll spare you the details), which gave an insight into all the different bacteria living in our gut microbiomes. Cameron's was better, again annoyingly. Basically, we are all different in the way we react to different foods – innocent porridge can set people off on a high, for instance – and we should tailor our diets to foods that help us avoid the spiking highs and the subsequent energy flops, and instead keep us steady. Yes, it's smashed avocado and sourdough all round for me, with a sprinkling of chopped nuts.

Keeping your blood glucose steady is about more than just avoiding those sugar crashes. The more spikes you have, the less responsive your cells become to insulin, and insulin resistance can lead to Type 2 diabetes, so it's really important to try and keep things on an even kilter. As I got to grips with controlling the glucose spikes, I followed the @glucosegoddess author Jessie Inchauspé on Instagram, and after a few days of scrolling her graphs of different food combinations and glucose highs, I got the point. Aside from avoiding a Tunnocks' Teacake binge, the main rule at meals seems to be: eat your veg first, protein next, and carbs and sweet things last. Inchauspé is French, and of course that's what the slimmer French have always done, by putting crudités (salad and raw veg) first on the menu, and a tiny square of dark chocolate at the end with an espresso. Her website has some useful advice which I'll summarise:

- Eat a savoury breakfast, not a sweet one
- Add a plate of vegetables to the beginning of your meals
- Before eating, have a tablespoon of vinegar (any kind) in a glass of water or drizzled on your vegetable starter. (This lowers the spikes)
- Only have fruit whole, never juiced or dried
- Eat sweet foods at the end of a meal instead of on their own as a snack
- Go for a ten-minute walk after lunch or dinner

We also have to discuss nutritional Satan – sugar. No one has a good word to say about it. White sugar is sucrose, which is half fructose and half glucose, and it turns out that when fructose is broken down by the liver it creates uric acid, which can accumulate in the joints and cause inflammation and arthritis. Glucose is the primary energy for the brain and most cells in the body, but it's much better to get it from slow-release sources like wholegrains or vegetables. A spoonful of sugar does not make the medicine go down – it makes the spike go up. Fructose tends to be stored as 'visceral fat' around the stomach and organs like the liver and heart. That's probably why a quarter of Americans have non-alcoholic fatty liver disease, as the American diet is very fructose heavy. And not surprisingly, fructose is bad for your microbiome as it reduces the amount of beneficial bacteria.

Cameron ripped off his CGM early, but I carried on dutifully, although I was by now bored catatonic by my own body. I expect many people would enjoy and benefit from the follow-up conversations with the Zoe team, and the recipe and lifestyle advice, but I didn't find it particularly enlightening. Quite simply, Professor Spector says we all need to eat thirty plants a week, be they green leafy veg, nuts or even spices, plus the three K's that are so important to the microbiome's superpowers – the probiotics kefir, kimchi and kombucha, fermented foods where the bacteria party is already kicking off. Prebiotics like garlic, onions, asparagus, beets, cabbage, leeks, beans, peas, lentils and legumes are key to building a happy gut too. Beneficial monounsaturated fats like those in olive oil and avocado help your 'good' High-Density Lipoprotein (HDL) cholesterol fight off the 'bad' Low-Density Lipoprotein (LDL) cholesterol in fatty red meat and butter. LDL cholesterol can build up in artery walls, narrowing them, and high levels increase risk of heart disease and stroke. HDL cholesterol helps remove other cholesterol from the bloodstream and takes excess cholesterol to the liver for disposal, so higher levels are better for heart health. As someone said: 'Think of LDL as dropping off cholesterol in your arteries, while HDL acts like a clean-up crew.' You can up your healthy polyunsaturated fat levels with oily fish, shellfish, nuts and seeds. Coffee keeps the party going in your microbiome, increasing the diversity of the bacteria.

Fibre is essential too – wholewheat pasta and bread, kidney beans, lentils, peas. Professor Spector said in *The Times* that 'fibre plays a key role in appetite regulation and metabolism, harnessed by specific gut microbes'. The amount of fibre this time? 30g. So we're being told, variously, to eat 30g of protein, 30g of fibre and 30 different plants. Clearly thirty has some magical power – or do they just pick these numbers out of thin air?

After I'd done the Zoe experiment, the company brought out the 'MenoScale' calculator where you could rate the severity of your menopause symptoms – brain fog, sore joints, hot flushes etc. – and get nutrition advice to help. According to the Zoe website the average score was 23, but long-suffering menopausal women were scoring as high as 63. I got a much happier score of 2, almost as low as you could get, since on HRT I didn't have any of the symptoms, except for slightly dry skin. Often more vegetables and fibre and less alcohol in the diet can help reduce menopause misery, and Zoe customers said following the diet suggestions had improved symptoms generally by a third.

When my kids were small, one of their favourite films was an American documentary called *Super Size Me* (2004) (we were quite a weird family) in which the late Morgan Spurlock ate nothing but McDonald's three times a day for a month, and any time he was asked by the server 'Do you want to supersize that, sir?' i.e. have an extra-large portion, he had to say yes. By the end of the experiment, his blood tests were appalling and a doctor told him, 'Your liver has turned to paté.' My boys particularly loved the bit where Spurlock has to eat a burger,

Coke and supersized French fries and suddenly throws up out his car window into the McDonald's car park – a stark reminder that what we think of as 'comfort food' is really discomfort food, in the long run. His calorie intake was around 5,000 a day, and he tried everything on the menu. He also walked 1.5 miles a day. By the end of the month, he felt terrible, he'd gained 24lbs and his cholesterol was nuclear. As Spurlock said at the time: 'Everything's bigger in America. We've got the biggest cars, the biggest houses, the biggest companies, the biggest food, and finally, the biggest people.'

The *Super Size Me* experiment revealed how quickly the body could change – for the worse, but also for the better. A 2024 study led by Nikola Srnic at the University of Oxford confirmed this, showing how people could improve their 'good' HDL cholesterol by an amazing 10 per cent within 24 days and increase energy reserves in their heart muscle by eating a diet high in polyunsaturated fats, like olive oil, mackerel, salmon and nuts. The study gave two groups of people the same calories, so no one put on weight, but those in the high-saturated fat group, munching away on butter and croissants and sausages, had a 20 per cent rise in fat in their liver and around 10 per cent higher 'bad' LDL blood cholesterol levels, compared to three weeks previously when they started the diet. Reporting the story, one newspaper referred to 'lethal croissants' due to their high fat content. What I realised, as I dumped the butter and dipped my bread into olive oil, was that change is encouragingly swift. Now I just have one lethal croissant a week, with my mates in the café after our Saturday-morning swim.

However much nutritional science you understand – and

everyone knows a lot nowadays – it's still hard to motivate yourself to make change. With that in mind, I consulted an empathetic figure, the menopause and midlife dietician Nigel Denby, who is very much against dictatorial diet regimes and shaming people. He explained why he was driven to work in this area: 'It was watching my mum, Audrey, who had battles with her mental health most of her life. But in her mid-forties, I saw it begin to spiral, and her anxiety grow. She just got labelled as a woman that was "struggling with her nerves", and she never, ever lost that. Although I didn't understand that was menopause, I knew things were going on because she had four sisters, and I used to listen to them all shouting.' Audrey also struggled with her weight, and as a boy Nigel said he was 'a little bit chunky', so one day she took him with her to her Weight Watchers in Buckinghamshire. Somehow, aged five, he ended up sitting in a corner wearing a paper pig mask – the mask that was given to shame women in Weight Watchers who had gained rather than lost weight that week. 'Oh my God' was all I could say, twice, when Nigel told me that.

But, in a fine example of post-traumatic growth and courage, Nigel became a nutritionist himself, and twenty years ago, well ahead of the latest menopause movement, he started working with senior consultant Professor Nick Panay, past president of the International Menopause Society, who realised then that HRT alone was not going to solve women's problems. Nigel very much believes that women should get their hormones sorted out first, and then tackle nutrition. He takes me through how he approaches his clients. 'We know this isn't going to be easy. The art of it is finding a way that works for you. My job isn't really explaining five fruit and veg a day. It's working out: where are you now? What do you need to do to change? How are you going to keep that going? And that's the bit that's exciting. So you know somebody is on two fruit and veg a day, so where can you find the gaps to improve that, and how are you going to shift a change in behaviour until it starts to feel normal? Whilst I don't know what it's like to be a midlife woman, I know exactly what it's like to be addicted. I'm an alcoholic. I've been sober for fifteen years. I know that we have to make hard choices every day to change.'

I like the simplicity of Nigel's regime – three meals a day, no fancy fasting, and some planned snacking mid-morning and mid-afternoon if you want (not Mars Bars). 'Ideally snacks should be made up of two food groups like carbohydrate and protein, or fruit and protein. Good combos include Babybel cheese with two oat cakes, an apple and peanut butter, fruit and unsalted nuts, banana on one slice of toast. You get the picture?' When it comes to mealtimes, Nigel's plate plan is equally simple: 'At every meal, make sure half your plate is made up of vegetables, fruit or salad. One-quarter should be made up of protein and the remaining quarter from carbohydrates, preferably wholegrains.' Er, that's it. And when there are days when you're eating out, he suggests a small portion of fish, a small portion of chips and a ton of mushy peas. We cannot always be perfect, but every little helps.

The other simple hack Nigel suggests is groupthink – a supportive community. 'I got off my high horse at the beginning of lockdown and realised me sitting in a clinic in Harley Street seeing women on a one-to-one basis and micromanaging that wasn't necessarily the best way of delivering what I could do.' So he started with providing advice and creating WhatsApp groups of around ten women who wanted to change their diet, and kickstarted a supportive community. Nigel also does this for groups of women on the NHS, but you could set up your own WhatsApp group. 'I kind of let them learn a bit, and put it into practice, and then add on a bit more and a bit more. And then they come up with their own plans. So it's almost like doing a self-build house. Everybody's building their own house at the same time in the same street, but each house is slightly different. But everyone needs help – show me someone in their forties or fifties whose microbiome hasn't taken a kicking.' The women all looked after each other, provided encouragement and solutions, and started posting pictures of new meals, or dog walks, or recipes. 'They would say, "I used to struggle with that, but now I do this, and that really helps."' It wasn't fat-shaming at Weight Watchers, circa 1980. 'It's really celebrating,' said Nigel. 'This fits real women living real lives, and actually they can do this.'

I have actually been thinking far more about food since I researched this chapter, and knowing the science, rather than just having a vague sense of good and evil in my shopping trolley, has helped. What's so hopeful is how quickly your gut microbiome and cholesterol levels change for the better within a few weeks, and also that you can self-diagnose the menopausal or midlife mayhem going on in your gut, and tackle it. Handfuls of spinach all round!

SPIRIT

CHAPTER 13

Women and Wine

Coming from Glasgow, I grew up in a culture which has a rich alcoholic vocabulary. Just as the Swedish have many words for snow, so the Scots have many words for the various states of drunkenness: blootered, bladdered, guttered, hammered, steaming, mortal, paralytic, stocious and miraculous. Despite a history of alcoholism in my family, I always approached a drink with enthusiasm and joy, and generally could hold it rather well. My student job as a barmaid in the Western Bar on Great Western Road never really felt like work. I've never considered myself an alcoholic, though I could feel the pull of addiction at one point in my forties when rarely a day went by that I didn't have a drink. My career back then as a film critic was professionally oiled by rosé and champagne at premieres and film festivals (the worse the film, the better the free cocktails). It was a way of life, and for a long time I didn't see any problem with this, although I was aware of the sobering story of a veteran movie critic who had gone direct from a review to rehab in an ambulance.

Then, unavoidably, midlife entered the party, and started to disrupt things. At some point I went from 'social drinking' – a couple of glasses of red wine was good for the heart, wasn't it? – to 'grey-area drinking', when a choice becomes an ingrained habit. My ex-husband and I often finished a bottle of wine together over dinner at home most nights, and I always drank when I was out. So did everyone else I knew. In my forties, I was using drink as an evening decompressor, as many of us do at this complicated time. It's a time when we are under immense pressure, not merely multitasking, but fulfilling expected roles in our own, our children's, our parents', our partner's and our colleagues' lives. We are helpfully omnipresent, yet we can never be omniscient or omnipotent. Trying to control or even compute other people's chaos and needs is constantly stressful. And so we look to external relaxants which will let us be momentarily beyond time in a timetabled life, and instantly deliver that dopamine hit that we might be struggling to get from elsewhere. The first drink is delicious, and reliably effective, every night. We even describe it sometimes, semi-ironically, as 'self-medicating'. We self-medicate for so many reasons at this time: fear of ageing, fear of being supplanted at work, fear around disintegrating relationships, fear of the unresolved past, all encouraged by the hormonal firestorm in our heads. We might be trying to recapture a time when life felt less pressured, hoping that an Aperol Spritz or three will bring us back to the highs of a long-ago holiday in Italy, but instead we feel sickly, an orange warning light for the morning after, which becomes more and more of a burden.

Then there is the fact that culturally, women are often

encouraged to drink and women's drinking is often trivialised. The 'Mummy Wine Time' habit encourages daily decompression drinking, and makes mothers the butt of jokes: glasses labelled 'Wine not Whine', or in America, 'Mommy's Sippy Cup'. Problems are apparently solved by drinking, and not the recalibration of an often-unfair domestic burden. From early on we are fed 'female-friendly' advertising for pink gin like Gordon's 'This gin looks pretty in pink!' and Kylie Minogue Pink Prosecco – all very Instagrammable, giving the impression these drinks are fun and insubstantial, despite their very real alcohol content. I'm sure this doesn't happen quite so much to French women, in a country with a sophisticated attitude to drinking and neat little wine glasses in cafés – I don't think I ever saw anyone really blootered when I lived there. But it does happen in the UK, US and especially down under in Australia, where a fifth of middle-aged women confess to being 'binge drinkers'. In a Newson Health survey in 2023 of 1,200 perimenopausal and menopausal women, one-third said they were drinking more heavily than previously and 12 per cent admitted to drinking more than the suggested government limit of fourteen units a week. This might be in part because the effect of falling hormone levels on the brain can lead to an increase in addictive behaviour – a drop in estrogen levels leads to reduced serotonin and affects the pleasure receptors in the brain. Essentially, we find ourselves chasing highs that seem harder and harder to achieve. Replies to the survey were not just about alcohol, but substance abuse too, including Class A drugs like cocaine as well as more accessible and 'socially acceptable' over-the-counter drugs. The cost was staggering among these middle-class respondents, a relatively narrow demographic: they were spending nearly £3,000 a year on alcohol and over-the-counter medication in a bid to cope with menopause – and life.

But physically, we simply cannot drink as we did in our younger years, and far from helping, alcohol actually compounds the physical symptoms of menopause. Our ability to process alcohol changes as we age, particularly for women in their forties and fifties. Wine is a particularly bad culprit, and after just a couple of glasses of wine, hangovers unfortunately take on unexpected proportions. This is because wine contains sulphites, histamine and tyramine. Changing estrogen levels in midlife can increase histamine release, and inhibit its breakdown. We need histamine, but in excess it can cause histamine intolerance, including headaches, digestive issues and skin reactions. Alcohol also messes with our carefully curated stomach microbiome, killing good bacteria. The wine-no-longer-fine discovery is very common in midlife, but the good news is that many people find 'clean' spirits like vodka much more tolerable, and a bottle of lager tends not to cause a hangover. But red wine, whisky and brandy are more difficult to process for some of us. I have a dashingly fashionable friend who programmes film festivals, and thus permanently survives on wine and canapés, and she has an old-fashioned 'poison' ring from which she discreetly squirts a potion containing sulphate-suppressing and histamine-neutralising drops into her wine glass. I like her style, and determination to keep on partying. She swears by this method, and you can buy these wine drops, filters and purifiers online, but I haven't tested them myself.

Unfairly, this increasing intolerance seems to affect women more than men. As women age, their ability to metabolise alcohol decreases, so there's slower elimination of the toxins, and the ethanol in alcoholic drinks is technically a poison which we handled better when we were younger. I talked to Dr Fatima Khan, an Australian menopause expert at Epworth Hospital in Victoria, and she explained that 'women generally have less of the enzyme that breaks down alcohol, dehydrogenase, which makes us more susceptible to its effects. So we absorb more into the bloodstream than men do.' There are other inequalities that also make women more prone to getting drunk: 'Our bodies have a higher ratio of fat and a lower ratio of water, and we often have a smaller liver. The knock-on effect is bad sleep and a disrupted night as alcohol irritates the bladder.' This may be perfectly OK a couple of times a week, but daily drinking is more damaging: your liver metabolises alcohol, and it metabolises hormones too, so when things are already hormonally unstable around the menopause, that overload can intensify mood swings and hot flushes.

The change in how our bodies process alcohol at midlife can be even more serious than this, as Siobhan Crompton found out, rather dramatically. Siobhan is in her early fifties and works as an insurance underwriter. 'There's lots of entertaining and alcohol at dinners with clients, and over the years that has very much been a factor of my job,' she told me. And her body seemed to always process alcohol really well – she never really had a hangover. Then as hormones changed in midlife, so did her reactions to drinking, perhaps because she is asthmatic, which means you are more sensitive to histamines and other compounds in wine. Suddenly, the Prosecco took its revenge. Siobhan went to a barbecue at a friend's house and had a gin and tonic and a couple of glasses of Prosecco. 'But when my husband picked me up at 10pm, he was like, "What the hell have you been drinking?" I was absolutely out of it. Could hardly get in the car. I couldn't remember getting home. And I'd literally had three drinks. The next morning, I found myself on the bathroom floor, blood everywhere. I'd banged my head on the toilet and passed out. It was a really violent reaction.'

Two weeks later, Siobhan went to a friend's 50th birthday, and decided she'd just have one drink and stick to soft drinks after that. 'I thought, I'll just pretend I'm drinking, and it'll be fine.' But people kept offering her more, and she then drank what she thought was a weak, slightly sour punch. 'I was having a great time. We were dancing on tables and then I was dancing on the dance floor with somebody I didn't know. We were spinning each other round and I pushed her. She pushed me. And then I was face down on the floor and I'd really hurt myself.' Siobhan had broken her wrist and was in plaster for sixteen weeks. She also discovered that the punch was 'pure Bacardi and lime and no mixer'.

The accident called for a tough reassessment of her life. 'It's very difficult to actually look after yourself; this time of life is a bit of a perfect storm. I've got an elderly mum, a 13-year-old girl and a 19-year-old stepson, and a full-time job and two dogs. And then you have menopause and hormones . . . ' Alcohol, previously simply a part of her life, had become so unpredictable for her it was frightening, and eventually she had some tests done that showed she was allergic to fermented products. 'You don't know what the chemical re-action will be in your body anymore to this stuff.' She now drinks much less: 'One gin and tonic, maybe two. And then my brain literally goes, "You're done." Because if you drink any more, it's not going to be good. It's going to be dramatic.'

For Siobhan, it was a combination of the pressures of her life situation, and a shift in the way her body was unable to handle alcohol, that caused drinking to go from being a release to being a problem. She decided to make intentional changes to her life, so it revolved less around alcohol, and friends who only went to the pub, and to draw boundaries with alcohol at work – midnight karaoke sessions with younger work clients are on her 'just say no' list. She's found new ways to unwind and help her cope with the overwhelm. 'I do cold swimming. I do meditation. I've got a very short attention span, but I manage five or ten minutes in the morning. I'm trying to come back to me, because I'm not sure who me is or what I even want. But once you start embracing it, it gets easier. I'm still in the transitional bit of understanding where I come from.' She goes cold swim-ming with girlfriends in a lake near Knutsford. 'We go on little road trips and find a lake or a reservoir or a river and then have a bit of fun. It helps. My dad died recently as well. So I needed something to bring the stress levels down.' Siobhan now has a cold tank in her back garden, for daily icy plunges. It's a great new addiction. 'Everyone thinks I'm nuts, but when I get out, I know my brain will be in a positive place.'

*

Siobhan took action to consciously reconfigure her relationship with alcohol. This will look different for everyone, and for many of us, these midlife changes may mean it just works better for us to drink differently, or less. Personally, I have given up drinking almost completely, but for a couple of glasses a year at birthdays or Christmas. When I left my first marriage and went to live alone for a while, I dropped the daily drinking at home – with the memorable (or perhaps not so) exception of the evening I knocked back an entire bottle of wine by myself and live-tweeted building an IKEA Malm chest of drawers. If anything's going to drive you to self-medicate with alcohol, it's probably building flatpack furniture (just make sure you stick to Allen keys and avoid power tools). Now, I've been basically sober for six years because my partner Cameron doesn't drink, and when I met him I wanted to be in sync with him, on the same planet: the planet of full colour, full-feeling reality, even when that was a bit tough at first. But it got easier very quickly, and there is a lot going for it. I think I had rarely had sober sex until I met him, and I can very much recommend that, for starters.

Personally I'm not keen on the word sobriety; it's used enthusiastically and with pride everywhere, from Alcoholics Anonymous (AA) to other twelve-step programmes, but for me the term still carries the weight of the other dictionary definition: 'the state of being staid or solemn'. Stopping drinking has not been a solemn process for me but a joy and a relief, one less thing to worry about. It also totally played into what was left of my midlife vanity, because my skin improved. It was clearer, and within a week the eye bags had become less capacious, and I was sleeping better. I felt much healthier. Cath Cookson, a Pilates instructor from Norfolk who gave up drinking, told me: 'I just felt puffy and pale. I find old photos of myself with lines down my face and I look different now.' But she also found public sobriety a trial: 'I asked a barman for sparkling water, and he just looked down at me and said, "This is a *bar,* madam."' She also finds alcohol-free wines have the same bad effect on her, so 'it's about finding a grown-up drink that suits you'.

The market for non-alcoholic 'grown-up' drinks is growing and has now improved so much from the days of a warm glass of water, though I will still draw the line at a girly Gordon's Pink 0.0% Gin. As with every mental and physical health trend, sobriety has met capitalism head on, and there has been an outbreak of alcohol-free events, people with 'soberglow', mocktail bars and drinks. There's a whole 'California sober' discussion that entails vaping weed, probably an equally bad idea. I love an alcohol-free lager, although I do find the craze for celebrities to jump on the bandwagon a little irritating: Blake Lively's Betty Buzz, Bella Hadid's Kin Euphorics, Lewis Hamilton's non-alcoholic tequila, Katy Perry's De Soi, Tom Holland's Bero and even, God forbid, Jeremy Clarkson's Hawkstone Spa non-alcoholic lager. But the new 'clean' drinks taste far better than they did, and have ended the embarrassment of asking for a non-alcoholic drink in a bar, and being hassled about it by friends. Plus the packaging means soft drinks are almost impossible to spot among the hard stuff.

For about a year, I still had to force myself, armed with elderflower spritzer, into any large room filled with partying strangers, and feel the fear, rather than numbing it with an instant, euphoric serotonin hit of alcohol to loosen all my inhibitions. As Ernest Hemingway once said: 'I drink to make other people more interesting,' and somehow I feared I was also less entertaining stone-cold sober. 'I worried about that too,' said Cath, the Pilates instructor. 'I worried that I wouldn't be funny anymore, but then I realised it's not the drink that makes me funny. My real friends completely embraced it.' In fact, once I was talking to people, the craving fell away, and I found I was enjoying myself as much as before – if not more. A long time ago, I interviewed American Mary Karr about her terrific memoir of growing up with an alcoholic mother, *The Liars' Club*. She was very welcoming at her house, and fed me tuna sandwiches, and I loved this quote from her: 'When I got sober, I thought giving up was saying goodbye to all the fun and sparkle, and it turned out to be just the opposite.'

For me there was, and will always remain, the problem of forced eight-hour drinking, initially foodless marathons at weddings, New Year's Eve if there's no dancing, and 'peak dinner party insanity' around midnight when the food has gone, the conversation is rampant and the bottles are empty. While I usually love the early part of the evening, and I do miss joining in the later screaming political arguments, I sometimes have an out-of-body sensation in the room, and I feel utterly exhausted and have to leave. At that point I can just drive myself home, of course, which is a bonus.

While the first sips are great, most of us find that once we are a few drinks in, alcohol is a depressant, although studies show some addicts can stay higher for longer, which makes stopping even harder. A few more drinks and some people start having blackouts, when their body still functions but their memory stops working, and some might even pass out as the room starts to move of its own accord. That's at the extreme end, but even if you're not on a complete bender, regular alcohol use changes your brain patterns, and raises cortisol and stress levels, and then, of course, you want to drink more to chill out. This is the scary science bit, because uncontrolled cortisol levels and stress over time can lead to long-term health problems like obesity, increased risk of infections, insulin resistance and metabolic syndrome. Plus, menopausal women who drink more than two units of alcohol a day increase their chances of getting breast cancer by 20 per cent. I'm not saying we should all be giving up alcohol, but in midlife we need to give it a long, hard stare and maybe change our consumption patterns. I know so many women who have thrown in the bottle, mostly because they can't physically tolerate it anymore, and on the whole they don't regret it.

For me, it's been, with a few hiccups, a pleasure and a revelation. However, I am not in any way dismissing the lifelong struggle so many others have with alcohol, drugs and other addiction – the unspeakably hard, soul-bearing, past-eviscerating work and the relapses they may have to overcome to get to that safe place of sobriety. As mental health and addiction expert Dr Gabor Maté explained: 'Don't ask why the addiction, ask why the pain. To understand people's pain, you have to understand their lives. In other words, addiction is a normal response to trauma.' Fortunately, there is a lot of help out there for those who need it. While I've only gone along as an observer to twelve-step meetings (and those in Alcoholics Anonymous are not supposed to go public about anything, including being a member – the clue's in the name), I have learned a lot from friends in the last few years about how these kinds of programmes work. The twelve steps provide a steady, almost psychotherapeutic framework over months for self-assessment, growth and personal transformation, and your 'higher power' doesn't need to be a god of any kind – there are all kinds of spiritual paths. There are anonymous twelve-step groups for everyone, whatever their problem: those with eating disorders, codependents, gamblers, debtors, adult children of alcoholics, drug addicts, cocaine addicts, technology addicts and sex and love addicts. There is also Smart Recovery (smartrecovery.org.uk), which is more secular, not about unearthing the past but about setting goals for the future, and uses techniques like motivation, achieving a healthier life balance and cognitive behavioural therapy. It also does not strictly require abstinence.

Alcoholics Anonymous was started by Bill Wilson in America in 1935, and the original works are dated, but the philosophy of community and abstinence still holds in self-regulating local groups and seems infinitely adaptable. Some people find the acknowledgement of admitting powerlessness over alcohol, setting aside ego, submitting to a higher power and making amends difficult, and books like Holly Whitaker's *Quit Like A Woman* have a more modern feminist take. There is some fascinating questioning of the twelve-step method in the play I saw recently, *People, Places and Things*, starring Denise Gough as an addict entering rehab: 'You want me to conceptualise a universe in which I am the sole agent of my destiny and at the same time acknowledge my absolute powerlessness. It's a fatal contradiction and I won't start building foundations on a flawed premise.' Gough was herself an addict in her twenties and got clean, so her delivery of this from on stage was all the more convincing: 'Drugs and alcohol have never let me down. They have always loved me. There are substances I can put into my bloodstream that make the world perfect. That is the only absolute truth in the universe.'

Gough's character eventually makes it through the twelve steps, staggering and relapsing along the way. I won't go into detail here, but you can read about a typical twelve-step programme at alcoholics-anonymous.org.uk. The only criterion for membership of AA is that you want to stop drinking. I had a look round the AA website, since there are now dozens of in-person and online groups around the country and abroad. You can pop into the English-speaking Paris meeting while on holiday. You can also be at home in your pyjamas and hang out with your favourite group – and you don't have to speak unless you want to. There's an online meeting in Marseille in France you could tune into, or 'Black Country Ladies' (hard to know what that may mean), the 'Oxford-New York West Village Exchange', the Lowestoft 'Cos We're Worth It' Women Online, as well as lesbian, gay and trans meetings in Soho and Edinburgh. In America there is 'Put a Little Gratitude in Your Attitude', beaming from Greenwich Village, Manhattan. For those in suits in London, there's 'City Breakfast' before work.

I went with my partner to a twelve-step retreat for

recovering addicts and friends at a barn in Norfolk one weekend in spring, mostly drawn by the gorgeous stone stable buildings and wild swimming in a chalk-stream pool. What I also found in all the group meetings, meditation and yoga was this intense, unshockable and utterly supportive community of people, who could deliver hard truths about themselves with gobsmacking courage – and often wit. Over a couple of days there I met Carys, who is 55, was a nurse in London for thirty-eight years, and has also been sober for eleven years. She has reddish-brown hair, a big smile and is full of oomph, and has now trained in Reiki massage. I told her about this book, and she said she was happy to share her whole experience, with honesty, for other women. She finally became sober at 46, in the throes of perimenopause too, and her story is a web of life circumstances and rogue hormones that build up into a midlife bomb. Carys remembers her mother taking her to the doctor for regular headaches when she was 18, and he saw something else was wrong. 'He said: "I think your daughter is suffering from clinical depression." From that day on, it was never mentioned. There was no help sought – because *she* was the problem. My mother was an alcoholic, and she knew that deep down, but she couldn't actually do anything about it.'

Genes relating to the metabolism of alcohol can be passed down, but it's not a given. What is a given is that early family trauma was baked into Carys. She got on with her life and career as a nurse, marrying and having two sons, but she thinks her later drinking might have been triggered by the hormonal and mental crash of post-natal depression, also untreated. 'I didn't drink throughout my pregnancies, which is unusual for an alcoholic. I couldn't wait to stop breastfeeding. And as soon as I stopped, bang! That was it. I was drinking again. That was my reward.'

When her boys were at primary school and she was working as an NHS nurse, her social drinking started to increase, but she never actively drank at work – she just had to handle the morning-after hangovers. 'Actually, I was hyper-vigilant. I was paranoid – I had to go back and check the patients' records on the computer. I didn't make any mistakes, but it was exhausting.' Later, perimenopausal brain changes and forgetfulness added to the strain, triggering intense anxiety. As time went on, her alcohol use grew heavier. 'A couple of glasses of wine, then a bottle, then the bottle went to two bottles. And then, by the end of my drinking, I was on three bottles a day.' She used to get dropped off drunk by girlfriends in a taxi after a night out. 'I'd just get out of the taxi and try to sleep on the drive, saying "I'm in bed now" so they'd have to take me in or get the key from the neighbours if my husband was away.'

The breaking point for Carys was at a school parents' event – always a trial for anyone, but infinitely worse if cheap wine is available. Carys got so drunk she had to leave the room. 'I aimed for the door and found an empty classroom and promptly fell asleep. They locked up the school for the night and my husband drove home thinking I'd gone awol and taken a taxi.' When he realised Carys wasn't home, her husband drove back to the school and woke up the headmaster, who lived in a house on the grounds. The headmaster came out in his dressing gown and slippers, and they unlocked classrooms until they found Carys and woke her up. 'I promptly threw up on the headmaster's slippers.'

We start laughing, because it's both the worst thing but also very funny. But the shame and gossip afterwards added another layer of agony. 'There's a point where you fall on the floor and just cry out and say, "I can't do this anymore. I cannot carry on like this." Basically, you're surrendering to your rock bottom, and everybody's rock bottom is different, and I know many people who have harder stories than me. But that was mine.' Carys's husband, who is a practising Catholic, intervened, and drove her to a religious retreat in the country, and told her she needed to make a decision. 'It was all crucifixes and Mary and Joseph. He dumped my case on the floor and marched off. The marriage was not in a good place back then. So I went in, and what he hadn't told me was it was three days of absolute silence. Oh, shit. All that noise going on in an addicted head. It was not easy. But something happened to me that I really can't explain. I felt the presence of something. I don't know what it was. And I got through the three days. I didn't stop drinking immediately, but that seed had been sown. I just thought to myself when I got home, I'm going to have to do it.' She found a twelve-step programme, went to daily meetings, and that's how her recovery started.

'No other human being can get you sober. I didn't get sober for my kids. I didn't get sober for my husband, even though they were begging me to. I finally realised, you have to get sober for yourself, and it has to come from inside. You have to have that gut-wrenching feeling that you have to surrender and throw the towel in. It's all about change and no other human being can do that for you. That's the gift of desperation.'

It took Carys a few years to do the twelve steps of recovery and her sponsor was a woman and a Quaker, so there was a spiritual element to their regular conversations. Carys had converted to Catholicism earlier, and going to Mass regularly helped at first, and she still prays every day. Therapy was part of the work she did too. 'It just helped to right-size my thinking. I was in overwhelm. And somebody was giving me a different perception on how to look at things, and how to manage things that were actually getting on top of me.'

Like most women at this stage of life, Carys had a lot going on, and her job was particularly tough. We know the NHS is underfunded, and that means patients who have waited months for medical appointments have even higher expectations. 'Every day, people were hoping I would rescue them. Every ten minutes. Of course I tried, but it's quite a lot to bear.' For a while, she worked as a menopause prescribing nurse, but she didn't recognise the symptoms in herself when she was perimenopausal. But then she got sober and found more clarity. She started hormone replacement therapy. 'That took care of the insomnia. That was brilliant. Hot flushes, night sweats, they went fairly quickly. The joint pains took time. But they're better now than they were. So taking HRT was a life-changer for me. I mean, I can differentiate drinking from the symptoms now, and it was all messed up.'

For Carys, and so many people I've met who are in twelve-step programmes, the therapeutic work continues for herself, and she also sponsors and helps other women new to the group. The weekly conversation with the recovery community is still much needed. Maybe it always will be needed. 'So your shell comes off in layers and layers. You're left with the core of who you are. You're the frightened soul that's been left when the drinking gets taken away. But it's a good thing. It's a good thing because you've now got something you have to build on.' I felt very emotional after talking to Carys that day: she's straightforward, honest and funny, and she'd shared just about everything. You don't meet people like that very often.

If only we talked about this more: the hopes and expectations around alcohol, and were more honest about the downsides, rather than it being hardwired into almost every social and after-work event in our culture. Future generations are doing better: Gen Z drinks much less than Millennials, and so on. This chapter is a tentative step into the complex and serious world of alcohol, addiction and recovery, and I'm no expert, but it's important that we have these conversations, inform ourselves, and break down the taboos around talking about alcohol. Women are the fastest-growing demographic becoming alcohol-dependent, and this is – or at least should be – a big topic in the midlife conversation. It's not perhaps as easy as bestselling therapy guru Brené Brown puts it – 'Sobriety isn't a limitation . . . it's a superpower' – but I am very curious about it all (I believe #sobercurious is the Instagram term). I also wonder what looking through sober glasses in midlife brings to us and our relationships with the world. When the comfortable padding of alcohol has gone, do we then confront ourselves and others and change the way we live for the better?

The debate is starting to pop up in surprising places. I regularly listen to the You Are Not Broken podcast on hormones, menopause and sexual health by the brilliant Dr Kelly Casperson, and there she was doing a surprise 'sobriety special' with her brother Hans – both of them have been off liquor for three years. They were really enjoying it, and she told listeners: 'Alcohol is so normalised yet so incredibly destructive. Here's to your personal growth, whether that for you is decreasing or stopping your relationship with alcohol completely or something else. Getting to know yourself on a deeper level as we age is truly precious.' I like that.

CHAPTER 14

Digital Detox

I came across a cartoon in *The New Yorker* of a gravestone, with the comic engraving:

50% LOOKING AT PHONE
50% LOOKING FOR PHONE

Ouch, I thought. That's an only slightly exaggerated summary of our lives because I spent four hours on my phone today, and one hour looking for my phone *in my own house* until I found it carefully filed with the unopened mail. I once unintentionally laundered my partner Cameron's phone, putting it in the washing machine in the pocket of his bathrobe. Alerted by the rhythmic clunking, I was pleased to have found his phone, but then I had to sit watching it go round and round, panicking and unable to intervene mid-cycle. It actually dried out OK, but don't try this yourselves at home.

When I check the types of usage on my phone, a lot of

it is professional: answering emails, campaigning on my @menoscandal social media, and work WhatsApp groups, plus a certain amount of reading the papers and chatting, looking for upcoming sales on the Finisterre eco-outdoor clothing and wetsuit website (the older you get, the more excited you get about equipment rather than fashion) and seeing what my friends, neighbours and children are up to. It's professional, it's social, it's necessary – but it's still addictive, particularly the social media, and some days I have a jerky, sleazy, overstimulated feeling if I go on it too much.

It was interesting, and a little uncomfortable, to see how I spend time on my own phone, but I've also become a phone spy while thinking about this chapter. On the bus on the way to the British Library to write, I try to sit behind people scrolling on their phones to see what matters to them. They're mostly younger, and if they're not texting, they're on TikTok and Instagram. The average engagement with a TikTok post is three seconds, so it's bish bash bosh through the For You livestream, with only the occasional halt for puppies, tornadoes, miracle skin creams for tweens, and Taylor Swift. The randomness and stupidity of the algorithm is painfully clear when you track a bunch of people in mid-TikTok consumption – mostly they are getting stuff they really don't care about, with about a one-in-ten engagement rate in posts. What a waste of time in the scroll hole. I expect the people plugged into podcasts or music are getting something much better. But most of my fellow passengers are doomscrolling or sifting through phone garbage. Of course, it's all about *how* we use these resources; a well-curated Instagram or X feed is a useful thing if you have some specialism or obsession. I learn a huge amount from the medical, midlife and menopause community on my Instagram, and feel very supported there. It's also a great vox-pop research tool. But there's a time and a place for our phones, and I think we're all aware that most of us are getting it horribly wrong.

On my house-swap holiday in Portugal this year, I watched children and teenagers and twentysomethings not strolling but scrolling on the beach and in restaurants, unable to read books, or be playful, or engage in conversations with their families. Often, they photographed only themselves and not the new worlds or people around them. From their feed, you wouldn't know where they'd been, raising the question: 'Did you go somewhere nice on holiday to look at your device?' I wondered how this generation of phone addicts would learn expressions, emotions, visual cues, debating skills and irony from other humans. How would they live with this agitating restlessness, difficulty in focusing and craving for endless stimulation? Like any other addiction, phone dependency leads to falling dopamine highs and lack of impulse control, with the addition of the anxiety machine that is social media.

This potential mental health crisis is being acknowledged in upcoming legal battles, as more than a dozen American states began the process in 2024 of suing TikTok for creating an app designed to be addictive to children and teenagers 'while making false claims to the public about its commitment to safety', according to the *New York Times*. These states claim that TikTok relentlessly designed features – 'the slot-machine effect' – to encourage compulsive use and that many children were using the app instead of sleeping. Many adults I know are doing that too, basking in the evil blue screen light at 4am; in fact, around 20 per cent of us regularly look at our phones in the middle of the night, foolishly lighting up our insomniac synapses. TikTok is owned by the Chinese company ByteDance, and over there the Chinese version of TikTok Douyin restricts nighttime scrolling with a cut-off from 10pm to 6am for under-14s, and puts a forty-minute limit on daily use. Eton College and various academy schools in the UK have banned smartphones altogether. As well as the mental health ramifications, there's a physical health crisis looming. While I was talking to doctors about osteoporosis and midlife bone density for an earlier chapter, a couple of them mentioned they had been surprised to see an increase in younger people with weak bones too: the only jumping teenagers were doing was from post to post on TikTok.

It's tempting to portray this as an epidemic affecting young people – which it is – but it's also having a huge and profound impact on us grown-ups who ought to know better, but whose phone use has grown year on year. In a small American survey of 1,000 adults by Reviews.org, 57 per cent confessed they were addicted to their phones, 60 per cent slept with them, and in 2023, people spent two months on their phone per year on average, checking their phones 144 times per day. If that's not obsessive-compulsive disorder, I don't know what is. And here's something you always hoped wasn't true: 75 per cent use their phone on the toilet. John Lewis now sells a £40 silver toilet roll holder with a phone shelf above it, and this is very much a trend. Just say no.

It's easy to lie to yourself about how much time you spend on your phone. An hour a day maybe? Surely no more. Go onto 'Settings' on your phone and scroll down to 'Screen Time'. I just did that. I have a 25-hour-a-week, three- or four-hour-a-day habit – and that's since I started to pay attention to and curb my phone use. I don't use it at night, so I spend just over *two days a week* on my phone. And for some, that's nothing. I interviewed a woman who works in PR, and a man who's a trainee lawyer; to some extent they use their phones for work but her 3.5-hour-a-day habit was topped by TikTok. When the lawyer opened his phone analytics, he covered his eyes. 'Seven and a half hours yesterday,' he confessed. That's probably a 40-hour week in total.

There was a time when I lived mostly alone that I was much more of an addict. A midnight scroller. A notification junkie. A drunk online shopper. A Slacker. I slept with The Devil and took my phone to bed. I lost hours down internet rabbit holes. My various WhatsApp groups were also breeding like rabbits. I sent work emails after six o'clock and at weekends. I had no shame and no boundaries. That was me until a few years ago, although now I have a partner, and I take him to bed rather than my phone, which is a huge improvement in so many ways. But despite cutting down, I still have the digital DTs some days, the itchy need to know the news or have another little dopamine hit checking my latest post on Instagram or LinkedIn. There's that moment when you've just glanced at social media, and then realise shamefully you've been there for ages. This is called 'the 30-minute ick factor'. There's also a new word for an acute case of phone deprivation syndrome: 'nomophobia' – no mobile phone phobia – which can, at its very worst, apparently cause anxiety, disorientation, sweating, agitation and even heart palpitations. Plus, there's 'textaphrenia' – panic at not being able to send or receive messages. Some people even experience 'phantom vibrations' – a feeling that their phone is sending them alerts, when it isn't.

These are perhaps at the more extreme end, but we're all suffering the effects of constant phone use, and most of us have not taken the time to confront and understand them. The overstimulation from TikTok, texts, Instagram, emails, WhatsApps and Slack messages causes sensory overload and panic. Your body and brain think you're in danger and this can all build up to a flight, freeze or fight feeling at peak notification time. Your prefrontal cortex goes from rational and reflective to rattled and reactive. When we're stimulated in a soulless digital way all the time, the default mode network in our brains gets neglected; what seems like boredom and silence, walking without a podcast playing, is in fact the time when your brain is at wakeful rest, daydreaming and mind-wandering. The default mode network – time out or time off – is the quality time when we plan and imagine the future, when we remember the past, build our own autobiographies and engage in moral reasoning. It's also activated when we are looking at landscapes, beauty, architecture. The Italians have a perfect phrase for the default mode network – 'il dolce far niente' – the sweetness of doing nothing. Nothingness matters. It's the neurological basis for the self.

We are resorting to ever more extreme methods in order to claw back some of this phone-free nothingness. You can restrict your time on certain apps or buy a 'phone jail', a timed device that keeps your phone under lock and key. One sells for £14.99 on Amazon, with real bars and the slogan 'Reconnect with the Real World!' Here's the advertising blurb: 'In the middle of a game with your family but keep getting distracted by your phone? Been waiting for hours on end for someone to text back? Lock up your phone for a few hours in this mobile phone jail and enjoy some screen-free time! Interact with the world around you as your phone serves its decided sentence.'

It's a question of control, and the balance has shifted, dramatically, in favour of the phones. You think you are pressing your phone's buttons, but you quickly realise that the phone is pressing your buttons. As we know, The Devil suits his temptation to the sinner, and one particular app will probably be your weak point. When your device is not around, you have a constant yearning, a smartphone-shaped hole in your pocket, and soon there will be a smartphone-shaped hole in your heart if you're not careful, as the algorithm and the apps take away the last shred of your human interactions. As Gore Vidal once said: 'The brain that doesn't feed itself eats itself.' By abandoning the real world and relationships for the online world, you are serving yourself the digital equivalent of ultra-processed food. You are cannibalising yourself to profit Meta.

Over 90 per cent of us in the UK and US have a smart-phone. So what do the experts say about what that's doing to our colleagues, our families and our souls? What happens when you exchange hours of real life for the ersatz version? In her book *Dopamine Nation: Finding Balance in the Age of Indulgence*, Stanford psychiatrist and addiction specialist

Dr Anna Lembke took a hard line: 'The smartphone is the modern-day hypodermic needle, delivering digital dopamine 24/7 for a wired generation.' She compared compulsive overconsumption of social media with other addictions. Prolonged use of drugs causes huge surges in dopamine, so that can cause the brain to shut off some of the receptors that the neurochemical acts on. That tolerance means we need more to achieve the same high, and for some of us it could be the same with our phones. She wrote: 'The paradox is that hedonism, the pursuit of pleasure for its own sake, leads to anhedonia. Which is the inability to enjoy pleasure of any kind.' Dr Lembke is keen for people to lock their phone in a drawer for twenty-four hours, and return to reality. 'Stop, and turn, and face whatever it is. Then I dare you to walk toward it. In this way, the world may reveal itself to you as something magical and awe-inspiring that does not require escape. Instead, the world may become something worth paying attention to.' Phones can still be part of life, but we need a detox to recalibrate our relationship with them.

How do we recalibrate? I interviewed a digital wellness expert, the encouraging Laura Willis, whose job is to provide her clients with tools and techniques to make their tech habit manageable. While a digital detox is fashionable, and intermittent digital fasting is healthy, aiming for daily digital health is a more practical idea in the long term, accepting the real world where phones are essential tools for living, working and communicating. 'I always say, "The tech is not there to pull us apart from each other",' said Willis, who believes in using tech wisely, for connection rather than a disconnect from real life. That we now have the acronym IRL – in real life – is kind of sad, and her ambition is to integrate the two worlds, ringfencing reality.

Willis was working as a self-employed PR and marketing consultant when her own tech crunch moment came. 'I was on the brink. I was on my email all the time. Slowly things got out of control. I couldn't stop looking at my work. My daughter was about nine months old, and I sat in the kitchen one night and I realised I was a complete insomniac. I was never without a bloody phone. I went to sleep with it, I looked at it to check the time, I woke up with it beside me. I wanted to run away because I couldn't cope anymore, and I was having panic attacks. Honestly, I was at my worst point, and that's when I went right, I need to do something.'

Willis went to her GP and was diagnosed with severe insomnia – a typical new mum, apparently. He put her on sleeping tablets for ten weeks, but she didn't want them. She changed GPs and got a different opinion. 'He just said to me, you're overwhelmed, what's going on? He recommended mindfulness meditation, and put me on a CBT course for insomnia.' Everything got better. 'It was about taking the time to have space, and to meditate. That created the headspace for me to understand.' That default mode network making a comeback. Willis also got an old-fashioned watch to tell the time, rather than her phone.

As a social psychology graduate, Willis became an early questioner of tech's deleterious effect on our brains, and began to make adjustments to her own digital behaviour: working offline so she could concentrate, batching her emails to three hits a day, coming off social media, and suggesting anyone who wants to email her after six o'clock can call her mobile in an emergency. Guess what? There are no real email emergencies. Most can wait until tomorrow. After Willis made personal changes and threw the digital shackles away, she said: 'The clouds parted and I was like, that's what I'm meant to do. I'm meant to help people with this.' She set up her business Shine Offline – now Laura Willis Digital Wellness. I met her because we both sometimes do workplace wellness events for Thriving London, rescuing people from menopause and hormonal hell (me) and digital hell (her). She also keeps a close eye on the digital habits of her two children, aged 8 and 12.

'Right,' I challenged Willis. 'Let's take your typical multitasking midlife woman. I will suggest how to solve her hormone problems, but how are you going to solve her digital problems? She's a working woman, and colleagues email her at night. She's got phone-hungry kids, and the frankly terrifying demands of the school mums' WhatsApp group. She is also a late-night online shopper, with many ill-chosen orders and returns, and an Instagram lurker, with an addictive TikTok habit of watching time-lapse garden transformations. Her whole life is bound to her phone. She is literally losing sleep over it as perimenopause ramps up. How does she cope?'

Willis grins. 'It often feels like a massive mountain to climb. I find it easiest to break it down to her working time and her personal time. When she's waking up, she may be using her phone as her alarm clock, in the bedroom.' First, she has to get an alarm clock to follow the no-phones-in-bed rule. In the Willis household, they plug their phones into a socket in the coffee cupboard at night, 'and the phones don't come out until after everybody's eaten their breakfast. Let's be present in the moment.' Another useful tip is to have a home phone and a work phone if you can afford it, or swap home screens. Especially for those of us working at home, Willis suggests not checking emails on the phone. 'Instead, sit down at your desk and open your laptop and make it as if you're in the office. That's the start of your working day.' She also insists that everyone needs to take breaks, particularly a lunch away from the desk or workplace, 'but don't have a cup of tea or go outside and just scroll through your social media. Take a break from all screens, or your brain will never go into default mode and it will get really exhausted. And then you get really, really stressed out.'

Since meeting Willis, I've learned not to look at my email first thing in the morning. 'Instead, I like to suggest a morning mission,' she advised. 'You've got one thing that needs to be done today that's really quite hard, so give it your full, fresh, undistracted brain power.' Other people I know meditate for five or ten minutes before starting the day, but I'm often too harebrained (how great is that word for modern times?) and scatty for that, and I have to write down an idea if I've had it on waking up. This is where the great anti-phone weapon comes in: 'Get a notebook,' said Willis. 'Carry it everywhere. It means you can stay away from your phone, even make a note if you wake in the night, so you can go back to sleep.' Staying away from our phones in order to concentrate is crucial. I realised I was having problems when writing with 'continuous partial attention'. Willis explained this happens because technology is around us all the time, in multiple streams. We work with our in-boxes and Slack notifications open, in a constant state of doublethink, even if we believe we are concentrating on a task. And this is true of our leisure time, too. Willis told me that scriptwriters in the writers' room for a Netflix drama series have to make sure the story works for 'double screen viewing' – that's someone watching television and scrolling on their phone at the same time. About half of people look at their phone while watching television, so screenwriters now have to repeat bits of the plot so the phone-junkies can keep up. The same is true socially: around 20 per cent of people scroll while eating with someone. Manners anyone? More seriously, about 17 per cent still look at their phone occasionally while driving, despite it being a criminal offence. Continuous partial attention is affecting every area of our lives. And our brains simply aren't built to double-process in this way. 'If your phone is even within your sightline while you're working, it has a brain drain on your cognitive capacity,' says Willis. 'It doesn't even have to be turned on. Just seeing it has a negative impact on your ability to use your brain, because it causes a distraction, because you know something's going to come in.' I'm now trying to leave my phone in solitary confinement in another room if I've serious writing to do.

Some readers here will be in leadership or management positions, and Willis finds that senior leaders worry about not being available to their teams all the time if their phone is switched off or in another room. She advises on tech use (and abuse) in business and big organisations: 'You need to understand that if you want to do good work, you've got to be mentally present in that time, but not *all* your time, and you have a role to demonstrate that you're in control of that. If you're a leader who's just constantly reacting and responding to emails and expecting other people to do the same, you're not going to get very far.' It's about setting boundaries: turn off notifications and banners, write an email when you like and then schedule it to send at a sensible time, put do-not-disturb settings on your phone so only certain numbers can get to you, like school or your partner. And it's also about setting an example to your colleagues – and family. Good digital leadership really matters at work, at home and in education. 'I'm interested in the influence of people at the top on everyone else around them,' Willis says. 'It's all one story – leadership matters in business and by parents, because when we start to discuss use of smartphones and screens together, we begin to question our habits.'

Leaders also owe it to their staff to pay real attention, particularly on Teams or Zoom meetings, and Willis tells me about a head of HR she'd been mentoring at a law firm: 'She had a mentoring update with a junior lawyer in her firm, and realised she'd spent the whole time looking at her inbox, not even thinking quite what that was doing to that young person. Demoralising them. Making them feel rubbish. So be mindful that you've got young people who are looking to you, who respect you. Your guidance is having a massive impact on them.' I think we can apply that to parents too. I'm not aiming to tackle parenting much in this book – this midlife investigation is about paying attention to ourselves – but some of what Willis says about how she handles digital behaviour around her family is worth hearing.

They use an Alexa in their kitchen, so they can make basic enquiries without having phones around, and she also lets her son play computer games with friends. 'They're doing stuff together. As long as there's laughter, I'm OK with them being on technology. And it's bringing some sort of connection, it's bringing them together. It's bringing joy into their lives. Technology has got to play a role, and we've got to live in harmony with it, rather than demonising it.' And that harmony will look slightly different for everyone. She explained: 'I'm trying to show people at work and home that it's about creating that harmony for yourself, but also understanding the way it works for you may not be how it works for your partner or your child, your colleague, your boss, or someone who's neurodiverse. We need to get people to talk about their digital preferences.'

So technology has a role to play socially, but let's be clear: we need to fight the demons, and this requires conscious effort. It can sometimes feel draconian, but boundaries need to be set, in conversation with all those involved. While my friends are digital dinosaurs and far too polite to use their phones at dinner, at university my daughter Molly and her friends used to put their phones in a pile in the middle of the restaurant table at the start of a meal. In a situation where phones are going to actively inhibit connection, they need to be removed from the picture. But phones are glorious too, and when you hit that sweet spot of digital harmony, it's about connecting with the people and things you love.

One of the things in life that makes me happiest is having a meandering WhatsApp video call with Molly, who lives in New York. She calls me when she's cooking, props me up on a recipe, spatters the screen, or brings me to the mirror in her messy bedroom to vote on some dubious item of clothing she's picked up in a second-hand shop. At my end, Skye the dog is often featured, cruising the London streets as we converse. Molly and I just hang out together for half an hour at a time, rambling. We talk when we're up, we talk when we're down. Sometimes I walk electronically alongside Molly as she goes to work, chatting about the price of coffee in Manhattan ($9, and a tip!), looking up simultaneously at the bottom of her chin and the ice blue skyscraper skyline passing above. Such are the gifts of technology at its very best.

CHAPTER 15

Divorce, the Moneypause and the Couplepause

'I love my husband, but sometimes I watch him through the prongs of my dinner fork and imagine him in jail.'

That anonymous comment perfectly expresses the frustration – and love – that many of us struggle with in a decades-old marriage or relationship. Which way will it tip for each person? Will the future hold acquiescence or anarchy? What if you no longer want to be half of a couple, but your whole self instead? What if your time together just happens to be up? Some people grow together with their partners, some grow out of their partners, and others grow up and find their partners. I'll try to address those possibilities here. Obviously, this subject is so complex that a single chapter cannot hope to answer everything, but what we can do here is look at the Spaghetti Junction of midlife relationships, menopause, mothering and labour – and consider ways not to crash the car.

We know by now about the unpredictability of menopause's dastardly little sister, perimenopause, and how hormones don't just drain away in your forties, but behave badly and unpredictably before finally leaving at the average age of 51. The calming hormone progesterone goes on strike, ramping up anxiety and anger, and mood-enhancing estrogen leaps and plunges by the day or week, creating a dangerous combination of sexy highs for some, and miserable lows, all of which ramp up the likelihood of arguments, affairs and separation, especially if the cracks were already there. Not surprisingly, the average age of divorce for a woman in the UK is 44, right in perimenopause central.

That could also be due to The Rage we discussed earlier, during which perimenopausal irritation boils up into volcanic anger, usually directed at family or colleagues, often when they are committing such heinous acts as eating crisps loudly. This anger is not easy to live with for everyone else because it can be sudden and apparently unreasonable. I mentioned The Rage in my previous book on the menopause, but it's worth recalling here precisely which items I threw, in my forties, when I was dealing with three children, a sick mother, a dog and a full-time job at *The Times*. In no particular order, the following ended up hitting the kitchen wall: blue poster paint, broccoli, a butternut squash, a full butter dish and a copy of *Nigella Christmas*. No one was injured, I cleaned up the mess (the bits of broken china in the butter were particularly trying), tension was released, and everyone felt better and behaved better afterwards. Previously I had never shown signs of a volatile temper, and I don't have one now, probably because I'm on calming HRT, but I share this with you as a window onto the fact things change in midlife – *we* change in midlife – and that has a profound impact on our relationships.

You can also see why, aside from boredom and growing apart, a menopausal woman might not be easy to live with. Family and divorce lawyer Farhana Shahzady, who has personal experience of same-sex relationships, has also often worked with clients who have two sets of hormones going awry at once. 'We deal as lawyers with same-sex relationships, and I can tell you without any measure of doubt, that the situation is amplified when you have two women of similar age going through menopause, separation, or relationship difficulties. It can be horrible. I have some very close friends in that kind of position. It's difficult because I've seen couples where one woman has sought HRT and treatment for menopause, the other hasn't. And there's a lot of friction and tension around that.'

In both heterosexual and same-sex relationships, midlife brings a devastating combination of factors: many women have lowered libido, or don't want to have now-painful penetrative sex (and don't know about rejuvenating vaginal estrogen), so that can result in rejection and anger issues, often on both sides – or worse. There is an increase in physical violence and domestic abuse towards women around the time of menopause – from coercive control, to threatening behaviour, or psychological, emotional or financial abuse – and a 2020 report by the charity Against Violence and Abuse stated there was a 'two-way relationship' between menopause and domestic abuse. It highlighted that almost 40 per cent of women killed by men in the UK are in the 36–55 age range. Women undergoing the menopause can be more vulnerable to lack of confidence and low self-worth, putting up with the abusive treatment, but everyone should know that help and advice is available from charities like Refuge and Women's Aid in the UK.

The hormonal and physical changes of menopause also often intersect with a particularly challenging set of life circumstances that put a lot of strain on a relationship as each partner has to reconfigure their role, and the pitfalls of inequality and resentment can be hard to avoid. The magnificent Margaret Atwood, author of *The Handmaid's Tale*, once defined menopause as 'a pause while you reconsider men' – and that's not merely as lovers, but part of your shared enterprise of work and family. As we start to have children slightly later in life, the triangular rack of mothering, perimenopause and career can stretch a person, and a marriage, to breaking point.

Fiona (name and identifying details have been changed) agreed to talk to me about her recent journey through marriage and divorce. She is now in her early fifties and used to work as a senior executive in a large media company, and has three children. She got married when her son was a few months old, and decided after that to take some time off the brutal demands of her full-time work while her children were very young. 'I went into parental mode. I really, really wanted to be with the kids when they were young. I chose to take three and a half years off. I probably was ready.' Her husband agreed. 'It was kind of "she's retired". And I think he enjoyed the sense of providing – until the real costs of child rearing on one income started piling in.'

As the family grew, they decided to move from London and take on a huge house they planned to renovate in a village in Scotland. Fiona had help with childcare, and was planning on going back to work. There was some conflict even then over money and childcare, but suddenly her husband was offered a job overseas. 'To begin with, I was like, woo! Yeah, let's do it. We'd taken on this big old house. It was a money pit, and I kind of thought, great, let's do that on a sizeable salary. I'll come back for a holiday in the summer. And so I turned down jobs in the UK and went there.' But the 'dream of streets paved with gold' in a foreign city ended up being more of a tedious Stepford Wives' life in the suburbs. Fiona was planning on finding work, but she didn't have the necessary industry contacts abroad. The combination of that with unreliable, expensive childcare meant she had no choice about continuing to be a full-time carer for her three children. Her career was withering, while her husband's thrived and his lack of support started to take its toll. Moving for one partner's work almost inevitably creates these imbalances which can lead to tipping points for anyone.

After a while, Fiona really missed using her creative brain – fingerpainting was not enough: 'I found constant parenting the hardest job in the world. It's so much based on repetition and routine. Pretty much 90 per cent of it is domestic labour. It's the hardest job and the least respected. And obviously that's part of the patriarchal system, isn't it?' There's an unwritten financial contract in some marriages that undervalues the worth of work in the home and prioritises that of the parent working outside the house. As a result, there is little consideration from the earning partner that the main parent might want to take a few hours off at the weekend – after all, they've not been at 'work' all week. This can lead to the needs of the at-home parent being trivialised and the desire to spend 'family time' less appealing than that of working. Fiona also found that being the default parent began to extend beyond her children. 'The role of "mum" is one that can easily creep into our adult relationships too – as the carer, the organiser, the cleaner. I'm okay to parent, but I am very passionate about *not* having to parent grown men,' she told me. 'Especially as he started referring to me sometimes as "Mummy" when the kids weren't even there.'

As the distance grew between her and her husband, Fiona began to feel increasingly isolated. In the UK it might have been different, but in her new conventional 'Stepford' community, the iconoclastic Fiona stuck out. 'It was all, "Hi, welcome. How have you acclimated?" But they didn't get me.' She was just miserable, unfulfilled and lonely, having given up her home, career and support networks.

The time zone meant that she couldn't call her friends in the UK when she wanted. 'Everyone was asleep, so I'd have a gin and tonic and cry. I was just so isolated. I was probably depressed for nine months.' She also felt resentment about the inequality and power-shift in the relationship: she'd come to the marriage in her mid-thirties with her own house and income, and now her husband held all the purse strings. She tried to be neighbourly and literally keep her spirits up: 'I like drinking, I get giggly and fun, and I would go beyond three and not be the only one who had done that. But it was when one of them said, "Oh, someone enjoyed the mama juice last night!" I thought, no fucking way, I'm not being that person. So I stopped drinking.' At about that time, Fiona also read Glennon Doyle's self-help memoir *Untamed – Stop Pleasing, Start Living,* which came out in March 2020, just in time for so many unhappy couples going into Covid lockdown. 'I read three pages of that. And I texted the friend who had recommended it and said, "I think by the end of this book, I'll be getting divorced." And sure enough, I was.'

In the first Covid lockdown abroad, Fiona was home-schooling the children 'and he was working from home. With seemingly minimal calls and the football (when it came back) on the big screen permanently. Living his best life. I mean, I've worked as an executive and the mother of three. I know what hard work looks like. It doesn't look like that, watching telly and a couple of Zoom meetings a day. I had to ask him to take an hour off at lunchtime with the kids to make them food and take them out to give me a break. I needed an escape. I had become this thing that was no longer Fiona.' By the time the second lockdown came, it looked like school hours would still be reduced, and that was the breaking point for Fiona. 'We were stuck in a scary situation away from friends and family, not knowing what would happen next.' She decided enough was enough, got on a plane with her children and returned to Scottish schools and the half-renovated house in the village. 'The kids were tearful at first. I wasn't tearful at all. I was actually free. I felt free. I felt that I was coming back to my heart, to the house that I love. I was wandering around the field at certain points, just wandering around naked, burning, like a woman gone absolutely mad. But it was really healing.'

Thinking about Fiona's breaking point brought me back again to my favourite book of 2024 – destined to be a forty-something separation classic – Miranda July's *All Fours*, and the moment when her protagonist boils over. 'I imagined . . . finding out that all the women in the neighborhood were also leaving their houses. We were all running to the same field, a place we hadn't discussed but implicitly knew we'd meet in when the tipping point tipped . . . Start the revolution here now in this field? Or drive back and slip into the fold. She finished: 'Our yearning and quiet rage would be suppressed and seep into our children and they would hate this about us enough to do it a new way. That was how most change happened, not within one lifetime but between generations.'

Fiona's own revolution in a field in Scotland has reached a place of calm after her swift exit. Her husband eventually returned to the UK, the divorce went through, and Fiona is now primary carer of her children during the week, where they attend local schools, and her ex and his new partner have them two weekends a month and for a few holidays per year. So Fiona is still very much the main parent – but on her terms, and she is now paid maintenance by her ex-husband. She is also working on a book which aims to warn women about losing their power as dramatically in marriage and parenting as she did. 'I definitely want my voice to be out there. Because that's when you get power, isn't it? My humour's back, my passion's back. And no one's holding me back now. You know, I'd like to change things for our kids. I'd like more women to be more empowered in this area, financially, and in successfully combining caring and career.' Fiona feels a strange sort of grief for the original family she has now lost, and is sad that her kids have had to endure the pain of divorce, but said: 'I'm also proud of the way they're building resilience.' She is building resilience too. Obviously, as head of the household you have to be sure you can tackle all those household jobs, said Fiona. 'There's a big, big spider. And you are the one who goes, "I tackle the big, big spiders."'

As a London divorce lawyer, Farhana sees many cases which are similar to Fiona's: the upending of marriages as the domestic burden shifts and expectations of equality fall away. A failure to share parenting is one part of the divorce grenade, but another is menopause and men's midlife dissatisfactions too. Farhana started to understand her work differently when she had an early menopause in her forties, and began to notice the effect of hormonal dysregulation and brain fog on her menopausal clients' divorce outcomes, emotionally and monetarily. Divorce and dealing with the custody arrangements around children is tough enough at any time, but this seemed worse. 'I realised some of my clients were struggling to give a witness statement in court. Clients panicked over the hostile correspondence and completing lengthy and complex documents. They were tearful and unable to cope with or process all the procedures which they could have handled before, and that the onset of perimenopause often mirrored the onset of difficulties in their relationship.'

Despite the fact Fiona had dealt with hundreds of complex contracts in her work, she found the divorce process overwhelming. 'It was terrifying at times. At each stage, I researched or found out what was the counterplay, and I played it. But it's horrible facing delays and not feeling you have the right to move things on.' And there is a peculiarly transactional element that can feel uncomfortable, as you have to monetise roles that are traditionally valued in non-financial terms. Sorting the deal on child maintenance, Fiona's lawyer added up what it might cost to replace her with a full-time nanny; putting a price on domestic and emotional labour. This act in itself has in some ways been weaponised against women, a quiet insistence that we shouldn't put a financial value on childcare because that in some way devalues it. But it's important that women are financially literate when it comes to the value of their work in the home and family, because this can be a major barrier when it comes to leaving a marriage that is no longer working.

Even if women (or men) want to walk out of the door, childcare and economics sometimes leave them trapped – you cannot run two households for the price of one, and to some extent choosing divorce can be a privilege of the rich. As part of the Family Law Menopause Project, Farhana wanted to consider whether there are financial barriers for midlife and menopausal women that are routinely being ignored. She has named the intersection of hormones and divorce 'Moneypause', and explained: 'For years women have been reporting feeling short-changed as they go through financial remedy proceedings or financial negotiations. Although Moneypause is not an inevitable symptom of hormonal transition, it's all part of the cultural, structural, health and institutional inequalities women face at this time.' Farhana has been in the profession for over twenty years, and talking to her fellow solicitors, she felt menopause was not being considered, and had no legal currency. When she did an online survey of almost a hundred family law practitioners, she found 68 per cent of their divorce clients were in the 40–55 age group. 'Many of the women I see are incredibly worried about their finances and don't know how to cope. They often have abdicated financial responsibility to the husbands who are taking care of things, while women raise the family. So when they come to see me as a divorce lawyer, they're in disarray. They don't have a handle on their finances. They don't know how they're going to survive and very often they are still responsible for older children living at home.'

While a 'clean break' final settlement, often 50/50 depending on childcare needs or not, works well for some couples, many women are already on the back foot financially, having worked part-time or taken a career pause for caring for children or sick parents, which means they have lost out on promotions and building up a pension over the years, so they need more than half of the capital and maintenance as well in a settlement. It's not easy to catch up when re-entering the midlife employment market. Ageism is still a barrier, and we know one in ten women leave their jobs due to menopause symptoms, so in some cases spousal maintenance can be a life-line. 'But it's legally unpopular and offered begrudgingly for the shortest possible term, if at all, because the legal system simply has no concept of menopause or the related problem of Moneypause.' Many of the lawyers in the survey concurred with this: 'A clean break can come too early, not recognising the long-term health impact of peri/menopause on working capacity,' said one. 'I think this is a reflection of society in general having a limited understanding of what effects the menopause has on a woman's ability to earn,' said another. 'Judges have very little if any thought or understanding about the condition and its impact.' Two-thirds of the family lawyers thought women were disadvantaged in financial settlements by a lack of understanding of the menopause, but many also found it tricky to bring the subject up with clients. Another solicitor observed: 'I feel women are very vulnerable around the time of menopause, may often be depressed and not functioning as well as they might have done. I worry they do not take on board advice and settle too low, just to rid themselves of one problem.'

Farhana has occasionally suggested to some of her clients that they visit their GP and discuss menopause before getting further embroiled in a legal battle. 'It's important to help clients stay sane as they're buffeted by what can be stressful financial negotiations.' Farhana also did a survey of over 400 midlife women who had gone through divorce. Bear in mind this was not a diverse poll but one done through LinkedIn and social media, but over 70 per cent of respondents felt that their menopausal or perimenopausal symptoms played a role in their relationship breakdown, and 86 per cent of those who had used a lawyer said they did not raise the issue of menopause or perimenopause. Farhana said: 'My fear is that if we don't talk about menopause and if treatment isn't sought, we are not going to move forward very positively. And I'm a divorce lawyer, so my job isn't to save marriages, but I think marriages could sometimes be saved with this.'

Pensions are another area of inequality, and women need to think about the future and not just the here and now when agreeing their settlement, to avoid retirement poverty, Farhana explained. The Fair Shares Report into financial arrangements around divorce showed that only 11 per cent of divorcees had a pension-sharing order and it was usually the woman who lost out. 'They tended not to pursue pension sharing, preferring to retain all or more of the matrimonial home, often because of the immediate needs of raising children.' Despite years of supposed equal pay, the pension gap is massive: on average, women retire with pension savings of £69,000 compared to £205,000 for men. Many women also, in an old-fashioned way, left the household finances to their partner, and it's worth gaining full knowledge of bank accounts, pensions and insurance policies before even mentioning the word divorce.

'The Moneypause is not inevitable,' said Farhana. 'But these systemic and deep-rooted barriers make it hard for many women to achieve a good standard of independent living after divorce or separation. On top of that, women now have their first baby around 31, which means they may have children in puberty as they enter menopause.' She summed up: 'Menopause is like water; it can seep into almost everything with varying degrees of damage and can intersect with socio-economic background, ethnicity, sexuality, gynaecological health and education in a unique and sometimes devastating way. Lawyers have an important part to play in changing this.'

Only 40 per cent of those divorcing use lawyers to help reach financial and custody settlements, and others turn to mediation or do-it-yourself divorce packages. 'At the moment we have a system which is very litigious, and litigation doesn't suit many women,' said Farhana. The survey showed that 60 per cent of women prefer mediation. 'But there are caveats to that, a risk of an imbalance of power, which the survey did also address. We need to be careful that we don't deliver settlements for wives which are lopsided.' Mediation is great for less complex and less acrimonious cases – it's much cheaper and it helps clients set clear goals and make fair decisions together for the future. There are also great support groups on Facebook, like The Divorce Hive, where the women's experiences (anonymous or not) are simultaneously soothing and hair-raising. When I was getting divorced, I also drew on the experiences of my friends, about half of whom were already divorced themselves. That helped both emotionally and economically, but if you don't have a wise and sensible friend, it may be worth paying for a chat with a divorce coach – there are lots online that can take you through the process step by step, advertising 'education, strategy, preparation, resolution, healing, and transformation'. You may be able to do this with dignity and fairness.

Nora Ephron once said: 'You should never marry a man you wouldn't want to be divorced from,' and that's worth bearing in mind. Perhaps this seems cynical, but divorce is also a result of some very positive changes. 'Divorce is a product of long life,' said Farhana, who has done a deep dive into research and has now set up the Family Law Menopause Project. 'People died long before they had a chance to alight upon divorce, and between 1700 and 1857 there were only 314 Acts of Parliament in relation to divorce, most of them initiated by husbands. Divorce rates only really gathered pace in the middle half of the 20th century, helped by increased lifespan – we died on average at 69 in 1955 – and a change in attitudes.' Now there are around 80,000 divorces a year in the UK, two-thirds of them initiated by women. But understanding the perfect storm of divorce or break-up and menopause is relatively new, and there are positives to be found here too; losing those softening hormones is not all bad – it sometimes lets women see more clearly the compromises their caring instincts have been masking, and just decide that enough is enough.

When you think about the aeons we stay together in marriages or partnerships these days, remaining in the same equanimity and balance as two ever-changing humans is nearly impossible. I met my former husband aged 25, and was in a relationship with him for 25 years, and who is fully formed at 25 years old? Not me. Unless you do the work along the way and consider questioning your relationship and giving it regular maintenance, it will rust. There's a word for this disconnect in midlife, the couplepause, and that's giving a nod to the hormonal, mental and physical changes in both genders. Of course, much like menopause, some lucky couples will sail through the couplepause untroubled, and many more will hit its turbulent waters but want to make it through, together. And the only way to do this is to work at it – constantly. Maintenance isn't only needed around menopause. Relationships, like cars, should have regular MOTs and constant room for improvement as we grow up (and I wish someone had told me that too).

I've brought back the wise Dr Kalanit Ben-Ari here, who first appeared in Chapter 1 on mental health, because I wanted to ask her more about her work as a couples therapist, running weekend group workshops for couples, and an eight-week online course too. She emphasised how worthwhile it is to see a therapist early on, to get the tools to strengthen love and understanding, when you can still put energy back into the relationship. 'Unfortunately, people are waiting for too long before getting therapy. So the conflict escalates until it really cannot be bearable. And then they reach out.'

Dr Ben-Ari also underlines the importance of consciously putting yourself in your partner's shoes. Therapy is not about apportioning blame, but about coming to an understanding. 'As a therapist you are not there to be judge. What we want to do is help you to see each other and yourselves more clearly, to bring the unspoken into the spoken, to put the unconscious into the conscious, thereby increasing empathy, connection, and intimacy.' Obviously, this entire book is reported with my own peculiar female bias, and every chapter could have a male equivalent or riposte. But at least for a moment, talking to Dr Ben-Ari, I got an inkling of a different point of view. 'If only women knew what went on in the heads of their husbands,' she said. (She works with many men as individual clients too.) 'The fact that your husband goes calmly to sleep in bed five minutes after you've had a terrible fight, doesn't mean that when he wakes up, and is doing other things, that he is not thinking about how upset you are, or is feeling shamed or blamed or not good enough for you.' And the only way to know what someone else *is* thinking, is to communicate. As we say to angry toddlers throwing toys – you need to use your words. And often, men and women don't.

While women feel the domestic and emotional burden discussed in this chapter, Dr Ben-Ari points out that men have their own burdens. 'It's in their DNA to worry about finance, and that's a mental load too.' Also, as women we often don't appreciate how a simple statement can be devastating. 'When women say to men, "I don't trust you," for some reason, which just could be, say, about a one-off incident when they are unable to pick up the kids, it feels like a huge statement. It's basically saying, "I cannot trust you emotionally that you will be there for me." Men often hear and internalise this as "You are not trustworthy; you are not enough," or "I cannot trust you – emotionally, financially, or in being present – that you will truly be there for me." And we women don't appreciate how painful it is for men to hear that.' A vicious cycle dominates childcare for men and women: women bear the bulk of the work, so men get less practice at childcare and more criticism for their failings, so women don't trust them. And so it continues, unless you make an intentional change.

There's so much to discuss here it would fill enough books to fill a whole library, but Dr Ben-Ari pointed to the book by Harville Hendrix, *Getting the Love You Want* (Simon & Schuster, 2020), which is a classic couple-rebooting resource, based on the Imago Relationship Therapy she uses in her practice, which dissects how attraction works and how to address the hidden issues that cause conflict – in particular, replicating the same problems in every relationship you enter, because those patterns are often shaped by your relationship with your parents. It turns out that the 'opposites attract' cliché has some truth in it; someone very different can bring you a sense of completeness.

I also asked Dr Ben-Ari about that midlife perennial, the affair, and the possibilities of the relationship recovering from one – or two. 'An affair is, by definition, taking the energy out of the relationship. You're taking part of you outside of the relationship and you're always closer to the person that you have a secret with. It's exploring parts of yourself you may not want to bring into the relationship. It's sex. It's connection. It's how you feel about yourself in the presence of someone new. It's the glow of the secret.' In the last few decades, we also have developed secret lives online: texting, or just quietly pressing 'like' on an Instagram post. That might develop into a full-blown affair, or it might just be a bit of fun. Dr Ben-Ari said it depends: 'For some people, something online will feel really awful, a betrayal. But this is for the couple to figure out their own boundaries. If you're doing the equivalent of flirting with someone in the lift, and you won't see them again, maybe it's OK. So each couple needs to have that dialogue.' In novels, and in real life, people are constantly discovering secret affairs when they pick up their partner's phone by mistake, and then there's the public fallout. And that's only the beginning – then you have to decide which route to take next. Dr Ben-Ari said that many couples try to hold a relationship together after an affair and come for counselling. 'One party says, "I will do everything that is needed to bring that partner back." And there is a way to work with that, but it is also my job to bring people to the consciousness of how long they would be able to hold that position, and coach them on how to rebuild trust and exercise patience during the process. It's so delicate. We often start out thinking that we can change someone, then, over time, we realise that the person is not going to change.' But, she explained, often couples who come to therapy after an affair, with the intention to repair the relationship, end up with a relationship that is much stronger and more intimate than it was before. 'While there are no quick fixes, I've repeatedly seen how healing, growth, and a stronger bond are possible.

Of course, some couples decide at this midlife stage that sex is one thing and their long relationship and companionship quite another, and they can hold those two points of view simultaneously. Midlife is a time, as we've seen in previous chapters, when couples' libidos become out of sync, be it decreased sex drive, or the perimenopausal sex surge, or lowered testosterone and erectile dysfunction. Or there's the sheer boredom. 'Suddenly they are not satisfied with the sex that they are having. And they want to work on it and demand more, and their partner finds it shocking or upsetting on some level,' said Dr Ben-Ari. There are other reasons for having an affair; obviously falling passionately in love is a good one, but some women just want to be *seen* again.

'They like someone that sees them as a sexual being. It's an identity issue: women are often looking for something in themselves, whereas – and it's a bit of a cliché – I have sometimes found for men that affairs are often with people who admire them, look up to them.'

There is still some shame around these social norms that the man wants more sex, and the woman doesn't. 'It's a very old story. We think that we've progressed, but it's still there. You know, a woman might find she's not so tired, and doesn't have a three-year-old, and wants more sex, has more energy. In middle age, I hear about women reading more erotica, fantasising more or having more dreams. Things that they didn't explore. Some women never even masturbated. And then midlife, they are open to exploring.' But does that exploration take place at home, or away? For the whole relationship, not just sex, the magnificent and terrifying question in midlife is whether you are going to start that journey of discovery together – or separately.

The last time I had dinner with Fiona, she had started online dating, and had not only been clubbing, but, grippingly, had dated both men and women. She doesn't feel she needs another half right now. 'I'm being as unconventional as possible and rebellious, just being true to what I want in the moment. So that might take me in places I'd never even considered before.' The fulfilment she feels now – and she's done a lot of work to get there – is a massive contrast to the emptiness she felt inside 'with the big house and the husband and the job, all those ticks. But I had a big hole inside then. Now that big hole is filled. With me.'

Divorce changes everything, and it is particularly

profound if you have children. As Fiona said: 'It will change every relationship that you have in your life, and you will change forever. They will change forever. Your path is changed forever, you know. So it's not for the faint-hearted, is it?'

I don't think it's that easy for most of us. Divorce is one of the hardest things I've ever done, and it doesn't ever turn out the way you expect it to. The last decade of my life has been both the worst and the best, but it's taken a while to realise that. Women who take the first step in separation have to deal with overwhelming levels of guilt at exploding the family unit, and I was horrified to realise I had left my three children, and former husband, with permanent scars, inflicted by me. When people say 'heartbroken', they can't imagine the carnage or the anger. I assumed we would be two parallel families, with my sons on a gap year or at university, and my 15-year-old daughter passing back and forth each week, but it turned out to be much harder than that. There was never going to be a family again, and I suppose I didn't really grasp that properly. I was slashed apart by a deep, aching love for my children, and an instinctual, animal need to escape and be alone, with an affair hopelessly pasted across the cracks. It took me years to atone and heal, and I have very different, more adult and honest relationships with my children than I might have had. I know it's clichéd, but time (and therapy) does heal, and my children, my former husband and our new partners all had drinks together last Christmas. Gracefully and gratefully.

CHAPTER 16

Renovating Relationships

There's nothing we all like better than watching a house renovation on telly: the futuristic dreams, the organic raw materials, the upcycled countertops, the haemorrhaging of plumbing and cash, the peril and the persistence, and the ultimate unveiling, a year late, of a well-considered object of beautiful intention and design. It's a bit similar when renovating your relationships and friendships in midlife. They require rebuilding and upcycling, especially if you are slowly becoming a different person inside while relationships remain static outside. Rebooting doesn't just happen. It takes thoughtfulness, time, courage – and work. This is true of both romantic and platonic relationships. Midlife is a time when relationships in both camps may have suffered – perhaps because our focus was on children, or work, or some other endeavour. And on coming back to these relationships, we find cracks have appeared.

When we are comfortable, we often take our friendships for granted. Then, in this time of midlife eruption and deconstruction, we may suddenly notice that some friendships are up for renewal, and remember how important they are for our well-being and joy. I never really analysed my friendships properly until there were two seismic events in my life: leaving my marriage and leaving my job. Until then, I just floated happily along, part of a successful couple with a group of similar friends and colleagues. But when trouble hits, you really find out who your friends are. Mine rallied round like protective tigers on Prosecco. I'm an only child, my parents are dead, and having no brothers or sisters in any crisis is tough. But as I sat on the floor that first day a decade ago, having left my family home and moved into an echoing flat, the doorbell rang. It was my friend Robin Hunt, also an only child and a writer. He came in, sat on one of the unopened boxes containing the IKEA Stocksund sofa which I had yet to build, and we had a cup of coffee. He was absolutely no help at building the sofa, but he just was *there*, like a brother, the only-child support network at its finest. I've done the same for my other only-child friends in divorce or crisis too, paying it back. Perhaps that was the first lesson of many that I learned in the metamorphosis which was to come. Just be there.

I still keep one of the £1 blue spotted coffee mugs I bought in an emergency the day I went solo; it reminds me of the bittersweetness of that strange time. It's bloody lonely when you leave a marriage, particularly when you instigate the break-up, feeling that you're on low moral ground, and that you're causing unnecessary hurt. You're alone after decades of companionship and shared children and a shared language of living. And the effect of uncoupling on your friendships is shocking: lots of social settings and events are suddenly closed to you, either because of self-censoring in case the other person will be there, or because the invitations have stopped. It's hard for your joint friends, often other couples, to be seen to be fair and equally supportive; sometimes they favour one side over the other or there's a brutal cut-off, saint versus sinner. There can be a real sense of grief over friendships lost. In hindsight I can see that it would have been sensible to openly discuss the difficulties and embarrassments faced by friends of a disintegrating couple, to work out ways around this, and acknowledge it was a shitshow that time might heal, rather than pretending everything was normal. I so appreciate the couples who kept inviting me round, even on holiday, when I was at rock bottom. And I want to namecheck Karen Brown, a friend and artist who is ten years older than me, and a great deal wiser, who just took a walk with me every week when I was in the throes of divorce, and listened.

When I was interviewing Emma Sayle of Killing Kittens for the sex chapter, she also wanted to talk about decoupling from other couples post-divorce. 'It's the way your couple friends work as a double unit, like two atoms together, and now you're just one atom and it doesn't function anymore. It's like you need a relationship to be allowed to be invited round to a dinner party. And it really doesn't happen to the men. They're just lovely single men, you know?' A newly single woman is, we agree, a challenging presence in the room. 'Some couples are pretending to be in these happy relationships, and the fact you've questioned everything is threatening the dynamic. Everything about you probably disrupts their vibes in some deep sense that they don't want to admit to themselves. You're a happily divorced woman who's going about her shit and is doing amazing things and that can really upset her old female friends who are still exactly where they were. You are a dangerous rocket passing through their lives and they go, "Should I get on it?"'

Leaving a job, an industry, or a whole world you've been in for decades, also brings grief and hurt. Did people like you for yourself, or because you were powerful, useful to them? Were they only interested in exploiting your knowledge and connections? Or is it just that the river of a workplace moves on, and you're left behind, out of the flow? Again, it may be worth being honest with colleagues and yourself. Do you have that much in common now? Does your friendship extend beyond the workplace? When I finally left my job at *The Times* and the world of film criticism, I realised in retrospect how incredibly sociable it was – festivals, cocktails, premieres, screenings in fetid cinemas at 9am on a Monday morning – and that life was work and vice versa. In fact, I've stayed good friends with lots of my fellow critics, less so with people I worked with at *The Times*. But it's worth consciously analysing why these changes happen, and what they mean to you, and which relationships you want to nurture now work has gone. It might even be useful to journal about it, to help order your thoughts and diffuse the more paranoid ones. As the person leaving – whether that's a marriage or a job – you can feel very powerless, the self-imposed outsider, and being intentional and proactive about how you continue those relationships brings the power back into your hands.

It's also helpful to interrogate your own expectations of friendships. As a teenager, my entire aim in life was to be a writer like Dorothy Parker, known for her devastatingly caustic remarks, poems and screenplays, as well as her witty, Martini-oiled presence at the Algonquin Round Table in New York in the 1920s. Her expectations of loyalty were high: 'Friends come and go, but I wouldn't have thought you'd be one of them,' she once said to fellow critic and writer Robert Benchley. But the coming and going sometimes leaves you with a better set of friends, more in tune with your present rather than your past. Is it in any way logical to assume our schoolfriends should still be our best friends? For some women this has worked out, but others have grown up to be different people, and are still growing up. We feel guilty when we move on from a group of friends, and we shouldn't – it is probably best to graduate from the school mums' WhatsApp group (why never the school dads?). There are friends that fit perfectly into particular times in your life – the breastfeeders, the 10K runners, the revolutionaries, the book group – but they are not there to be friends forever. And that's fine – we can treasure those friendships for what they are, incredibly important connections at a moment in time, rather than mourning what they're not. I have delighted so much in the intellectual stimulation of making new friends with each period of my life – I never thought I'd hang out with so many radical doctors, for a start.

Some friendships you may have expected to stick around, but it's not to be. Because people change, and it's OK to reassess even a long-standing friendship. An authentic friendship is reciprocated, but if people suck the life out of you and never give anything back, or just talk incessantly about themselves, that's a burden that you should not have to bear. Ditto anyone in their anecdotage, usually a man who self-importantly tells the same self-regarding story again and again. Ask yourself if they are a radiator, bringing warmth and comfort, or are they a drain, sapping your energy? Because at a time in your life when your energy is finite, and demands on you are heavy, it's OK to walk away from a drain. I'm as guilty as anyone else of having friendships I couldn't sustain, got bored by, or no longer had time for as my work ate my life for long periods. Because as you head into the next half-century or less of life, quality rather than quantity really matters – and sustainability.

And there are the friendships you don't walk away from, the ones you work on however hard it may be, because they are the friends-for-life, who make your world bigger rather than smaller, who are there at those crisis points regardless of where they are in their own life. Because we also have to acknowledge that even in these friendships we will sometimes simply be in different places, and you can allow the friendship to be asymmetric for a while – we all have needs that need mopped up. Sometimes your life circumstances, or life choices, leave you out of step with friends for a time. I still party and holiday with a big group of friends from Glasgow University, forty years on. I dog-walked my great friend Portia Kamons through her divorce, and when the time came years later, she dog-walked me through mine. We're still walking and talking. As Parker once said: 'Constant use had not worn ragged the fabric of their friendship.'

What about romantic relationships? We looked in the previous chapter at what happens when the renovation falls through. When the cracks are not superficial, but foundational. In which case, you might find yourself back on the market – and the market has changed. Let's talk about beginning again at relationships, specifically dating, online. Quite rightly, many people will wish to remain single and indeed celibate, but for those of us looking to re-find passion in midlife, the first hurdle is getting over the fear of dating apps. Online is really the only way forward now, unless you have an extraordinarily large group of ultra-social friends, some of whom wear labels that say, 'Yes, I'm single!' In 2024, 61 per cent of couples met online (compared with 25 per cent in 2012), and only 13 per cent still met through friends, and 8 per cent through work.

The fantastic Erin Keating has thoroughly investigated the online dating scene for her American podcast, Hotter Than Ever, which I recommend, and she says meeting in real life is extremely unlikely these days. 'So I'm going to say that if you are using the apps, the number one tip is – this is a marketing project.' Of course, some people market themselves better than others, and there are a few questionable marketing techniques out there. There's one question that comes up whenever you look at dating-app pictures of men, and that is: why are so many of them holding a big fish? This is not just the older generation – my daughter in America sees this among twenty-somethings on Hinge too.

While you might instinctively swipe that fisherman away, Erin said to make allowances: 'Don't reject him for holding a fish in his photo. A lot of times men are really proud of the fish they caught. I think there is a whole doctoral thesis to be written about why men do this, what it symbolises. But he wants to show off to you something he's accomplished and unless you are a vegan . . . or hunting or fishing of any kind is a deal-breaker for you, give them a break.' It's the same with men posing with motorbikes, often not their own. Perhaps it's best to look upon dating as an entertaining anthropological experiment, not a dead-cert romantic meet-cute, and spread your net wide. You never know whom you may find in these new-fangled times. I have a friend in Alcoholics Anonymous who was talking about dating people who are also in recovery (which is not always advisable when things are still raw), but he had this great line on sober romance: 'In AA we say, "The odds are good – but the goods are odd."' After being conventional for years, maybe an odd one is the one for you? That said, it might be best to proceed with caution; reel as many potential suitors in, and then weed them out with verbal calisthenics by text, followed by a phone call, or even a Zoom, before meeting them for a coffee or a drink or a walk in a public place, armed with a get-out time. Don't do a dinner date at first – it could be hours of expensive hell.

Three years after my marriage ended, I started dating online, and I bravely decided to go out on one date every week, hoping that sheer numbers and persistence would bring me luck. My weekly reports of failure also provided rich entertainment for my friends. I went on a dating site which has now, sadly, closed, Guardian Soulmates, which was affiliated to the newspaper, and very much not a swipe-left-swipe-right instant match. Weeks of witty emails were required, and people posted pictures of themselves reading Victorian novels and lounging in dark jazz bars. Awful, but exactly what I wanted. I love finding out about people, and I dated some smart, entertaining guys: a writer with a sideline in Italian cookery (self-obsessed), a psychotherapist (smug), a university librarian (dull), a Scottish Nationalist (bonkers), a travel company owner (Quaker), and a documentary maker and deep-sea diver (interesting). God knows what they thought of me; usually we had one date, although occasionally more. But eventually being on Guardian Soulmates did unearth my soulmate, my new partner Cameron, who recognised my photo on the website, despite my daft pseudonym 'Ironically' and not having seen me since we left Glasgow University, where we had first met, aged 17, at law school. I'll finish our story later.

But what we can learn from this is that there is a freedom in online dating, even for those of us who had not been out there for 25 years. It can be fun! And while Cameron may have recognised me, it can also be delightfully private. No one cares what you're doing, no one knows who you're hooking up with, no one knows if you've had ten one-night stands – or none. You can be with women or men or experiment. You can safely ignore or block people you don't like, and you have the freedom to be a new version of yourself, or perhaps a more authentic version.

Dating apps change all the time, so it's worth signing up for a few. My neighbour, the writer Nina Stibbe, is on Hinge, which at least has some words as well as pictures, and her daughter created her profile (just a tip). 'But I keep getting men who just want to have Sunday roast,' Nina said, less than excited. Tinder is the Wild West, as we know, and involves a massive amount of sifting and swiping. On Bumble, women get to make the first move, Feeld is 'the dating app for open-minded individuals', and there are other sites like eHarmony and Match, as well as more niche sites like J Date for Jewish singles and LoveHabibi for Muslims. I think there's still a better website or app to be made, with more crunchy detail and communication, for people in midlife or older, and SilverSingles just isn't it.

'I realised the years were passing when an internet date cancelled because one of his teeth had fallen out. If it had been me, I would have kept quiet about it. When you're older and looking for love, rule number one is to give the appearance of being hale and hearty. Nobody wants a wreck – keep that for marriage.' These are the wise words in the *Guardian* of another of my neighbours, Deborah Moggach, aged 76, who is the doyenne of literary late-life romance, as the author of *The Best Exotic Marigold Hotel*, which became a film starring Bill Nighy, Maggie Smith and Judi Dench. Debby's latest novel is *Little Black Dress,* in which the heroine, abandoned by her husband in 'smugly coupled' North London, decides the best place to meet new single men is at the funerals of their wives, before they're snapped up by anyone else. Debby is now adapting the book for television – perhaps more a coffin-com than a rom-com. She also went on a *Guardian* Blind Date when she was 75 with Mike, aged 76, a mathematician and physicist. They enjoyed some intelligent and amusing conversation, shared plates in a restaurant, and gracefully exchanged phone numbers. But Debby wasn't that keen and confessed: 'I think it was a slight relief when I said: "Here's the killer: I not only love dogs, but I like them sleeping on my bed." (I didn't add "*In* my bed", which is also true.)' Cookie, the dog she shares with her grandson, is delightful.

Twice-married Debby is rather exceptional, a leader in this generation of later daters. Recently, I was sitting typing in Sam's Café in Primrose Hill, and I looked up from my coffee and suddenly saw a huge portrait of Debby looming above me, with wild blonde hair and a bejewelled bra, holding a glass of wine, part of an exhibition photographed by Eva Stibbe, Nina's daughter. Inspired and impressed, I went round to Debby's house for coffee to ask her to impart her hard-partied wisdom. 'Most of my female friends have given up,' she said. 'They're quite happy leading independent lives and not stepping into the treacherous dating swamp. Anyway, by our age the possibilities are thin on the ground. The men have either copped off with a younger model or become too stuck in their ways. Even the notorious adulterers have hung up their spurs and returned to their long-suffering wives, who'll see them out. Besides, if they left home they'd miss the grandchildren. And they adore them. Because you do. I do. Because there's nothing like it. It's absolute heaven.'

The available pool of mature men is smaller too, although the odds are decidedly better for lesbian love. There are roughly 1,680,000 women over 75 living alone, compared to 786,000 men. 'And so many of them are gloomy,' said Debby. 'Gloom is not on. You can't be a grumpy old man or complain about your ailments.' When Debby went on a date with bruised arms after some blood tests she made sure to wear long sleeves. 'You know, damaged goods is quite attractive when you're young, but damaged goods when you're old isn't.' We discussed the movie *Le Week-End* in which Jim Broadbent and Lindsay Duncan play a long-married couple questioning their relationship on a trip to Paris. Every day, they have an allotted 'Ailment Hour' where they can talk about what ails them, but then they have to shut up about their health for the rest of the day.

Debby and I wondered if the next generation is going to be different, creating new ways of living and building relationships, bolstered by HRT, vaginal estrogen and Viagra. She said: 'I think so, because your body is telling you certain things. You know, the man can't get it up, and the woman can't get it in, because it hurts so much. It could be so much better.' As Debby said: 'I'm totally up for another crack at it. What's there to lose?'

Of course, not everyone is interested in re-entering the dating game, and there are other ways to find companionship in later life. I told Debby about some research I had been doing into the revival of communes – a bit like her ensemble in *The Best Exotic Marigold Hotel* back in 2004. I asked her if she drew on personal experience. 'Yes, I've always lived in a sort of communal way. When I was living in Hampstead, I was living with this Hungarian, and his wife, and my children were living there too, and there were a couple of other Hungarians – and their girlfriends – living there as well, coming and going and working on the house.' Debby has always had a variety of lodgers and her children and grandchildren come and stay too. She thinks the success of the *Marigold Hotel* as a book, two films and a musical was because 'it didn't look at the ages of 75 and over as incipient dementia and strokes and death and things, although it acknowledged that. It looked at this time as a new chapter, and emphasised the fact that we're the same people we always were. When you're young, you think old people are all the same, and we're not. We're reinventing it all.' The inhabitants of the Marigold Hotel are giving a new spin on communal living in later life, rejecting the stereotypes of the retirement home with its institutional carpets and plastic-covered armchairs in favour of something more vibrant and thrilling.

As we get older, isolation grows: over three million people in England and Wales aged 65 and over live alone, more women than men, and by the age of 75 there are twice as many women living alone than men. Humans were not designed for this. Loneliness leaches years off your lifespan. Plus economics and the gender pension gap alone make communal living, perhaps a house-share with good friends or empathetic lodgers, look enticing. Why be alone if you can continue to contribute – and party? Becoming part of a commune or a co-housing group is a growing trend for people who have reached the half-century mark or more, and for some families and younger people too. As marriages – heterosexual and same-sex – smash in the tsunami of midlife, partners die, children move on, lovers leave, expectations change, and online dating proves profoundly irritating, many people are left living alone who just don't like it very much. They don't necessarily want a lover, but they want to befriend, to not be bored, to be a useful part of a creative community. The word commune is losing traction, perhaps due to seventies' stoner connotations, and the 400 or so groups round the UK tend to call themselves 'intentional communities'. Many of these communards are perfectly sane, even rather conventional. What they offer is actually closer to how humans have lived for thousands of years, in small groups, sharing resources and companionship.

If the terms 'retirement village' or 'golf community' make you want to shrivel up, this is not what this breed of communes and co-housing projects are about. The diggersanddreamers.org.uk website, a hub for intentional communities across Britain, is a gripping read, with much discussion on Big House, Spiritual, Urban and Co-housing communities. The photographs of the beautiful big houses around the country are enticing: Georgian rectories, 'Strawberry Hill Gothic' mansions, and farming co-operatives with stable blocks – oh, and The Temple Druid Community, a therapeutic centre and sustainable farm with the ethos 'Earth care, people care, and a fair share for everyone'. Diggers and Dreamers say: 'This is the classic idea of the commune in a big old house where everybody shares everything. There are some places like that but there are also quite a lot of places where the big house has been divided up into lots of self-contained units. And, of course, not all communes are in the country!' Some of the co-housing projects are multi-gender and multi-generational and include couples and families, like Centraal Wonen Delft in the

Netherlands, cool social housing designed for a hundred residents with large, shared kitchens, which has been around since the 1980s. Others, like New Ground in North London, are women-only with a strong feminist ethos and focus on the later years: the youngest resident there is 58, the oldest, 95. Some women work, others volunteering, others writing and painting. The modern glass and brick buildings include communal eating, gardening and meeting spaces as well as private kitchens and studios, and a guest suite for overnight visitors, so brothers, friends, lovers and grandchildren can stay over – but they can't live in.

It's an amazing privilege to curate your own community: 'For so long we have all been slaves to the housing market, and it's really hard to create intentionally cohesive communities within that. People who are attracted to co-housing usually want purposeful closeness to their neighbours as a big part of their lives,' English co-housing architect Mellis Haward told the *Guardian*. 'It's not just about alleviating loneliness – it allows people to become part of an ecosystem of families and individuals.' Haward's latest co-housing project is a diverse, multi-age, mixed community called Angel Yard, being eco-built in Norwich. In America, there are now Mommunes, single mothers joining forces and living together, splitting bills and childcare, sharing the pleasures of parenting. The UK Cohousing Network has a website with alerts about new projects, and advice on how to begin what seems to be a complex legal, architectural, planning and negotiating process to start building your own utopian community. Developers are also creating purpose-built co-housing.

In midlife, some people want not just to shrug off conventional living, but to dump the bricks and mortar too. In Chloe Zhao's film *Nomadland*, my favourite actor on earth Frances McDormand takes to the open road in her van to look for adventure and work after her husband dies and her job prospects crash in the dead-end town of Empire, Nebraska. Her van is affectionately named Vanguard, and somehow McDormand's character manages simultaneously to be defiantly alone and part of a bigger, welcoming, unquestioning community at campsites and meet-ups. The film was based on a non-fiction book by Jessica Bruder about her own experiences in her van, Halen (after the hard-rock band – see what she did there?). In the film, when McDormand is asked if she's homeless, she demurs: 'No, I'm not homeless. I'm just house-less. Not the same thing, right?'

In the States, three million people live in vans, often continually travelling, sometimes due to poverty and sometimes attempting a later-life *On the Road* Kerouacian dream. There are 'snowbirds' who migrate south across the States in their campervans with the weather in winter, and north in summer. Another trend over there is 'Tiny House Communities', where people downsize into studio-sized houses with a communal element. Jane Campion's New Zealand television series *Top of the Lake* anticipated this by featuring a community of women who lived in isolation by a lake in a circle of old shipping containers, with Holly Hunter playing their feminist guru: 'Everything you think you are, you're not,' she says. 'What's left? Find out.'

During the Covid years and onwards, people became digital nomads, working and living abroad, renting or swapping homes, and the travelling van trend also took off during lockdown. Having a van meant freedom and escape, and on holiday on the Scottish islands of Skye and Gigha during that strange time, I met couples and single people who had not just bought motorhomes, but done it brilliantly on the cheap, fitting out old post vans or Ford Transits with mattresses, water tanks, mini-kitchens and bookshelves, and touring the Highlands. What better activity was there in lockdown? Around Bristol, there were 150 van-dwellers before lockdown, and now there are over 600. Van living can be long term, or just seasonal, when the weather is good. What if you could just rent out your house for a while – a week, a fortnight, a month – and drive away?

Unable to personally test living in a commune or indeed taking off in a van for a year, when researching this I canvassed the opinions of my friend, writer-photographer Anita Chaudhuri, who has unexpectedly become rather an expert on co-housing after being assigned to write about three different housing projects for the *Guardian*. Anita and I met last century at university, when we both worked on the Glasgow University *Guardian* student newspaper, and we'll see more of her in the next chapter on Creative Renaissance. Anita began her commune-odyssey at New Ground. 'When they asked me to go visit the feminist co-housing collective in Barnet, I thought it might be boring, but the minute I got there and saw the design, I thought, well, this place is incredible. A lot of love and emotional investment had gone into it. They spent twenty years bringing it to fruition and some of the women who had been the original visionaries were no longer alive by the time it finally got off the ground.

I could see that these women were just a bit ahead of the path I am on, and that they were basically like slightly older versions of all my friends. But what struck me about this group of women was they were at this stage of life where they were post marriage and post family. Many of them were widows, and some even had children living nearby. But they didn't like that sort of relationship of dependence with their family.'

She found that the residents envisioned a different way of life, and even as they grew older they wanted to keep going out. 'One woman who's 95 is still working as a book editor. She went through the Holocaust, an incredible woman. She regularly goes to the theatre and the hairdresser with another younger woman in the community. And they've been great friends for some time.' That's brilliant, but I imagine there are also some complexities: those who don't pull their weight, those who are downright annoying. Diplomacy matters and rules and boundaries are probably rather important to settle upon early, especially if residents buy rather than let their flats or houses.

The interview process to join such communities is as thorough as it is mysterious, with people invited in to cook a meal or spend an evening. Anita reported this from the Dutch co-housing group, Centraal Wonen Delft: 'I wouldn't exactly describe it as an audition, although I did have to sing at my interview,' says Marten, who moved in after a relationship broke down. 'That was unusual, and it happened because I told the housemates that one of my hobbies was singing. Understandably, they said: "Well, let's hear what you sound like before we say yes."' The communal kitchens and shared bathrooms in the Delft community housing might have been the breaking point for me. I find it hard enough to share a dishwasher with my own family. As we know, there are people who stack dishwashers like a Scandinavian architect, and there are others who stack dishwashers like a racoon on crack. I am the latter.

Of course, you don't have to actually be friends with everyone in the community – it's more of an intentionally interconnected village. Anita explained: 'Community is having people around you who have this thing in common. Previously it used to be the church or whatever, so you're not going to be best friends with everyone. You're going to have your particular friend, and there'll be other people you really value because they're very knowledgeable about certain things you know about – or because you just feel they're *not* your comfort zone. And I think that's quite a valuable thing. And maybe later in life it becomes a lot more important to actually have extra bodies around to help, neighbours, so people don't get siloed in their own little bubbles and go out less.'

I ask Anita if she fancied the communal life, after she made a final visit to Cannock Mill, an eco-village in Essex created by a feminist architect, intended to simultaneously tackle the climate crisis and loneliness in later life, among other advantages. There was a communal allotment, a fire pit, community chickens and beehives. It sounded idyllic. 'I'm not sure it's for me,' she said. 'I grew up around the Indian half of my family who live in communal households anyway. All my cousins and everyone in Calcutta are sort of cool about it, having multi-generations coming and lolling around together,' she said. 'It depends how much you like your individual life, your own stuff, and I can see people might not want to give up on that so easily. I can't imagine having breakfast with this random group of people, but I could imagine sharing with extended family or friends.'

Co-housing makes massive financial sense, particularly in cities like London where renting and buying is extortionate. Why live in a one-bed flat when you can escape to the country and communally own a village? Anita was also attracted to the co-owning of community cars and domestic items. 'I mean, why on earth does every household have to have a lawnmower to use once a month? It struck me that there's a huge cost saving and environmental saving for the planet.' I liked that too. Being from Glasgow, we both recalled the tradition of 'the steamie', the communal laundry room where women gathered gossiping at the bottom of every tenement building, next to the drying green at the back. I still remember my mum saying, 'You'll be the talk of the steamie!' when I did something reprehensible.

A quarter of older people in the UK are 'house millionaires' – their houses are worth over a million pounds, and many of them are living alone, like Dickens' Miss Havisham, frozen in time with all their possessions. Some people are starting to find that stultifying, and there is a growing fashion for Swedish Death Cleaning, explained by eighty something Margareta Magnusson in her bestseller, *The Gentle Art of Swedish Death Cleaning*. 'It sounds a little morbid, but you can remove the burden of decluttering for your loved ones after you've passed away, so you're left only with the

essentials and those items that have the most meaning ...
While it was initially intended for those later in life, it can be
relevant at any age when clutter has started to accumulate.'
It's nice to go a bit Marie Kondo on your stuff at any time,
streamlining your life. Divorce can bring losses, but also
clarity around possessions – you often find you really don't
need most of them. You lighten up.

What if you do clear out a couple of bedrooms and rent
them out to friends or entertaining lodgers, perhaps a cross-
generational experiment featuring Gen Z and Millennials
co-mingling with Gen X and Boomers? What could possibly
go wrong? My friend Deborah Moggach rented her spare
room to Nina Stibbe (and suddenly found herself featuring
in a year-long diary of Nina's life, *Went to London, Took The
Dog*. They are still friends.) I can see a Friends Co-op might
be fantastic to live in at some point as one grows increasingly eccentric. Of course, it wouldn't equal the excesses of
student and twenty something flatshares, but who has that
epic stamina now? I'm still good friends with many of my
teen and twentysomething cohabitees from Glasgow and
London. The friend whose dad kept bringing us rubbery
fish he caught in the Clyde for curries. The friend who
carefully took out my contact lenses when I was blootered.
The friend who needed a joint and hugs after an abortion.
The friend who lay in bed watching, too surprised to move,
as I unwisely chased a burglar downstairs into the street,
screaming. (I was naked at the time.) The friend who arrived with his mattress and moved into the hallway for
months, where he created an art magazine called *The Dog
Blanket*. The friend who lent me his umbrella to open to

catch the drips from the leaks in the ceiling. (An umbrella is much quieter than the 'ping' of a pot.) The friends who stayed up all night talking, until eventually we all changed time zones, rose in the afternoon, and were in sync with New York.

Communal living is hardwired into our natures, and the friendships (and stories) that we can get from it are to be treasured. I love the idea that as we move into midlife, we can choose the kind of communal living we might want in future: the cast, the crew, the props, the location – whether it's an eco-village in Essex or the Best Exotic Marigold Hotel. It's a liberating sign.

CHAPTER 17

Creative Awakening

There were copious creative renaissances and dreams unfurled during the Covid lockdowns, but for most of us, oil painting, tap dancing, memoir writing, home hairdressing, learning Klingon and maintaining a sourdough starter all faded to black once we returned to reality. But others gave their lives a more permanent shake-up, leapt off the office treadmill, and never returned – like my friend Anita Chaudhuri, who unexpectedly found her vocation, half a century into her life.

Anita was working full time as a freelance writer, mostly for the *Guardian* and *Psychologies* magazine, when Covid hit. Photography was something that interested her, and she had taken a photography evening class at City Lit the year before Covid, but it had remained just that – a hobby. Then the first lockdown arrived with its empty space and time. 'It was the Great Pause. The weather was absolutely gorgeous. I remember walking out and simply taking pictures, not particularly exciting pictures at the time, of just everything I saw. And then the next day doing it again and again, not having so many demands, so I got to devote an hour a day. I started going back into my office near St Paul's, and the streets of the City were all utterly deserted. Photographically this was incredibly exciting.' She erased all colour because she felt like we were living in a black-and-white world. Her eerie images look like a film set the morning after a mass-extinction disaster movie. In 2021, in the winter of the second lockdown, she started taking early-morning photographs, which became her series 'The Sunrise Watchers of Primrose Hill', backlit almost-druidic shots of figures overlooking the London skyline. She felt inspired enough to enter them for an *Evening Standard* photography prize – and she won.

The shrinkage of life that we all experienced in lockdown also brought laser focus. 'Right here on my doorstep were secret gardens and wonderful urban trees. Gradually, I began to observe and consider my surroundings and community differently. When you slow down, guess what? People are more likely to stop and chat. Something had shifted and, far from being short of words, as I had been at first when lockdown happened, I had much to say. I would share my images with rambling captions on Instagram. This habit of photo-journalling had an immediate positive effect on my mood.'

There was an enthusiastic response when Anita shared some of her photos online, but it still remained a high-grade hobby which she was doing for escape, to enjoy the immersion of being in the present. 'But I do remember a distinct moment when I woke up and the thought came into my head: I need to apply to art school to do photography.' And that was what she did. She started googling and was astonished there was still time to apply, and she had earned some money from recent work. Destiny called, and she was accepted. By the end of 2022, she had graduated with an MA in Documentary Photography from University of the Arts London, and she now divides her time between writing and image-making.

Growing up in a Scottish-Bengali family in Glasgow, Anita had a hankering for photography because her dad was a keen amateur. 'He always carried this big camera round his neck. Nobody had proper cameras then, so he was often mistaken for a press photographer, partly because he was always taking photographs of things you shouldn't. I made him give me a go, and my early efforts were rubbish. He just said, "No, that's not for you." And he was usually such an encouraging man,' she said, laughing.

Anita, who is now 61, also has some difficulties with her eyesight, so picture-perfect clarity was not what she was interested in. 'I think what you're trying to do with photography is capture an emotion.' The meaning of the art was what mattered, and that comes over powerfully in her series *migraineland* (look it up on her website anitachaudhuri.com). Anita suffers from migraine headaches with aura, which is where the migraine is accompanied by visual disturbances, in Anita's case seeing halos of vivid colours. During lockdown, when she could only really photograph herself, she began this project as an exploration of the everyday reality of living with migraine aura, featuring black-and-white inkjet prints that she has then hand-coloured. Throbbing blues, yellows, pinks and greens subsume the landscape and Anita herself, in what looks like a painful psychedelic trip into another world. In one shot, she's pictured in bed with a bird pecking at her head.

The cathartic and artistic results of her new work were such that Anita wanted to teach people to use photography the way she had during lockdown, and she wrote a year of well-being columns for *Psychologies*. 'Each month we would have my photographs as illustrations for a different topic. Sometimes, when words don't come easily, an image can express so much.' She explained the joys of photo-journalling for mental health and well-being, teaching readers to make their own photo journal, 'documenting for posterity the rocky times, as well as the happy ones'. It's something we could probably all benefit from. In the process of photo-journalling, the visual and literary halves of Anita's brain sparked connections: 'Studying photography made me a different type of journalist. I was now much more interested in paying attention to details, what people were seeing themselves, not just looking from outside and describing.'

Going to university again brought Anita a creative peer group of other professional photographers, and an understanding of different techniques and editing post-production. She is currently exploring photography with analogue prints and watercolour paint, as well as interviewing and shooting portraits of other migraine sufferers. 'Part two of my dream for that would be that the Wellcome Foundation would take an interest, and we could do a whole exhibition about migraine with different artists and art forms.' I love the ambition. And why not? We are hardly more than halfway through our lives at this point, and there's so much to do next.

I am inspired by the way that Anita was possessed by the need to become a photographer – more an instinct than a choice – and the way she listened to her inner voice. When we talk about midlife creative renaissance, it doesn't just mean art. Perhaps it just means letting the authentic, questioning part of you come back up to the surface, after years of being busy, sensible and dutiful. Although it's become a bit of a cliché, Julia Cameron's famous workbook *The Artist's Way* is a useful (and fun) tool for daily self-discovery, encouraging journalling, connecting with your creative side and discovering new talents, with a series of tasks to do along the way, including taking yourself on 'artist dates'. Her advice is: 'Leap -- and the net will appear.' Midlife is a time when we might feel more able to follow that instruction – when we are no longer directly responsible for children (or perhaps a partner), when we don't necessarily have to do the 'responsible' thing, when we might find we care less about the arbitrary constructs of 'success' and 'failure'. Now we have stopped keeping up with the Joneses, we can undermine the Joneses.

I've been listening to an entertaining audiobook, *The Art of Creative Thinking*, by Rod Judkins, who is a lecturer at Central Saint Martins art school and a creative consultant, and what comes through his investigation is generally that the madder and more obsessive you are, the better. He explores how accidental events become art, why failing again and again is good, and the idea that playfulness has creative power in itself. He hated creativity-suppressing traditional school, but he loved it when he arrived at art school, 'All around me there were people experimenting for the sheer hell of it, doing things that made no sense – or rather, doing things because they made no sense. There was an air of freedom and release. While all around in the world outside, people were being thoughtlessly reasonable, doing something because it was what everyone else was doing.' Midlife is very much a time to stop being reasonable, and who gives a damn about what anyone else thinks? And this is not just about art. 'Creativity is not about creating a painting, a novel or a house, but creating yourself, creating a better future and taking the opportunities you are currently missing.'

Strangely, my own renaissance involved learning about science, hormones and how to understand medical papers and communicate their contents to a wider public. It awakened a part of my mind that had been offline since double physics at school. Once I found out how hormones worked and their profoundly positive effect on long-term health, it was literally a calling to get the message out in any form of media (sometimes an irritating one; there have been times when I never, ever want to hear the word menopause again). I became involved in a political, digital and scientific revolution with thousands of co-conspirators.

My friend Nicole Verity, who's 63, had a similar midlife political awakening when she started working for the radical climate change campaign group Extinction Rebellion (XR). This was quite surprising when I think back, given that I met her by chance in 2001 in the kids' uniform department at John Lewis Brent Cross when we each had three small children and were in back-to-school hell. But I knew instantly that she was different from the other mums stuffing unwilling arms into too-big blazers. Nicole had long, wild hair and a wildly iconoclastic attitude to life. We both grew up along with our children and became different people. Nicole soon started training to be a psychotherapist, with a leaning towards Buddhist practice, and started taking clients in 2009. But by 2018, the climate emergency became something she could no longer ignore, and she joined XR. I asked her why, and whether it was a calling. 'It's a compulsion. It's not just finding a purpose. It's my duty as an elder. I've had to give everything. I have at least to try to make change.' By way of explanation, she directed me to a poem, 'Hieroglyphic Stairway' by Drew Dellinger, which begins:

> it's 3:23 in the morning
> and I'm awake
> because my great great grandchildren
> won't let me sleep
> my great great grandchildren
> ask me in dreams
> what did you do while the planet was plundered?
> what did you do when the earth was unraveling?

Nicole took a break from her therapy work to become a full-time activist, holding space at XR meetings, working the phones, and alerting friendly lawyers during protests where XR members were arrested for blocking bridges and roads in London, and making sure everyone was accounted for. 'I found myself on the street in a hi-vis jacket. I liked it, too.

Carrying stuff, talking to people. I didn't go with anybody. I often did the back-office shift from two in the morning to six in the morning, because that's the only time I could be out of the house.'

She is still campaigning on climate change now, but has returned to client and group-based therapy in a different form, including eco-psychotherapy in her practice, and is part of the Climate Psychology Alliance. There was a disconnect for her with the small scale of personal therapy and the huge issues the world is facing. On the Alliance website she wrote: 'My climate-related work focuses primarily on seeing grief, depression, despair and apathy as appropriate responses to welcome into being, so that we can understand their root is in the longing for life to flourish.' She now prefers to work outdoors with her clients. They get to choose a park bench with a view.

Nicole experienced three major changes in midlife: becoming a climate campaigner, becoming a therapist, and becoming menopausal. It turned out she had been somewhat depressed looking after three children at home (although as a chaotic mum working part-time, I always was deeply envious of her genius at calm, organic parenting, and always found her wonderfully easy to talk to even before she trained as a therapist). But the weekly personal therapy you have to undertake when training as a psychotherapist was life-changing for her. 'You know, you go on a journey with it. It's a privilege to be able to do that, because of the new awareness of yourself, the forgiveness of yourself. The kind of heart opening. Practising as a psychotherapist is a hell of a place to be. It's also a really extraordinary privilege for a client to come in and to some degree trust you. Sometimes you have to wait for certain souls to feel they can trust you. There is such reciprocity in the relationship. You meet each other all the time. I don't want to sound like I'm getting therapy from my clients, but I am getting so much from being present to them.' As a journalist I find that too, in an ordinary way, talking to women intimately about their bodies and minds, connecting on a deep level. Often when I'm interviewing women, I have a sense that they're giving me this huge gift back that I have to do something very good with.

Nicole went through the trials of perimenopause and menopause while she was a therapist herself. She decided not to take HRT, and instead managed the white-knuckle ride. 'Menopause is actually quite a complementary place to be as a therapist, because the menopause draws you inward. It's a time of deep reflection, an isolated time. I think it was cleansing, helpful.' But while the emotional and relational part of her brain was working, she had some technical glitches. 'I struggled when I offered to do the website for the place where I was working. I just could not pull that together. It was embarrassing. I had completely lost my confidence. Sometimes I couldn't put sentences together. It's interesting how you become almost non-verbal for a while.' And as hormones drained away, she felt angry sometimes too – just the psychological disquiet of living life in the same place, in the comfort of North London, while her views were changing. 'Sometimes I feel like I'm choking on the contra-dictions in my own life, the cognitive dissonance needed to get through the day, to be with loved ones, and watch them shop, seduced into consumer manipulations. All I can do is try to attend to the quality of my presence in this time that has arrived, and I find land-based and spiritual practice very helpful.'

Actually, I've rarely seen anyone handle the menopause and revolution with such grace as Nicole. 'I think it was a huge relief, a different journey. You arrive in a place where you're not responsible. The milk dries up. It's literally that.' Many women talk about no longer needing to nurture and be responsible for a family, and that can be the moment when they have renewed energy to take responsibility for the world, to look outward into the community, or in Nicole's case, the planet. 'I think we have to step into it, being of service and being of value. If we're up for it.'

Often we crave the precise opposite of whatever we have experienced so far, and while many of us who have raised families turn to face outwards into the world – travelling, relocating, volunteering, marathon running, learning new skills – there are others who find themselves nurturing deep domesticity for the first time. This is not just about gardening cat ladies, or becoming a dog parent with a fur baby, terms I detest. This could be about becoming a fantastic grandmother or aunt – or, it turns out, a mother. A somewhat astonishing example of this late development is Julia Peyton-Jones, the celebrated director of the Serpentine Gallery for 25 years, who became a first-time mother when she retired at 64. The announcement was met with surprise, but as we know, men do late parenting like this far more often – because they can. It's not clear how Pia, the baby, arrived, but what was clear was Julia's joy in her new role, and at creating a book of daily sketches of their family life in lockdown together, which she described in an article she wrote for *Vogue*. 'When I thought back even to a few short years earlier, it seemed impossible to comprehend how my world had altered. Even now, when I consider what brought me at the age of 69 to be publishing a book (*Pia's World*) about my four-and-a-half-year-old daughter, who has changed my life in every conceivable way, I feel newly amazed. Until she arrived, I was completely free to see whoever I wanted whenever I wanted, to travel as the spirit moved me, or as my job as director of the Serpentine Galleries required, to immerse myself in running one of the world's foremost cultural institutions, surrounded by brilliant, stimulating people. What made me jump off the train after it had already left the station?'

Clearly Julia had a longing for a creative naissance rather than a renaissance, and who's to say this is not possible as we live longer and healthier lives? 'I learnt every day about motherhood, with much hilarity as well as tears,' she wrote. Her book of drawings is a visual diary of life with Pia in the intense bubble of Covid lockdown, their games and routines, and the intense need she felt to protect and nurture her daughter. 'I knew that I would draw on every conceivable resource that I possibly could to become the mother she deserves me to be.'

While Julia is enjoying late motherhood, my final renaissance interviewee Karen Arthur is powering into grandmotherhood at 61 with her first children's book, *Grandma's Locs*, just one of the multiple talents she has unleashed following a menopausal crash and resurrection. The colourful picture book came out in 2024, a poetic tale of hair, identity and family, celebrating Karen's Afro hair, worn in a variety of ways, and the hair of her mixed-race grandson. On the cover, there's an illustration of Karen by Camilla Ru wearing her signature Dame Edna Everage-style winged spectacles, which reminds me of when she became a model a few years ago for Specsavers – her huge, intense eyes all over bus stops and posters, following you wherever you went.

Karen's creative renaissance came when she hit rock bottom. We discussed Karen's experience of mental health in menopause in an earlier chapter, but to cut the story short here, Karen was working full time as a teacher and struggling under a leaden depression. As the stresses of life built up, she used sewing as an outlet – between taking marking home. 'It got to the point where the sewing bit became more important to me. I was on automatic pilot at school. At the weekends I would design and make bags.' Eventually, she made her first clothing designs for a local fashion show, 'and the buzz was amazing'. But soon after, her mental health started to plummet. 'I realised that something wasn't right.' One day when the fire alarm went off at school, she packed her bag, walked out, and never returned to her job. Karen felt she had hit rock bottom, but this was also the first step towards her creative renaissance, which would see her turn her love of sewing into a hugely successful fashion design business, as well as seeing Karen become a podcast host, broadcaster, activist, speaker and author – among many other creative endeavours.

I met Karen in 2021 in her fashion design studio in the old Catford Town Hall, when we were filming her (still wearing Covid masks) for the Channel 4 *Sex, Myths and the Menopause* documentary. She is keen on upcycling, and was creating skirts out of logoed coffee sacks, and wedding dresses and stunning coats from African fabrics and repurposed curtains. Even in lockdown, she sold a gorgeous array of masks online in African fabrics. Karen explained what changed for her in menopause: 'I always used fashion as an armour and a shield, as an outside validation, as opposed to it being what I wanted, and that's changed because now I don't give a shit. I always felt comfortable with my frocks and my earrings, and I always looked good, but I wanted to feel comfortable in my skin. I started to wear my aunt's clothes and recycled things I'd made, and I would post pictures of my outfits and put the hashtag #WearYourHappy and tell people the origins of everything.' Wear Your Happy also became a bespoke fashion advice service where Karen comes to your house and repurposes your entire wardrobe – and gives you confidence by focusing on the things you love most about your body, rather than the things you hate. And key to this is wearing what makes YOU happy. 'The menopause teaches you to set boundaries. You don't feel the need to people please. In fact, you sometimes have the need to people displease and consider yourself instead. It's the great unlearning. The awakening.'

The awakening of Karen's talents has not just affected her, but the world around her. Following the Black Lives Matter movement, she started her influential @menopausewhilstblack Instagram and powerful podcast series. She is now a broadcaster too, with a regular show on Gold Dust Radio. She became a sought-after interviewee herself, and was even featured in British *Vogue*. 'Menopause gave me my voice,' Karen says. 'It wasn't that everything was great once I came to terms with it. Quite the opposite. But my approach to my life is different, and so things that challenge me, challenge me in different ways.' She's started running the JOY Retreat, the first menopause retreat for Black women in Barbados, birthplace of her mother and family members: 'I wanted a space for Black women specifically to learn to rest, and I wanted a space to honour my mother's ancestors. My ancestors. Barbados has a rich, tragic history of slavery. I wanted to give back to that economy too. I wanted to create a space that people needed. They come and they sleep, and there's an itinerary that is scheduled, but the schedule isn't rigid because you can't tell menopausal women what to do anyway.'

That questioning of the colonial past also led her to take a commission to create a dress for a statue of Queen Victoria in Liverpool to reflect on the city's complicity with slavery. Karen's dress for the queen is made of swathes of African fabrics and printed sackcloth, and the project was featured in a Sky Arts documentary. Another dress, created for an exhibition of entrepreneurs in the Migration Museum in Lewisham, coupled a plain British cotton shirt with colourful Madras and Ankara fabrics. At the launch, she told africanews, 'It's important to me as a Black woman and as an older Black woman to let people know that I'm not invisible, I'm not about to disappear. And it's important to acknowledge the contribution of people like my parents and lots of parents of migrants who contributed to this country.'

You might think that Karen had made enough radical changes to her life and career, but there was one more to come: a move to from London to St Leonards on the south coast. Being by the sea has changed her perspective. 'Even though some stuff in life is a shitshow at the moment, I find I'm gentler with myself in terms of my mental well-being. If I feel like going back to bed, I do, but I recognise I won't remain that way if I watch the next sunset or listen to the sea. There are several things that I live by, and one of them is finding the joy in almost everything.' Perspective is all, and changing it sometimes takes years of struggle and intention. Starting with small steps into the unknown is the way forward, perhaps with a creative mate, a co-conspirator. But at the other side, there are the rewards of living an authentic life. All the renaissance women in this chapter – Karen, Anita and Nicole – have something in common, and that's vision of their place in the wider world: a shift from role to soul.

'Age is a privilege; menopause is a privilege,' said Karen. 'I've done more with my life in the last eight years since I left my career as a teacher, because I made a conscious decision to only do the things that I love for however many years I've got left on this planet. I am having the time of my fucking life.' There you have it.

CHAPTER 18

The Psychedelic Adventure

My journey ends with the maddest part of the midlife journey so far – a psychedelic trip. Come with me to a yurt in a forest somewhere in Europe. The space is minimalist and calm: thick fresh cream canvas walls, a polished wooden floor and a tented, cathedral ceiling. In the circle are eleven women all in white, some wearing long dresses. When they emerge from the dappled, green wood, they seem to have come from the lacy depths of a Victorian novel. I'm way out of my depth here spiritually, and sartorially too, in the white dungarees I got yesterday in the street market. I can feel my heart palpitating, jarring against the gentle sound of a stream nearby. I'm completely bricking it.

There is a lead facilitator and two helpers – or perhaps wise women or shamans – for this hard-core psychedelic and therapeutic experience, and eight more women sitting on large cushions around the room: a neuroscientist, a hairdresser, a psychotherapist, a horse whisperer, a writer, a yoga teacher, a midwife and a full-time mum of two. Some are on a return trip; others are neophytes like me. We are a mixed bag of nationalities and cultures – German, Dutch, English, Scottish, African, Indian – and we all speak English. We are in our thirties, forties, fifties and sixties. We are all here hoping to change the trajectory of our lives, to look into the future with elation, and to excavate and heal a past that we still cannot fathom. To aid us in this all-night task, we will be taking, under strict guidance, a large dose of the psychedelic plant medicine psilocybin. Our magic mushroom mix includes three different strains: Amazon, Golden Teacher, Jack Frost. What will they do to us?

Now that I'm out the far side of my own midlife crisis, I have come here to explore my unconscious, but I'm secretly terrified I'm going to have a bad trip, a total horror-movie experience, and while we've been told to try to mentally foreground the issues we want to explore, which we discussed in a previous one-on-one session with the lead facilitator, I'm just panicking that I will fall into a psychedelic pit and think about snakes. I have a serious snake phobia, which began as a child in Scotland in the Clydebank Odeon when I saw a brown boa constrictor appear from a hole in the tiles above James Bond as he lay naked in the bath in *Live and Let Die*, followed by that disturbing voodoo scene with the poisonous green mamba. To compound things, my dad often told me the true story of a cobra that roamed round the soldiers' tents when he was a young mechanic in Burma in the Second World War – until the sergeant major shot the snake and propped it up on a stick, which gave my dad another fright in the dark. (My dad was 46 when I was born, and this now seems like an astonishing tale from another era.) But the early phobia was planted in my mind, the damage was done, and I used to jump and recoil if I even saw a photo of a snake in a magazine. When I went to the zoo with my three children, I'd walk through the reptile house staring fixedly at the floor. When I was interviewing the hypnotist Paul McKenna for *The Times*, I got professionally hypnotised free of charge for my ophidiophobia (the technical term), which helped quite a bit, but I'm still not serpent-friendly. Worse still, in the taxi on the way to the yurt experience, I pass a huge billboard advertising an expensive snakeskin handbag, which sets me panicking.

But everyone in this psychedelic circle is reassuringly friendly. We've been told to detox beforehand and not eat too much or drink alcohol, as the large dose of mushrooms could make an unlucky few throw up. Sitting around sipping herbal tea, I get to know some of the women's stories. Once people know I write about women's health and hormones and the menopause for a living, they tend to tell me all sorts of surprisingly intimate things. I am a safe repository of the unspeakable and unrepeatable. The women in the circle know I'm a writer, but that I'm only reporting directly my own experiences, not theirs. These questioning women are here for self-healing, and multidimensional reasons beyond: spiritual longing, unresolved grief, repressed memories, oppressive marriages, secret addictions, parental shadows, entangled relationships, depression, anxiety, gender curiosity, revelation, or simply seeking a vision of pure joy. Our facilitator tells me about her own psychedelic plant medicine journey, which included ayahuasca and psilocybin, and helped her heal from past trauma: 'The more that I drank medicine and sat with the different plants, the more I learned. It was a decade of proper, deep work, pulling off every layer that I could get my hands on like an onion, every skin that I could shed.'

I begin to feel better about the snake phobia, safe in this circle of enquiring minds, and start hoping for the psychedelic enlightenment I've read about in academic studies – until I go for a walk up the hill beforehand with the neuroscientist, who has taken this trip previously with the same wise and reassuring facilitator. 'What's it like?' I ask her. The neuroscientist makes a happy-sad face: 'It's five years of therapy in one night.' Perhaps the hard stuff is not going to be some snake-based trip but eviscerating my unconscious. Peeling the onion. But I'm hoping the trip will be exhilarating too, an experience. I am taking the magic mushrooms partly in the rip-roaring tradition of 'Gonzo Journalism', named after Hunter S. Thompson who took mescaline, LSD, cocaine, weed, 'and a whole multicoloured galaxy of uppers, downers, screamers and laughers . . . and a quart of tequila' while reporting for his 1971 book *Fear and Loathing in Las Vegas*. I won't be going quite that far, but I'm still well out of my comfort zone.

I've taken magic mushrooms a few times before, once when I was 15 and got on the back of my friend's motorbike as the high kicked in. We headed like a 'Bat Out of Hell' (we liked Meat Loaf back then) out of Glasgow down the A82 alongside the River Clyde to Dumbarton Rock, with no regard whatsoever for our survival. It was a wild and very stupid ride. Since then I've had a few honey-pickled shrooms partying at home with friends, which made everything hilariously joyous and the moon enormous. But that was very much recreational, in lower doses, and a long time ago. The yurt experience, I hoped, would be much more profound; done with powerful group intention, powerful female intention, and therapeutic in some as-yet unknown way.

My positive experience of the major brain changes caused by taking body-identical HRT – a copy of my own natural hormones estrogen, progesterone and testosterone – has made me fascinated by the work of chemical messengers, drugs and plant medicines on the mind. I followed up on my own brain resurrection by reading the neuroscience on the extraordinary mental changes caused by hormones – or the lack of them – around menopause, as well as throughout the menstrual cycle, and this made me much more open to looking into the science of psychedelics, and eventually brought me here, to experimenting with mushrooms myself, some thirty years after my early trips. HRT had given me back my words, my memory, but what about the vision? How else could I explore my brain? Were there more connections I was missing?

I read the serious book *Psychedelics* by the appropriately named Professor David Nutt, who leads neuropsychopharmacology research at Imperial College London, and is particularly interested in the effects of psychedelics (ayahuasca, lysergic acid diethylamide or LSD, and psilocybin) on depression. Professor Nutt's fellow researcher, Professor

Robin Carhart-Harris, now in the neurology department at the University of California, initiated brain scans in 2016 on twenty volunteers taking LSD or placebo and said: 'We observed brain changes under LSD that suggested our volunteers were "seeing with their eyes shut" – albeit they were seeing things from their imagination rather than from the outside world. We saw that many more areas of the brain than just the visual cortex were contributing to visual processing under LSD, even though the volunteers' eyes were closed. Furthermore, the size of this effect correlated with volunteers' ratings of complex, dreamlike visions.' Exciting. Professor Nutt said: 'Scientists have waited fifty years for this moment – the revealing of how LSD alters our brain biology. For the first time we can really see what's happening in the brain during the psychedelic state, and can better understand why LSD had such a profound impact on self-awareness in users and on music and art. This could have great implications for psychiatry, and helping patients overcome conditions such as depression.'

There's huge hope around this work, and the research is professional, no longer the wacky era of Dr Timothy Leary's 'Turn On, Tune In, Drop Out' experiments with LSD in the 1960s when some of the scientists got extremely stoned too. Since 2018, the US Food and Drug Administration has granted breakthrough research status to psilocybin as a treatment for depression. Of course, the truth is that humans have known of these powers since the dawn of time. From the ayahuasca plant medicine ceremonies of the indigenous peoples of the Amazon in South America to my own hairy, short, damp Highland ancestors grubbing up magic mushrooms for ceremonies in stone circles, humans have always used psychedelics for healing and spiritual purposes.

Now the science officially confirms that psilocybin's chemical structure and action on the brain is in fact similar to those of the 'feel-good' hormone serotonin – but often better. A 2023 meta-analysis of psilocybin-depression trials showed 'promising potential for the treatment of depression, among other conditions. Some of the benefits include a rapid and exponential improvement in depressive symptoms and an increased sense of well-being that can last for months after the treatment, as well as a greater development of introspective capacity.' In a 2024 report in *The Lancet*, a researcher at Imperial College tested fifty-nine male and female patients with depression. One group were randomised to have two 25mg doses of psilocybin, and the other group were given six weeks of escitalopram, an antidepressant. The testers were also given psychological support, and both groups showed an improvement, but in terms of self-reported changes six months later, the psilocybin group did best on social functioning, psychological connectedness and finding meaning in life.

The spiritual element seems significant too: a randomised double-blind trial on fifty-one people where they were given a single high dose of psilocybin (versus a tiny placebo dose) produced substantial and sustained decreases in depression and anxiety in over 80 per cent of patients with life-threatening cancer. 'Participants attributed improvements in attitudes about life, self, mood, relationships, and spirituality to the high-dose experience.' The transcendental experience helped many of the patients handle impending death and grief more easily. The benefits were still there at a follow-up six months later. In 2021 the *New York Times* ran a story on the healing revolution under the headline 'Psilocybin and MDMA are poised to be the hottest new therapeutics since Prozac'. The news is getting out there, and lots of people are now microdosing daily, whether through official or unofficial routes, and reaping the benefits, although Professor Nutt's book seems to show that, when it comes to the low microdoses, a placebo does almost as well.

My own discovery of psychedelics as an instrument of psychological change rather than entertainment began when I was a film critic and went to a random screening of a documentary called *Magic Medicine* (2018), about that same team of researchers at Imperial who started a trial of psilocybin on a group of patients with treatment-resistant depression. The psilocybin seemed to allow people who had been on antidepressants and in therapy for years to access the memories which they'd closed off to protect themselves – early trauma too awful to bear – and to find more self-compassion. The scientists filmed patients talking honestly about struggling with suicidal thoughts and weighty, immoveable sadness for years.

The patients then took a carefully guided psilocybin trip in a hospital room, dimmed and relaxingly decorated, with calm music playing, and a therapist and a helper at either side of the bed, ready to reassure or hold a hand if need be. Patients wore an eye mask, to go deeper into their unconscious landscape. Many cried, some laughed, some grew agitated, but they all experienced change. In his heightened state, one middle-aged man suddenly realised a recurrent, nightmarish, dark figure in a garage had been an abusive relative, and afterwards started the process of understanding what might have happened to him as a child. One patient said: 'Though hugely difficult to accept at the time, these revelations, brought about by the psilocybin, maybe completed a psychological jigsaw to allow me to process this new knowledge which had prevented my ability to heal.' Psychedelics can make the unconscious mind available to the consciousness; brain regions communicate differently and there are more neural signals which indicate complexity of thoughts. There's less 'top-down' thought, and more sensory activity too. Reporting the study, the Imperial Centre for Psychedelic Research said: 'When delivered safely and professionally, psychedelic therapy holds a great deal of promise for treating some very serious mental health conditions.'

Those depression experiments were done with official permission to test the drugs for scientific purposes. But for ordinary psychonauts like myself, the big psychedelic trip is of course as fashionable nowadays as it is illegal. That's why I can't tell you which European country I'm in for this experiment, or the name of the wise and wonderful facilitator. In the UK, the psilocybin-containing magic mushrooms you used to be able to buy twenty years ago at stalls in London's Camden Market have been reclassified as a Class A drug, along with heroin and crystal meth and cocaine, which seems a bit daft, given the mushrooms' much better safety record and the fact they grow wild all around the UK. I do have some qualms about exploitation, the psychedelic-tourism industrial complex that Michael Pollan discusses in his fascinating book *How to Change Your Mind – The New Science of Psychedelics*. Tribal rituals can be exploited as Instagram fodder, as tech bros head to South America for luxury experiences on ayahuasca – a psychoactive plant brew which is a purgative too – and I've talked to people who have been left in deep paranoia, unguided and unsupported on trips. You want to make absolutely sure you are in safe and respectful hands before you take the leap. Our facilitator, who has worked with both ayahuasca and mushrooms, takes care with that: 'We need our rituals,' she says. 'They help us. Everything in the space needs to be considered and curated in a sacred way to create an experience where people feel held. They can arrive and safely drop into a completely new space where whatever needs to come up for healing, can come up for healing. You know that the person who's holding that space has got you a hundred per cent.'

From what I've learned, it seems the safe framework around the trip and the integration into your life afterwards through talking, thinking and journalling is equally significant, and certainly my facilitator interviewed us all beforehand in depth, asking about previous depression, loss, or suicidal ideation, as well as our families and past lives in general before admitting us to the circle. This is sensible, as there is risk in a psychedelic experience for some, especially those with severe psychiatric disorders or unresolved trauma. We also all did a group Zoom before we even set out for our destination, to get to know each other and share what we each hoped to gain from the experience. Of course, bad trips can still happen in a safe setting, but it is less likely. Professor Carhart-Harris said that psychedelic therapy is not just about the drugs themselves but a particular *way* of giving them, combining psychological preparation, supervision, music-listening and aftercare: 'How many people are aware that music-listening has been present in all of the modern psychedelic therapy trials?' Our facilitator turns out to have a visionary playlist, which will move us on from dreamscape to dreamscape throughout the long night.

As we prepare for that night's ritual, the facilitator (who might be better described as an earth mother, so rooted and reassuring is her presence) tells us that a lot of women come to her for plant medicine at midlife, on either side of menopause, and she explains: 'I almost feel like there's a recalibration as we move into our wisdom years. There's a bit of a sense of emergency too. And a deep questioning, going: "Wow, I've got how long left?" The midlife emergency brings on the emergence of repressed sides of your character, or at least it has for me. 'There is that finding of your dark half, your other half. And so many of these women are digging out this other person who has been very quiet and – oh my God!' She laughs. She goes on to talk about the mushrooms being 'plant teachers' that we can learn from, but I'm still in sceptical mode at this point, cynical about the so-called wisdom of shrooms and wary of a possible happy-clappy placebo effect. I am of strict Scottish Presbyterian DNA – instinctively, I don't dabble in the otherworldly. But I'm melting a bit, and the promising science has got me hooked.

In the spirit of proper enquiry, I dutifully make a list

in a notebook of some questions I want to ask myself – or perhaps the shroom, the goddess, the 'plant teacher' – on the psychedelic journey. Perhaps mine are typical midlife clichés: parental estrangement and death, a broken relationship, guilt and nagging self-criticism. In all, there's a sense of the unsaid and the unheard thrumming beneath my surface. I've done normal psychotherapy around these losses and changes, which was revelatory and useful. I've done anger, and exhumed my dark other half. Now I want to heal and feel happier, to not just intellectually dissect the reasons behind what happened but understand it emotionally. So here goes:

> How can I now understand my relationship with my mum Ella, who died ten years ago after a long haul through Alzheimer's disease, her pain sometimes frighteningly self-medicated by alcohol?

I've largely shut away this part of my past because it's a pile-on of grief, guilt, anger, loss and detachment for me, and I don't feel I can do anything useful about it. Those of you in midlife with ageing parents may know exactly what I mean. I did my duty as an only child visiting Ella regularly in Glasgow, hugging her, and making sure she was looked after by a sympathetic carer, and eventually in a good nursing home, but I never felt real love or connection with her as she diminished. Just an empty sadness. I felt I'd lost her years before.

I remember my mum being warm, loving and witty when I was a child, but she worked hard as a personnel manager in a department store in Glasgow, and from the age of eight I was alone in the house after school. My teenage years were somewhat rebellious (remember the shrooms on the motorbike), in deep conflict with my older parents and their safe, narrow values. I left for university aged 17 and I kept on moving: to Cardiff, London, Manchester, New York, Paris, Washington and London again. I returned to Glasgow a few times a year to visit my parents, but we weren't really close. I am 60, and my parents were late breeders for their time; my mum had me at 38 and was easily the oldest mother at the school gate. They were from a completely different generation – my mum was born in 1926, my dad in 1918. They led unbelievably tough lives themselves: my dad's sister was in and out of a mental hospital for twenty-five years; my mum's sister Irene died of tetanus from a barbed-wire cut when she was three; her dad lost his necktie-making business in the Depression and became an alcoholic; and my mum, who was really bright, gave up going to business college to support her father and her mother, who by then had multiple sclerosis. In short, it wasn't Happy Families.

Alongside raising me and working, my mum had to check in daily on her alcoholic father. When we visited him, my grandfather was alone and often blootered, and the tenement smelled of burnt kettle, but he used to entertain me as a child by getting his blue budgie Joey drunk on beer too. The budgie would stagger drunk down my grandpa's big nose. Wrong, but very funny. After my grandfather died, and once all that chaos and pain and working and caring for others was behind my parents, they found safety. They were the generation that believed in soldiering on, putting the past behind them – and talking therapy would never have been considered. I deeply respect their resilience, and I just wish we had spoken about it all. Instead, I helped them buy a nice two-bedroom flat with white carpets in the suburb of Bearsden, and they went to the library every week, took package holidays to Crete, enjoyed long walks in the Campsie Hills, and regularly went for coffee in Dobbies Garden Centre nearby. In their own way they were content, even happy. They deserved this calm. But I didn't want my world to be like theirs, to be smaller. I wanted my world to be bigger, less beige, less boring. I wanted to take risks and keep moving. And to do that, I had to disconnect as dutiful daughter to some extent. But in many ways, I am exactly like them. So the next thing I want to ask the shrooms is:

> Can I ever loosen that Scottish Presbyterian uptight, moral grip on my psyche, and let my emotions surface in more honesty?

Let's face it, the plant medicine has got a big task ahead of itself with this one, and no, I'm not expecting it to sort back through all those layers of my 60-year-old self, which themselves go back into the layers of my parents' histories. As the next generation, I've led a pretty privileged, middle-class life, I love my children and my partner, and I do work I really care about, so I'm not exactly suffering. Some people have far more raw and serious questions than mine; real trauma. But as our facilitator says: 'Every single person is going to go through their own extraordinary experiences. Some people are reconnecting and clearing sexual trauma, and other people are able to look at the dynamics with their parenting relationships for the first time in a different frame.' She explains that some people might be 'very triggered, in a very sensitive state, and that's why the facilitators are there: someone will come and be with you or sing with you and hold you through that'. Our facilitator has seen everything over the years. It's her vocation, and she sees results. (She charges very little, given the complexity of organising this.) 'I've seen people reconcile lost relationships. I've seen people grieve huge losses, like the loss of a child. I've seen people deal with a lot of body issues, confront their physical being and deal with bulimia and anorexia. They are in a dialogue with the body in that realm. Suddenly the body comes online.'

So let the ceremony begin. It's almost nine o'clock in the late summer evening in the vast yurt in the clearing in the woods, and we're about to lose track of time and space for at least six hours. We'll sleep here together on duvets on the floor afterwards until dawn. I put my watch away in my backpack and get out my water bottle, feeling more nervous nellie than Gonzo journalist. There is a firelight from a woodburning stove, the smell of sage and incense burning, and our facilitator singing exquisitely to bring us into the moment. There's an opening talk that takes us back deep into earthly wisdom, the roots of plant medicine, then some breathwork and a hapé ceremony. Two women assisting the facilitator get out bendy pipes, like straws, and we go up one by one to the front to have hapé – powder from a sacred Amazonian tobacco plant – blown up our noses. It rushes straight into my central cortex like ten espressos at once, bringing a sense of heightened aliveness. Now we are cleansed, very awake, and ready to return to what seems to be a sort of altar for a small ceremonial cup of mushrooms chopped up in cacao. It's absolutely disgusting. I'm a bit knackered, having not slept properly due to rampant snake paranoia the night before, and despite the hapé hit, I have a bit of a doze on my cushion, as we start in silence.

When I wake up over half an hour later, it's all kicking off for everyone – except the neuroscientist and me. A couple of people are crawling and groaning and throwing up discreetly in plastic buckets, but they don't seem to mind. Old hands at this. I observe how each woman seems to be sealed in a bubble of her own consciousness; some are rocking and speaking, one is crying, one looks ecstatic. Another is clearly seeing things in the fire we cannot see. I have a tiny inkling of being stoned as I look round all the women and can visualise their stories – their grief, their anger, their dawning perception – in a swirling cloud of emotion over each head. One woman's cloud looks like a storm brewing, as her long grey hair lashes around. It's all flooding out for them, release and relief. But I'm still being an uptight journalist, an observer not a participant. I'm still thinking about what the facilitator said: 'I just find it extraordinary and very heart-opening, this healing of the collective feminine. There's something about the women coming together, being in circle, in this ancient circle, and collectively healing and holding each other in a way that society does not encourage or allow, because usually we're pitted against each other.' I like that, but as I mull it over, I wonder if I'll ever let go and be a part of that collective healing, or if I'll always be slightly separate, a reporter, because that's my instinct, my job.

I feel free and comfortable with what's going on, but in truth not much is happening for me. Is that because *I'm trying not to visualise a snake*? I shut my eyes and look into the colourfield – they're called phosphenes, those lights and colours you see when your eyes are closed. And I notice the phosphenes are doing something very off. They're normally blobs of colour, like a Rothko, but now they've become like tiny cogs and interlocking wheels of brown Lego or Meccano, parts of a moving clockwork machine. They're weird but a bit dull. This is not what I'd call psychedelic.

Interestingly, a few months later, I open Aldous Huxley's *The Doors of Perception* about his 1953 psychedelic trip on mescaline, long after he wrote *Brave New World*, and I'm astounded to read something similar: 'The field of vision was filled with brightly coloured, constantly changing structures that seemed to be made of plastic or enamelled tin.' He feels he's below decks, and the 'five-and-ten-cent ship was in some way connected with human pretensions. This suffocating interior of a dime store ship was my own personal self; these gimcrack mobiles of tin and plastic were my personal contributions to the universe.' Oh cripes. Luckily, Huxley eventually trips, egged on by the sound of music, when he sees an ordinary garden chair. 'That chair – shall I ever forget it? Where the shadows fell on the canvas upholstery, stripes of a deep but glowing indigo alternated with stripes of an incandescence so intensely bright that it was hard to believe that they could be made of anything but blue fire … the event was this succession of azure furnace-doors separated by gulfs of unfathomable gentian. It was inexpressibly wonderful, wonderful to the point, almost, of being terrifying.'

Meanwhile back in the yurt, the facilitator comes over to me and the still-sober neuroscientist who looks like she might be having an equally dull, mechanical time. 'I think you need an extra dose,' she says. We knock back some more shrooms and cacao – and we're off! The tent walls light up, radiant orange and red, and I realise in delight that *I* get to choose the colours and where they go. I make the roof of the yurt pulsate green and turquoise, like the sea and landscape on the Scottish island of Gigha (on a good day) where I go on holiday. I arrange a fancy tequila sunrise for myself; at one point, I whimsically go for a chocolate chip mint colour theme. I'm having a lot of fun.

I eventually realise, as I should have from the beginning, that I am in control of this trip. There are no snakes. I'm deciding which doors I want to open in my mind and which I want to keep closed; I can now choose to play around in the psychedelic colourfield, to penetrate my consciousness as gently or as deeply as I want. As a bonus, I can still stand and walk around, and go for a pee and drink water. There's this blood-thrumming drumming throughout my body, as every cell is individually possessed by the psilocybin, but I also feel strong and rooted. I'm used to cold water shock and a big serotonin hit afterwards from swimming, and I can feel this building to be a much bigger mind–body high. I'm utterly suffused with love for my children, and my partner Cameron, and I bask in that for a while. I can't say I have the answers to all my questions yet, but right now, I think this trip is pure dead brilliant, as we say in Glasgow.

And then, with that thought, I am transported back to Glasgow. I am six years old, holding my mum's hand in the audience above a vast, empty circus ring at the Kelvin Hall in Glasgow. It is the first time I have been to a circus and there is a new, weird smell of elephant dung and horse dung from the white and grey ponies with red feather plumes that have left the ring. But now the circus is over, and the famous dancing waters are about to start! Fifty-feet-high fountains spring miraculously up from the floor, with changing-coloured spotlights playing on the columns of splashing water: orange, green, turquoise and pink. Then green, turquoise, pink, orange. We have a tiny black-and-white telly at home, so this is truly my first multicoloured psychedelic experience. There is even a tiny but noisy orchestra, violins and cellos vibrating. Music thrumming through our bodies. I've never seen a real orchestra before. The circus, the elephants, the fountains, the music, the colours – it's the most exciting thing that has ever happened to me in my six-year-old life, and my mum has brought me here. This is brilliant. My mum is brilliant. I hold her hand tighter. My mum has opened this big door to the bigger world out there, and taken me through it with her.

The morning after our psychedelic trip, we wake up bleary and ecstatic in the yurt, eat a huge breakfast of sourdough toast and eggs and farmyard butter, and write up what happened in our journals, filling a surprising number of pages, reporting back from the strange lands we'd visited that night. Then we all return to the circle and debrief for ten minutes together, part of the integration and recalling process, so we can continue to explore what we have unearthed long after we have returned to the real world. Everyone feels they have learned something previously hidden about themselves, or found deep release in letting grief, joy and other emotions flow out. I have uncovered and relived the magical circus memory – I fact-checked the truth of this vision afterwards because it wasn't in my memory bank before, and it seems to be largely true. It was simply a beautiful story I had for some reason hidden from myself. Aside from the healing power of reconnecting with a series of earlier, happier, surreal moments with my mum and my dad, I also have a strong sense for the first time that whatever had happened in the past, I am in the right place in life at the right time, doing something useful in the world. That feeling has remained with me, months afterwards, like stabilisers on my emotional bike.

Overwhelmingly, there was a sense of self-compassion rather than self-criticism felt by all the other women too, and a camaraderie among us – we'd seen each other at our maddest, most vulnerable and naked, in every sense. Some of us had taken our clothes off, and others had danced in the forest. I was in the latter group. (I do wish I could tell you more, but I agreed to write only about my own experience. Let's just say there were some gobsmacking scenes.) In the early hours of the morning, we had all danced ourselves to euphoric exhaustion. I love that psychedelics might be an unexpected (if sometimes illegal) tool in our midlife armoury, and I wanted to share this experience with you in the book because it has had such a profound impact on me, as a fast-track way to open up my mind. We need many tools, but knowledge is the most important one. Self-knowledge is even better.

I suspect you need to have done some useful therapeutic work beforehand to safely engage with the onion-peeling revelations a hefty dose of psilocybin can provide. And sometimes the trip might just be about pure joy itself, nothing heavy. Who knows? The unpredictability, even if you are in a safe space, might result in a truly terrifying roam in your own mind, and some of the women carrying recent trauma had a much tougher and deeper trip than me, and the support of the helpers was essential for them. I'm not sure I want to be a psychonaut again; it was so powerful and cathartic I think one trip is enough for me, and strangely it took a week to feel my body (not my mind) was my own again. I still felt the mysterious thrumming in my veins. Perhaps, to an extent, I always will. As Huxley says: 'The man who comes back through the Door in the Wall will never be quite the same as the man who went out. He will be wiser but less cocksure, happier but less self-satisfied'.

Psychedelics are at the exotic end of the midlife transformation toolkit, and are not for everyone, but that need for a psychological reset one way or another gnaws at most of us until it is satisfied. Physical changes like perimenopause and ageing bring psychological waves smashing in their wake. The effect is not merely felt in the cruel outer world of patriarchy where losing fertility means losing visibility, but there is an inner disconnect with our ever-young Dorian Gray picture of ourselves. Yet as we have seen in this book, these bodily changes sometimes result in something better too: a search for the soul, for a new purpose, for essence.

Conclusion

So, this is the end of my book – and perhaps the beginning of your magnificent midlife renovation project. Change for you might be small, slow and mindful – or it might be instant and nuclear. But whatever shape it takes, you are not alone. There's a glorious, growing wave of sisterhood out there, exemplified by the courageous women who have spoken out in this book. We've got a midlife safety net of other women who are sharing the same journey, urging us on: 'Go ahead. Leap before you look!' Not all of them are wearing dryrobes.

We are all questioning and transforming so that we can shape ourselves to lives which are longer. We have a new relationship with time – this next period is not of retirement, but of 'becoming' in our lives – and our relationships need to grow to fit that. We are also equipped with scientific knowledge and hopeful choices about our hormones and longevity that we didn't understand a decade ago.

When I found out about the positive powers of HRT in menopause, and the lack of information available, I knew I had to spread the word and make a documentary, even though I'd never made one before. Menopause campaigning then became my vocation for the next five years. It takes hard work and often failure until you see clearly, realising what it is you want to do, what it is that feels just right. Now I'm wondering what the next adventure will be.

While you may be itching to explore, discovering your direction can be daunting. Sometimes action comes before conscious thought, whether it's changing job, going back to education, creating, volunteering, writing, inventing, coaching, travelling or campaigning – and it's also a privilege to have enough money to be able to take risks in life.

There's a Japanese word, *ikigai*, which means 'your reason for being'. The concept combines what you love, what you're good at, what you'll get paid for, and what the world needs. *Ikigai* is worth playing with, chatting through, journalling around, and it's probably impossible to fully achieve, but why not try? As my favourite old bird role model, the French feminist and writer Simone De Beauvoir, said: 'There is only one solution if old age is not to be an absurd parody of our former life, and that is to go on pursuing ends that give our existence a meaning – devotion to individuals, to groups or to causes, social, political, intellectual or creative work ... In old age we should wish still to have passions strong enough to prevent us turning in on ourselves. One's life has value so long as one attributes value to the life of others, by means of love, friendship, indignation, compassion.' I'd also add fun and general fabulousness to that list.

What tools do you need to facilitate your second coming, to create your manifesto for change? Aside from journalling, plotting, throwing ideas around with friends and colleagues, I'd also suggest making a PowerPoint presentation, just for you, of where you are and where you want to go. I was listening to Erin Keating, a former TV comedy commissioner and mother of twins who presents the Hotter Than Ever podcast, and she revealed that before her divorce and change of career she made a PowerPoint presentation, just for herself ... It was titled 'Oh My God, So Much Bullshit' and detailed the unbalanced burden she was bearing as a working mother. She said: 'It was just for me to express all the things I had been lying to myself about in my life.' It went on for pages – and in the end the PowerPoint worked. She saw herself clearly, almost as an outsider, took steps to change her life, and found her authenticity again.

This is the moment, whether we're approaching or departing the half-century mark, that we can look into the richness and complexity of ourselves, something there's not been time for until now in our multitasking lives. In lockdown, I did an online memoir-writing course, just to give me some deadlines to produce some thoughts and loosen up some long-repressed personal history. The other students' chunks of memoir were absolutely gripping and getting autobiographical on myself turned out to be rather therapeutic. Of course, you can write a memoir for free too, without having to pay for a course. When he was in his seventies, my dad wrote me a hundred-page memoir on a typewriter using two fingers, and it was surprisingly revealing. I've talked to a lot of people who are interviewing their own parents for posterity and to learn more about what makes them who they are. I also want to say here that if you're in midlife looking after an ailing parent or perhaps two, I want to send you a huge hug because I know how hard it is when caring roles are untimely swapped. Talk about it, ask for help, share the weight.

Like writing therapy, talking therapy (if you can afford it) is also not just about repair, but life expansion, and I've learned about that from psychotherapist Dr Kalanit Ben-Ari, whose wisdom appears in earlier chapters. I have to confess here that, like a midlife cliché, I did a six-week pottery-throwing course with Kalanit (I was the worst in the class. Just deformed blobs. Loved it.). One day she sent me a paragraph explaining why there's so much more to therapy than trying to fix a problem, which I reproduce here: 'I believe we go to therapy to gain clarity about our relationships, our past, and ourselves. It's about having meaningful conversations. We go to therapy to know ourselves, and to heal ourselves. It's a unique experience to sit with someone and share our most shameful feelings, thoughts or behaviours, removing the masks you've worn for years. In therapy, we also reframe old stories that once created limitations or blocks in our way of being into stories that transform us and inspire us to become our true selves. Therapy helps us to build resilience, close the gap between the life we're living and the life we want, and ultimately fall in love with life – finding fulfilment, meaning, and joy.'

Coming out of my own midlife mess aged 54, I was lucky enough to fall in love with my new partner, Cameron. He had been working as a criminal barrister, but following his own midlife epiphany is now training to be a psychotherapist. We are both late developers. All the best books end with the words, 'Reader, I married him' and that's exactly what happened just as I finished writing this book. I suppose I never expected to do anything as conventional as marrying again, especially as I'm encouraging everyone else here to become wild disruptors of their own lives. Yet even after six years of living together, with eight grown children between us, getting hitched turned out to be incredibly moving, spiritual and hilarious. Cameron and I didn't want a big wedding so we decided to elope, and ran away to New York using our airmiles, planning to get married in City Hall – it's $35 for the marriage licence, and $25 for the short ceremony the next day. Bargain.

My daughter Molly lives in New York, so we stayed in a hotel near her in Williamsburg. It was an old warehouse with staggering views over the East River to the Manhattan skyline, and we were there during a warm November week when dawns were orange and the skies electric blue. The three of us started the wedding morning with brunch in the retro Baby Blues Luncheonette, 'A Good Place to Eat', in Williamsburg. Nico and Velvet Underground played in the background as we inhaled the Zorba Plate: two fried eggs, grilled halloumi cheese, Greek potatoes, tzatziki, heirloom tomatoes, followed by the Babycakes – blueberries and cream and maple syrup pancakes.

We went back to the hotel to get dressed in our wedding outfits – me in a blue tartan suit with mini-kilt, Cameron in a blue corduroy Agnès B suit – and walked through the streets past pizza parlours and cannabis stores in the sunshine to the L-train subway across to Manhattan. Despite the fact I was carrying a bouquet and Molly was snapping away like the paparazzi, all the other passengers, many of them masked, pretended this was not happening, because that's New York.

Our odd odyssey through the subway and streets reminded me of Cleo's meanderings in the film *Cleo from 5 to 7*, the poster for which I mentioned in the Introduction, and here we were at journey's end. We arrived outside the grand pillars of City Hall and joined the bride-and-groom queue: couples in emergency marriages renting bouquets by the hour; pairs of grooms, one with a lacy backless tuxedo; Polish tourists in jeans and jumpers; a bride from New Jersey in a meringue of white viscose. We felt right at home.

The ceremony probably lasted about three minutes, from 'will you' to 'I do' to the kiss, but it felt, for a moment, everlasting. Afterwards, we took photos under dappled yellow leaves on the traffic island outside City Hall and had the wedding lunch at a corner dim sum place we walked to in Chinatown. We could not have been happier. I didn't expect to be so lucky, so in love, or to have such a vast family, as well as work that I really care about at this point in my life. I didn't expect to be this excited about the future at the age of 60. But we are a generation of pioneers, reframing our lives. What are your plans?

Acknowledgements

This is not merely a book but the product of the hive-mind of hundreds of midlife women who have shared their experiences with honesty and humour. Thank you to everyone who is named, to all my friends who suddenly found they had become contributors, and to the anonymous interviewees who courageously brought me their emotional truth.

I rode into this investigation joyously, fired up by the knowledge and enthusiasm of the new menopause movement, which will change the future of women's health over the next decade. I am particularly indebted to the work and advice of these medical thought leaders: Dr Lisa Mosconi, Dr Radhika Vohra, Dr Louise Newson, Dr Sarah Glynne, Dr Bill Robertson-Smith, Dr Ceri Cashell, Dr Rachel Rubin, Dr Claire Macaulay, Dr Kelly Casperson, Dr Mary Claire Haver and Dr Vonda Wright.

Special recognition goes to Professors Jayashri Kulkarni and Arianna Di Florio for their insight into hormones and mental health, and to psychotherapist Dr Kalanit Ben-Ari for her wisdom. Dr Lauren Redfern, Dr Rachel Moseley and Dr Jay Watts opened up new ways of thinking to me, as did campaigning lawyer Farhana Shahzady.

Thanks once again to my agent, Sheila Crowley at Curtis Brown, for steering and encouraging these women's health projects, and to my brilliant and empathetic editors at Gallery Books, Michelle Signore and Kat Ailes.

Finally, I'm deeply grateful to my family for simultaneously teasing and supporting me as I work, and to my husband, Cameron Scott, for providing the happy ending.

Further Resources

Podcasts
Postcards from Midlife – Lorraine Candy and Trish Halpin
The Shift – Sam Baker
The Dr Louise Newson Podcast
The Liz Earle Wellbeing Show
Menopause Whilst Black – Karen Arthur
You Are Not Broken – Kelly Casperson

Mental Health and Addiction
The Samaritans – Samaritans.org
Alcoholics Anonymous – alcoholics-anonymous.org.uk

Support for Autistic Adults
Square Peg Community – squarepeg.community

Wild Swimming
The Bluetits Chill Swimmers – thebluetits.co
The Outdoor Swimming Society – outdoorswimmingsociety.com

Menopause
The Balance menopause app
Everything You Need to Know About the Menopause by Kate Muir (Simon & Schuster, London 2022)
The Menopause Brain by Dr Lisa Mosconi (Atlantic Books, Allen & Unwin 2024)

Psychedelics
The Psychedelic Society – psychedelicsociety.org.uk

Instagram accounts worth following
@menoscandal – Kate Muir
@menopause_doctor
@drnighatarif
@drvondawright
@drrachelrubin
@drkellycasperson
@drmaryclaire
@drcericashell
@the_pleasure_possibility
@dr_kalanit
@dr_mosconi

Notes

Introduction

p.1   I found the perfect quote on this from Miranda July's deliciously perverse perimenopause novel *All Fours*
July, M., *All Fours*, ch 6 (Canongate Books, Edinburgh 2024)

p.8   And why the extra decades that science has gifted us this past century changes the shape of life as a whole.
https://www.forbes.com/sites/avivahwittenbergcox/2021/11/10/lifes-4-quarters--and-how-the-map-shapes-the-road/

Chapter 1: Navigating The Mental Health Maelstrom

p.16   'Menopause depression: Under recognised and poorly treated'
https://journals.sagepub.com/doi/10.1177/00048674241253944

p.16   Professor Kulkarni and her team created the MENO-D rating scale to detect depression in perimenopause
https://www.monash.edu/__data/assets/pdf_file/0020/3503333/Meno-D-Rating-Scale-Sheet_HER-Centre-Australia.pdf

p.18   HRT had been a major player in psychological healthcare
https://www.ncbi.nlm.nih.gov/pmc/articles/PMC543946

p.25   The prevalence of suicidal ideation is seven times higher in perimenopausal women
https://www.sciencedirect.com/science/article/abs/pii/S0165032708004771

p.25   Di Florio's work with her team at Cardiff University, which appeared in the journal *Nature Mental Health* in 2024
https://www.nature.com/articles/s44220-024-00292-4

p.30   divorce rate at its highest between the ages of 40 and 49 for lesbian and heterosexual couples
https://www.nimblefins.co.uk/divorce-statistics-uk

Chapter 2: The Midlife Brain Reboot

p.38   'Women's brain health remains one of the most under-researched, under-diagnosed and untreated fields of medicine. Not to mention underfunded'
Mosconi, L., *The Menopause Brain*, p.23 (Avery, Penguin Random House, New York 2024)

p.39   The memory loss is temporary, as the brain's memory bank, the hippocampus, regains the volume that it lost in pregnancy
https://www.science.org/content/article/pregnancy-resculpts-women-s-brains-least-2-years

p.42   'Brain fog', reported by 73 per cent of women around menopause, is real
https://www.fawcettsociety.org.uk/menopauseandtheworkplace

p.44   one in ten women between 45 and 55 leave their jobs due to menopausal symptoms
ibid

p.45   'Men of the same age do not exhibit similar changes.'
Mosconi, p.9

p.45   'It's not just brain energy that changes during menopause but that the brain's structure, regional connectivity and overall chemistry are also impacted'
ibid, p.10

p.45   'Menopause impacts human brain structure'
https://www.nature.com/articles/s41598-021-90084-y

p.47   'It is plausible that possibly as the brain approaches menopause it gets another chance to become leaner and meaner, discarding information and skills it no longer needs while growing new abilities'
Mosconi, p.93

p.47   'The most powerful force in the world is a menopausal woman with zest'

Notes

Brody, Jane E. 'Personal Health', *The New York Times,
Section C*, 17, 29 July 1981

p.48 Poor sleep and hot flushes seemed to pose more of a risk
to the brain than mere low hormones
https://reporter.nih.gov/search/nU2_
RxFa7UCOhHWw4vMaCw/project-details/10119044

p.50 after at least eight weeks of meditation, yoga or
mindfulness
https://www.sciencedirect.com/science/article/abs/pii/
S0278262616301312?via%3Dihub

p.50 the amygdala, which helps with emotional processing,
often reduces in volume: as stress levels lower, you chill,
and it doesn't have to work so hard
https://link.springer.com/article/10.1007/s11682-018-9826-z

Chapter 3: Could I Be Neurodivergent?

p.55 Nobody who refused me my diagnosis ever considered
how painful it might have been for me
https://www.theguardian.com/stage/2022/mar/19/
hannah-gadsby-autism-diagnosis-little-out-of-whack

p.58 'Autism research is "all about the blokes and the kids":
Autistic women breaking the silence on menopause'
https://bpspsychub.onlinelibrary.wiley.com/doi/full/10.1111/
bjhp.12477

p.59 'The Night I Lost My Freedom, and Got It Back Again'
https://pubmed.ncbi.nlm.nih.gov/36605566/
www.rosematthewsresearch.com

Chapter 4: How Not to Disappear at Work

p.71 one in ten 45–55-year-olds admitted they had left their
jobs due to menopause symptoms
https://www.fawcettsociety.org.uk/news/
landmark-study-menopausal-women-let-down-by-
employers-and-healthcare-providers

p.73 big firms like Deloitte, KPMG and PwC, the triumvirate
that recently featured in a *Financial Times* article
exposing the misuse of NDAs
https://www.ft.com/content/
78f46a4e-0a5c-11ea-bb52-34c8d9dc6d84

p.82   'Gendered ageism in the media industry: Disavowal,
        discrimination and the pushback'
        https://pubmed.ncbi.nlm.nih.gov/37498310/

Chapter 5: How to Dodge Dementia

p.88   Alzheimer's disease and vascular dementia are the biggest
        cause of death for women in the UK
        https://www.ons.gov.uk/peoplepopulationandcommunity/
        birthsdeathsandmarriages/deaths/articles/
        deathregistrationsummarystatisticsenglandandwales/2022

p.88   Black women are nearly twice as likely to get Alzheimer's
        as white women, probably due to long-term racial and
        economic inequalities
        https://www.nia.nih.gov/news/data-shows-racial-disparities-
        alzheimers-disease-diagnosis-between-black-and-white-
        research

p.89   Hormone-starved women in early menopause or younger
        women who have their ovaries removed are more prone
        to early dementia
        https://www.ncbi.nlm.nih.gov/pmc/articles/PMC10095144/

p.89   The annual cost of caring for these patients is estimated
        to be over $100 billion
        https://www.ncbi.nlm.nih.gov/pmc/articles/PMC10480684/

p.89   By 2050, at least 14 million Americans will suffer from
        this disease, and two million in the UK
        https://www.gov.uk/government/publications/health-
        matters-midlife-approaches-to-reduce-dementia-risk/
        health-matters-midlife-approaches-to-reduce-dementia-
        risk

p.92   There's good news for some men too – low testosterone is
        also implicated in male Alzheimer's
        https://www.sciencedirect.com/science/article/abs/pii/
        S155252601302493X

p.92   Dr Mosconi's team undertook a meta-analysis of the
        effects of HRT on dementia published in the journal
        Frontiers in Aging Neuroscience in 2023
        https://www.frontiersin.org/journals/aging-neuroscience/
        articles/10.3389/fnagi.2023.1260427/full#ref21

p.93   The new body-identical or bio-identical HRT contains
        progesterone and has shown good results in some big
        observational studies

https://alz-journals.onlinelibrary.wiley.com/doi/10.1002/
trc2.12174

p.94 There's an important observational study of the effect of
HRT on the risk of Alzheimer's
https://pubmed.ncbi.nlm.nih.gov/34027024/

p.94 'It's not reversing disease; it's preventing disease by
keeping the brain healthy,' said Professor Brinton when
the study came out.
https://healthsciences.arizona.edu/news/releases/
researchers-take-step-toward-advancing-precision-
hormone-therapies-reduce-alzheimers-risk

p.95 There is also a tiny study over three months of forty-
three women in the early stages of Alzheimer's which
showed that transdermal estrogen improved cognition in
naming and visual memory
https://www.ncbi.nlm.nih.gov/pmc/articles/PMC3302351/

p.95 The amyloid immunotherapy drugs donanemab and
lecanemab were largely dismissed in a Cambridge
University report
https://www.cam.ac.uk/research/news/
far-from-clear-new-alzheimers-drugs-will-make-a-
difference-at-a-population-level-say-researchers

p.96 It's essential for neurologists and primary care physicians
to work closely with gynaecologists and monitor
treatment outcomes over time
https://pubmed.ncbi.nlm.nih.gov/34027024/

p.96 A small study of 244 healthy women in the journal
Alzheimer's and Dementia in 2022
https://alz-journals.onlinelibrary.wiley.com/doi/full/10.1002/
alz.12759

p.97 The Lancet Commission published a 'landmark' report in
2024 on all kinds of dementia
https://www.thelancet.com/journals/
lancet/article/PIIS0140-6736(24)01296-0/
abstract?mc_cid=9d4b08a8a6&mc_eid=UNIQID

p.97 Looking at 450,000 people in the UK Biobank database,
researchers found that higher lean muscle mass was
linked with a 12 per cent lower risk of Alzheimer's
https://www.mindbodygreen.com/articles/link-between-
alzheimers-risk-and-lean-muscle-mass-52934a

p.97 On nutrition, Dr Mosconi has also written a book worth
checking out, *Brain Food: How to Eat Smart and Sharpen
Your Mind*

https://www.qub.ac.uk/News/Allnews/2023/
Study-finds-a-Mediterranean-diet-may-reduce-risk-of-
dementia-by-almost-a-quarter.html

p.98   The Alzheimer's Society analysed sixteen studies and found that regular exercise reduces the risk of developing dementia by 28 per cent and, specifically, Alzheimer's by 45 per cent

https://www.alzheimers.org.uk/about-dementia/managing-
the-risk-of-dementia/reduce-your-risk-of-dementia/
physical-activity#:~:text=Physical%20exercise%20to%20
reduce%20dementia,studies%20into%20exercise%20and%20
dementia

p.99   A study of over 150 patients over six months showed that those who did high-intensity interval training (HIIT), rather than just daily exercise like walking, had quantifiable improvements in memory
https://www.aginganddisease.org/EN/10.14336/
AD.2024.0642

p.100   HRT through the skin can help keep the endothelium or the artery lining smooth, and one study showed it improved blood flow in postmenopausal women, both those in good health and for those with coronary artery disease
https://www.sciencedirect.com/science/article/pii/
S073510979700436

p.101   In an observational study of nearly half a million Finnish women over 15 years to 2009 (so mostly on the older HRT), the risk of death from vascular dementia was reduced by 39 per cent for those using HRT
https://academic.oup.com/jcem/article/102/3/870/3061928

p.101   But there are plenty of other studies which show that the older forms of HRT, particularly those containing synthetic progestins, have a higher risk of clots and strokes
https://bmjgroup.com/menopausal-hormone-therapy-
linked-to-increased-rate-of-dementia/

p.101   encouraging news around the use of erectile dysfunction drugs like Viagra and Cialis (generic versions are sildenafil and tadalafil) on vascular dementia and Alzheimer's
https://pharmaceutical-journal.com/article/news/
erectile-dysfunction-drugs-may-reduce-alzheimers-risk-
study-suggests

Notes

p.101   To some extent, vascular dementia can be slightly reversed by changes in diet
https://www.youtube.com/watch?v=wzH3oJVM66Y

Chapter 6: The Power of Wild Swimming

p.106   Nick Cave: 'This revelation began my love affair with cold-water swimming'
https://www.theredhandfiles.com/what-makes-you-happy/

p.109   a Dutch study found that people who showered in cold water from 30 to 90 seconds a day were a third less likely to call in sick at work, compared to a control group
https://www.ncbi.nlm.nih.gov/pmc/articles/PMC5025014/

p.110   diary entry by English writer Fanny Burney
https://archive.org/stream/TheHistoryOfFannyBurney/
TheHistoryOfFannyBurney_djvu.txt

p.110   Dr Heather Massey of the Extreme Environments Laboratory at the University of Portsmouth – how to cope with cold water swimming
https://www.port.ac.uk/news-events-
and-blogs/podcasts/life-solved/
s7e02-blog---the-truth-about-cold-water-swimming

p.111   'Loss of awareness and changes in vision are signs that someone is becoming hypothermic'
https://www.theguardian.com/lifeandstyle/2021/jun/27/
heather-massey-open-water-swimming-tips-dangers-
hypothermia

p.111   The Outdoor Swimming Society has good advice on all this
https://www.outdoorswimmingsociety.com/
warming-up-after-drop/

p.112   These coats should be left to those who *are* doing cold water swimming activities, not those roaming around London Fields with a matcha latte in hand,' she said in her column in *The Times*
https://www.thetimes.com/uk/social-media/article/
dont-humiliate-anyone-you-spot-in-a-dryrobe-especially-
when-its-me-xpwwmhhhg

p.113   Plus there's promising research on how cold swimming builds up good brown fat
https://pubmed.ncbi.nlm.nih.gov/34755128/

p.114   Brown fat tissue will also keep you healthy because it uses suspended calories in your body and increases your insulin sensitivity
https://outdoorswimmer.com/featured/what-happens-to-your-body-when-you-go-cold-water-swimming/

p.114   Brain scans show that even short-term head-out immersion in cold water increases connectivity between large-scale brain networks
https://pmc.ncbi.nlm.nih.gov/articles/PMC9953392/

p.115   'cold shock protein enables the brain to protect itself – in this case, against the damage to nerve cells in the brain'
https://www.cam.ac.uk/research/news/gene-therapy-approach-to-boost-cold-shock-protein-in-the-brain-without-cooling-protects-mice-against-neurodegenerative-disease

p.115   Wild-swimming guru and author of *Waterlog*, p. 4 Roger Deakin
Deakin, R., *Waterlog* (Vintage, London 2000)

p.116   NHS Sussex and the University of Portsmouth trial involving eighty-seven people with mental health difficulties
https://www.port.ac.uk/news-events-and-blogs/news/study-to-explore-if-outdoor-swimming-is-helpful-for-depression-after-successful-trial

p.117   Tension, fatigue, memory and mood negative state points in the swimmers significantly decreased with the duration of the swimming
https://pubmed.ncbi.nlm.nih.gov/15253480/

p.117   Study involving Dr Massey looked at magnetic resonance imaging (MRI) scans of brains of thirty-three adults before and after a five-minute, whole-body bath
https://www.ncbi.nlm.nih.gov/pmc/articles/PMC9953392/

Chapter 7: Ageproof Yourself With HRT

p.127   scientifically proven to lower your future chances of getting heart disease, brittle bones, dementia, Alzheimer's, colon cancer, joint pain, depression, Type 2 diabetes, urinary tract infections
https://www.themenopausecharity.org/2023/10/18/transforming-womens-long-term-health/

p.129   The American Women's Health Initiative (WHI) put out

press release which claimed that HRT increased your risk of breast cancer, clots and strokes
https://pmc.ncbi.nlm.nih.gov/articles/PMC6780820/

p.129   the study eventually showed a 23 per cent *lower* risk of breast cancer among women who took estrogen-only HRT
https://www.breastcancer.org/research-news/
hrt-and-its-effect-on-bc-risk

p.129   the lead author of that study admitted that it did not show a 'statistically significant' difference in rates of cancer among women who were on HRT versus placebo
https://www.nytimes.com/2024/09/19/opinion/
medicine-allergies-research.html?smid=nytcore-ios-
share&referringSource=articleShare&sgrp=c-cb

p.129   Two of the original WHI authors have published an apology for the misinterpretation of the study, admitting it caused many women to miss out on the benefits of HRT
https://www.ohsu.edu/sites/default/files/2019-04/CPD%20
IM19-Thu-01-Adams%20handout1.pdf

p.130   leading thinker in America on the menopause, obstetrician and gynaecologist Dr Mary Claire Haver, who is also author of *The New Menopause*, said 'This is what I call the old menopause, versus the new menopause'
https://www.theguardian.com/wellness/article/2024/may/
12/menopause-mary-claire-haver

p.130   Professor Robert Langer, said: 'Good science became distorted and ultimately caused substantial and ongoing harm to women for whom appropriate and beneficial treatment was either stopped or never started
https://pmc.ncbi.nlm.nih.gov/articles/PMC5415400/

p.130   the risks come mostly from the old synthetic combined HRT, and the new transdermal estrogen in a spray, patch or gel works well with 'natural body-identical progesterone which has a non-significant breast cancer risk'
https://www.chelwest.nhs.uk/professionals/
gp-hrt-advice-guidance

p.130   A number of large observational studies have shown natural progesterone has low-to-no breast cancer risk, and the old synthetic progestins like the medroxyprogesterone acetate are what caused cancer cells to proliferate
https://www.bmj.com/content/367/bmj.l5928/rr-3

p.134   menopause is not a compulsory education module in the Royal College of General Practitioners' curriculum
https://www.pulsetoday.co.uk/news/clinical-areas/womens-health/mandatory-menopause-training-for-gps-is-not-needed-says-government/

p.136   'Oral micronised progesterone has likely less risk of breast cancer and VTE [clot risk] than older progestogens [progestins]'
https://elearning.rcgp.org.uk/pluginfile.php/170662/mod_book/chapter/832/HRT%20NUB.pdf

p.137   We know that women who lose their hormones earlier in life due to hysterectomies and the removal of ovaries in surgical menopause are far more likely to die prematurely of cardiovascular disease and get dementia, due to long-term hormonal deficiency
https://pmc.ncbi.nlm.nih.gov/articles/PMC7231649/
https://pmc.ncbi.nlm.nih.gov/articles/PMC4581591/

p.138   HRT's protective effect against Alzheimer's – latest UK studies show it can half the risk
https://journals.sagepub.com/doi/10.3233/JAD-240646

p.138   The Menopause Charity's *Transforming Women's Long-Term Health* report
https://www.themenopausecharity.org/wp-content/uploads/2023/10/The-Menopause-Charity-Transforming-Womens-Long-Term-Health.pdf

p.139   One study showed eating ultra-processed foods, compared to a Mediterranean diet rich in fish, vegetables and fibre, could make your biological age over five years older
https://www.medscape.com/viewarticle/ultraprocessed-foods-linked-faster-biological-aging-2024a1000l7u?ecd=mkm_ret_241129_mscpmrk-OUS_ICYMI_etid7035031&uac=363153HZ&impID=7035031

p.139   simple summary of all the evidence on disease protection in *Transforming Women's Long-Term Health* on The Menopause Charity's website
https://www.themenopausecharity.org/2023/10/18/transforming-womens-long-term-health

p.140   'I've been on it since my forties and thank it for my energy and generally upbeat attitude. If I die, I die, but it's been a good life'
https://www.spectator.co.uk/article/we-oldies-cant-help-but-think-of-death/

Notes

p.140 'Doctors like to say "change your diet" or "do more exercise" or that HRT is a cancer threat, but that's nonsense – all the latest research shows that the risk is minimal. They don't like to prescribe HRT because of the cost of the drugs, but the benefits are incredible.' https://www.thetimes.com/article/prue-leith-interview-when-i-replaced-mary-berry-someone-said-oh-no-not-that-posh-bitch-d7bb29tzc

p.141 South Asian women have a higher risk of osteoporosis, and many don't know about the bone-building benefits of HRT https://www.nursingtimes.net/research-and-innovation/south-asian-women-in-uk-may-have-higher-osteoporosis-risk-21-03-2017/

p.141 Diabetes is also higher in Black ethnic and South Asian groups. https://www.diabetes.org.uk/about-diabetes/type-2-diabetes/diabetes-ethnicity

p.142 In fact, the more hot flushes you have, the higher your future risk of Alzheimer's disease https://www.contemporaryobgyn.net/view/hot-flashes-linked-to-alzheimer-s-disease-risk

p.143 The NHS says, 'There's no fixed limit on how long you can take HRT, but talk to a GP for advice. You'll usually have a review of your treatment every year.' https://www.nhs.uk/medicines/hormone-replacement-therapy-hrt/when-to-take-hormone-replacement-therapy-hrt/

p.145 Facial estrogen increased collagen production by 6.5 per cent over six months in one study https://pubmed.ncbi.nlm.nih.gov/10687834/

p.145 double-blind placebo-controlled trial on ninety women of a topical face cream containing estriol, as well as glycerin, Vitamin E and oleic acid, showed an 88 per cent improvement in skin https://www.myalloy.com/solutions/m4

p.146 New York dermatologist Dr Ellen Gendler confessed to *The Cut* that she had been successfully using the low-dose vaginal estrogen cream Premarin as an eye cream for the last *twenty years*, and she also suggests it is good for the back of the hands. https://www.thecut.com/2023/05/estrogen-face-cream-review.html

p.147 the item 'can help relieve, ease or support one or more of

the 48 menopause symptoms'. I don't think we want our menopause symptoms supported, we want them crushed, but that's what it says on the Gen-M 'Menopause Partner for Brands' website
https://gen-m.com/

p.147 'We call it the *MenoChain*, where every business, regardless of sector, has a role to play,' said Gen-M, and they charge big companies like Boots £25,000 to be a 'Global Influential Heavyweight'
Gen-M Partnership Info Pack

Chapter 8: Reclaiming Testosterone

p.153 Columnist Bryony Gordon wrote a spread in the *Daily Mail*, extolling her experience of taking the hormone along with her HRT
https://www.dailymail.co.uk/news/article-13663885/
daily-dab-testosterone-banished-anxiety-new-zest-life-
husband-BRYONY-GORDON.html

p.154 Testosterone for older women often receives negative press, with headlines complaining 'prescriptions soar'
https://www.thetimes.com/uk/scotland/article/
testosterone-prescriptions-for-women-soar-22j6q92n0

p.155 A survey of over 900 UK women showed that in almost half, the addition of testosterone to HRT 'significantly improves mood-related symptoms such as anxiety and irritability, as well as concentration and memory'
https://www.balance-menopause.com/news/
newson-health-announces-ground-breaking-research-into-
testosterone/

p.156 A deeper look into cutting-edge research indicates that testosterone might help protect us against dementia, cardiovascular disease, osteoporosis and even breast cancer
https://www.sciencedirect.com/science/article/abs/pii/
S104366182100342X

p.156 In 2019, a panel of experts from international menopause societies called for more clinical trials on testosterone's effect on osteoporosis, muscle and brain health in older women
https://academic.oup.com/jcem/article/104/10/4660/
5556103

Notes

p.157   The NHS says, 'women produce three times more
        testosterone than estrogen before menopause'
        https://www.guysandstthomas.nhs.uk/health-information/
        testosterone-low-sex-drive-menopause

p.157   Men with low testosterone are liberally prescribed top-
        ups for fatigue, depression, anxiety, low libido, muscle
        and bone health, poor memory, erectile dysfunction, and
        even night sweats – many of which mirror menopausal
        symptoms.
        https://www.kch.nhs.uk/wp-content/uploads/2023/01/pl-
        934.1-testosterone-replacement-therapy.pdf

p.157   half of women aged 45 to 55 say they had 'low to no
        interest in sex' in a Fawcett Society poll
        https://www.fawcettsociety.org.uk/Handlers/Download.
        ashx?IDMF=9672cf45-5f13-4b69-8882-1e5e643ac8a6

p.158   GPs or menopause clinics also carefully look into other
        health, relationship and psychological factors before
        prescribing, which is not the case for erectile dysfunction
        drugs, of which 4.5 million were prescribed to men in the
        UK in 2023
        https://click2pharmacy.co.uk/erectile-dysfunction-statistics/

p.158   Professor Susan Davis of Monash University in Australia
        published a major study in 2019
        https://www.reuters.com/article/business/
        healthcare-pharmaceuticals/testosterone-improves-sexual-
        function-in-older-women-idUSKCN1UP2JO/

p.159   Studies show prasterone, like local estrogen, is also safe to
        use for breast cancer survivors
        https://pubmed.ncbi.nlm.nih.gov/35343852/

p.159   When testosterone is combined with estrogen HRT it
        results in better bone density
        https://jofem.org/index.php/jofem/rt/printerFriendly/56/78

p.159   Similarly, testosterone can also be used to improve
        dwindling bone density in women living with anorexia
        https://academic.oup.com/jcem/article/90/3/1428/2836731

p.160   In a small trial in 1995 of thirty-two postmenopausal
        women over two years synthetic testosterone with
        estrogen HRT increased spine and hip bone mineral
        density more than estrogen alone
        https://pubmed.ncbi.nlm.nih.gov/10649811/

p.160   A 2022 investigation in *The Lancet* discovered that
        women over 70 who had low blood testosterone – but
        not low estrogen – had twice the risk of a cardiovascular

event than women with higher testosterone
https://www.thelancet.com/journals/lanhl/article/PIIS2666-7568(22)00001-0/fulltext

p.160 There's also a tiny but cheering study of women with chronic heart failure being given testosterone patches for six months – afterwards their walking speed and oxygen use improved compared to a placebo group
https://pubmed.ncbi.nlm.nih.gov/20888520/

p.161 women aged 55 and over who were using supplementary testosterone had a 50 per cent *lower* risk of breast cancer, according to an observational 2024 study of the American TriNetX healthcare database
https://academic.oup.com/jsm/article/21/4/288/7617174

p.161 Dr Rebecca Glaser, a pioneering physician in Ohio, has experimented with testosterone in menopausal breast cancer survivors for almost two decades
https://www.liebertpub.com/doi/full/10.1089/andro.2021.0003

p.162 A small 2013 study by Professor Davis shows that testosterone alone improves memory
https://pubmed.ncbi.nlm.nih.gov/24716847/

p.163 A 2024 study of over 500 women, comparing normal brains to those with cognitive impairment, showed that lower testosterone levels in those carrying the APOE4 gene (which can increase Alzheimer's risk) were associated with worse cognition, processing speed and verbal memory
https://www.researchgate.net/publication/381186514_Low_testosterone_levels_relate_to_poorer_cognitive_function_in_women_in_an_APOE-e4-dependant_manner

p.164 One study in the journal *Menopause*, following women whose testosterone was topped up after having a hysterectomy, showed improvements in muscle mass over twenty-four weeks
https://www.ncbi.nlm.nih.gov/pmc/articles/PMC6893124/

p.164 A panel of international menopause experts concluded that testosterone therapy in doses providing the natural level of a premenopausal woman might cause 'mild increases in acne or body/facial hair growth in some women'
expert consensus

p.167 If we all rush at once for prescriptions, it could cost the NHS around £40 per menopausal woman each year – and

it costs £372 for men who need a larger quantity
https://www.covwarkformulary.nhs.uk/docs/chapter06/
DPS098-Testosterone%20transdermal%20preparation.
pdf?UNLID=6973597372023623114226

p.167　The NHS cost of testosterone for women is probably
around £320,000 a year in total, using 2023 figures.
The NHS cost of erectile dysfunction drugs is £15.5
million
https://click2pharmacy.co.uk/erectile-dysfunction-statistics/

p.168　Dr Uloko has written a superb meta-analysis of
testosterone and libido in women, along with fellow, or
should I say sister urologist, Dr Rachel Rubin, and their
conclusions are very encouraging
https://www.ncbi.nlm.nih.gov/pmc/articles/PMC6486327/

p.169　Meanwhile, testosterone treatments for men were being
handed out like sweeties – by 2020, 31 products had been
approved by the FDA for men
https://pharmaceutical-journal.com/article/feature/
testosterone-for-menopause-why-women-face-difficulties-
accessing-treatment

p.169　Natural testosterone reaches a nadir at about 62 years
on average – and then, surprisingly, takes a turn for the
better for some women as they head towards 70
https://www.thelancet.com/journals/lanhl/article/PIIS2666-
7568(22)0001-0/fulltext

p.170　In 2024, the *Guardian* ran an article under the headline
'"Frightening" How Easily Women Are Able to Get
Testosterone, Say Doctors'
https://www.theguardian.com/society/article/2024/jul/
05/frightening-how-easily-women-able-to-get-hold-of-
testosterone-say-doctors

p.171　One of the most fascinating moments in Darcey Steinke's
book *Flash Count Diary* is when she considers how much
more gender fluid she feels after menopause
Steinke, D. *Flash Count Diary* (Sarah Crighton Books,
London 2019)

p.171　'Defeminization is not on the list of menopausal
symptoms. Even if ungendering were listed, it would be
framed as negative rather than as the rare opportunity it
is to finally slip outside the brutal binary system'
https://www.buzzfeednews.com/article/darceysteinke/i-felt-
confined-by-femininity-for-most-of-my-life-menopause

Chapter 9: The Importance of Being Cliterate

p.178 The peak decade for divorce for men and women is in their forties
https://www.nimblefins.co.uk/divorce-statistics-uk

p.183 In the UK in 2023, over 4.5 million drugs for erectile dysfunction were prescribed, costing the NHS £15.5 million
https://click2pharmacy.co.uk/erectile-dysfunction-statistics/

p.189 The Swell Sex Symposium in New York in 2024 (you can still access the talks online)
https://theswell.com/event/sex-symposium/ny/2024

Chapter 10: Viva la Vulva

p.197 The NHS death rate for hospital UTIs is 4 in 100
https://www.england.nhs.uk/south/2023/10/12/
older-people-across-the-south-west-urged-to-protect-
themselves-against-urinary-tract-infections/

p.197 According to the *American Journal of Obstetrics and Gynecology,* we can halve the risk of UTIs by giving women in perimenopause and menopause a safe, incredibly low dose of vaginal estrogen
https://www.contemporaryobgyn.net/view/
vaginal-estrogen-effective-against-recurrent-utis

p.199 I took advice from Professor Harding, who told me about the European Association on Urology guidelines, which researched lots of promising non-antibiotic options
https://uroweb.org/

p.199 Cranberry products and particularly juice, however, seemed to be marginally effective in scientific trials
https://www.sciencedirect.com/science/article/pii/
S2405456924001226Key findings and limitations

p.199 a major round-up in the *New Scientist* in 2024 said probiotics definitely help treat urinary tract infections
https://www.newscientist.com/article/2410096-probiotics-
help-treat-recurring-urinary-tract-infections/

p.199 Probiotics are living micro-organisms, live bacteria, and ones like lactobacillus crispatus, rhamnosus and reuteri, or bifidobacterium lactis and longus, are able to suppress the growth of urinary pathogens like E.coli
https://pubmed.ncbi.nlm.nih.gov/31990804/

p.200 Studies seem to show that the most effective lactobacilli
for controlling UTIs are lactobacillus rhamnosus and
lactobacillus reuteri
https://pubmed.ncbi.nlm.nih.gov/16389539/

p.206 With a simple swab, you're not only taking control of
your own health but improving research and treatment
options for women and people with vaginas everywhere.'
https://www.evvy.com

p.206 There's a massive female health gap around the need to
urinate all the time as you head into menopause
https://onlinelibrary.wiley.com/doi/full/10.1002/nau.25165

p.206 I looked these definitions up on the NHS Guys and St
Thomas's Hospital website – and they did *not* mention
vaginal estrogen in their list of treatments
https://guysandstthomasspecialistcare.co.uk/news/
menopause-and-urinary-incontinence/

Chapter 11: Pumping up Your Muscle and Bone

p.209 a third of those who break a hip will die within a year
https://www.nice.org.uk/guidance/qs16/documents/
draft-quality-standard-2

p.213 it is cheap and easy to offer HRT to those for whom it is
suitable, and it is approved by the NHS and the US Food
and Drug Administration for strengthening bones and
reducing breaks in menopausal women
https://www.nhs.uk/conditions/osteoporosis/treatment/

p.213 HRT can increase bone density by 7 per cent on average
over two years
https://academic.oup.com/edrv/article/23/4/529/2433275

p.213 'HRT has a consistent, favorable and large effect on bone
density at all sites'
https://academic.oup.com/edrv/article-abstract/23/4/529/
2433275?redirectedFrom=fulltext

p.213 In one study, HRT increased spinal density by 13 per cent
over a decade
https://pubmed.ncbi.nlm.nih.gov/8922661/

p.215 One study of over 700 women in Iran, where covering up
means women don't get much Vitamin D from sunlight,
showed 10 per cent of perimenopausal women had
osteoporosis
https://pmc.ncbi.nlm.nih.gov/articles/PMC5799602/

p.215   Testosterone protects bone strength in women too
https://pubmed.ncbi.nlm.nih.gov/19434876/

p.215   Men with low testosterone levels earlier on in life are more likely to get osteoporosis as they age
https://www.ncbi.nlm.nih.gov/pmc/articles/PMC7867125/

p.216   She is using what NHS menopause experts consider the safest option: estrogen gel or patch through the skin, and Utrogestan pills containing body-identical progesterone
https://www.chelwest.nhs.uk/professionals/
gp-hrt-advice-guidance

p.217   Lyon, Dr G., *Forever Strong* (Piatkus, London 2023)

p.218   In the American LIFTMOR trial, 101 women over 58 years old with osteoporosis or osteopenia were split into two groups and monitored over eight months
https://pubmed.ncbi.nlm.nih.gov/28975661/

p.220   Frozen shoulder affects 10 per cent of women in the UK at some point in their lives
https://www.ncbi.nlm.nih.gov/pmc/articles/PMC5741880/

p.221   Some Asian women are at higher risk of osteoporosis – smaller bone size can lead to lower area bone mineral density
https://pubmed.ncbi.nlm.nih.gov/38753886/

Chapter 12: Avoiding the Midlife Muffin Top

p.227   'Estrone activates pro-inflammatory genes associated with poor estrogen-receptor positive breast cancer outcomes', according to a recent study
https://www.sciencedirect.com/science/article/pii/
S1550413120302473

p.227   In the 45–64 age group, 72 per cent of women are overweight, and of those, 30 per cent are obese
https://commonslibrary.parliament.uk/research-briefings/
sn03336/

p.228   The majority of American women over 45 have high blood pressure or hypertension, which increases the risk of heart disease or strokes
https://pmc.ncbi.nlm.nih.gov/articles/PMC11150086/

p.229   'This drug will be very helpful to people who want to lose weight, need to lose weight, very important for the economy so people can get back into work.'

p.229 https://www.independent.co.uk/business/
weightloss-jabs-important-for-economy-so-people-get-
back-into-work-says-pm-b2629367.html
'Our widening waistbands are also placing significant
burden on our health service, costing the NHS £11bn a
year – even more than smoking. And it's holding back
our economy.'
https://www.theguardian.com/society/2024/oct/14/
unemployed-could-be-given-weight-loss-jabs-to-get-back-
to-work-says-wes-streeting

p.229 in the US, the cost is much higher: Wegovy retails at
$1,349 per month
https://www.theguardian.com/society/2024/sep/22/
health-productivity-losses-obesity-weight-loss-jab-costs

p.229 The effects on mental health are relatively uncharted, but
the warnings on semaglutide products differ
https://www.healthline.com/health-news/semaglutide-
drugs-ozempic-wegovy-mental-health-side-effects

p.230 One study found that people who stopped taking
semaglutides regained two-thirds of their weight within
a year
https://pubmed.ncbi.nlm.nih.gov/35441470/

p.231 American research has also suggested weight-loss drugs
could substantially shrink the opioid crisis by muting
addiction
https://jamanetwork.com/journals/jamanetworkopen/
fullarticle/2824054?guestAccessKey=67ec89b0-
a682-4fbf-97d9-1c0054b62d04&utm_source=for_
the_media&utm_medium=referral&utm_
campaign=ftm_links&utm_content=tfl&utm_
term=092524&os=vbkn42tqhopmkbextc&ref=app

p.233 In terms of bone and muscle loss, along with weight-
bearing exercise, combining semaglutides with HRT
seems to be a winner
https://journals.lww.com/menopausejournal/fulltext/
2024/04000/weight_loss_response_to_semaglutide
_in.4.aspx

p.235 more fibre in the diet may boost levels of the
hormone GLP-1
More fiber in the diet may help boost levels of GLP-1, an
Ozempic-like hormone: Shots – Health News: NPR Barley
porridge Scots

p.236 Husbands are also considered: *How to Take 20 Pounds Off*

Your Man tells readers to use 'stealth, subterfuge, trick and treat' because 'he alone cannot save himself'
https://www.self.com/story/vintage-diet-books

p.237 low diversity in the microbiome seems to be linked with higher levels of depression
https://www.nature.com/articles/s41467-022-34502-3

p.243 The *Super Size Me* experiment revealed how quickly the body could change – for the worse, but also for the better. A 2024 study led by Nikola Srnic at the University of Oxford confirmed this
https://www.bhf.org.uk/what-we-do/news-from-the-bhf/news-archive/2024/september/research-reveals-hidden-dangers-of-high-saturated-fat-diet

Chapter 13: Women and Wine

p.251 But it does happen in the UK, US and especially down under in Australia, where a fifth of middle-aged women confess to being 'binge drinkers'
https://www.georgeinstitute.org/media-releases/middle-aged-australian-women-drinking-more-than-they-have-in-decades

p.256 Stopping drinking has not been a solemn process for me but a joy and a relief, one less thing to worry about
https://www.theguardian.com/lifeandstyle/2023/apr/12/the-trauma-doctor-gabor-mate-on-happiness-hope-and-how-to-heal-our-deepest-wounds

Chapter 14: Digital Detox

p.270 more than a dozen American states began the process in 2024 of suing TikTok for creating an app designed to be addictive to children and teenagers 'while making false claims to the public about its commitment to safety'
https://www.nytimes.com/2024/10/08/business/tiktok-lawsuits-us-states-teens-mental-health.html?smid=nytcore-ios-share&referringSource=articleShare&sgrp=c-cb

p.271 around 20 per cent of us regularly look at our phones in the middle of the night, foolishly lighting up our insomniac synapses
https://www.statista.com/chart/15838/smartphone-addiction-in-the-uk/

Notes

p.271 In a small American survey of 1,000 adults by Reviews. org, 57 per cent confessed they were addicted to their phones, 60 per cent slept with them
https://www.reviews.org/mobile/cell-phone-addiction/

p.272 There's also a new word for an acute case of phone deprivation syndrome: 'nomophobia' – no mobile phone phobia – which can, at its very worst, apparently cause anxiety, disorientation, sweating, agitation and even heart palpitations
https://www.medicalnewstoday.com/articles/nomophobia

p.274 In her book *Dopamine Nation: Finding Balance in the Age of Indulgence*, Stanford psychiatrist and addiction specialist Dr Anna Lembke took a hard line:
Lembke, A., *Dopamine Nation: Finding Balance in the Age of Indulgence* (Headline, London 2021)

p.279 about 17 per cent still look at their phone occasionally while driving, despite it being a criminal offence
https://www.statista.com/chart/15838/
smartphone-addiction-in-the-uk/

Chapter 16: Renovating Relationships

p.310 Erin Keating has thoroughly investigated the online dating scene for her American podcast, Hotter Than Ever
https://www.hotterthaneverpod.com/post/
listener-mail-how-do-i-start-dating-again-after-60

p.316 over three million people in England and Wales aged 65 and over live alone, more women than men, and by the age of 75 there are twice as many women living alone than men
https://www.statista.com/statistics/531386/
people-living-alone-uk-age-and-gender/

p.318 People who are attracted to co-housing usually want purposeful closeness to their neighbours as a big part of their lives,' English co-housing architect Mellis Haward told the *Guardian*
https://www.theguardian.com/lifeandstyle/2023/aug/24/
we-have-brothers-sons-lovers-but-they-cant-live-here-the-
happy-home-shared-by-26-women

Chapter 17: Creative Awakening

p.330   Cameron, J., *The Artist's Way* (Souvenir Press, London 2020)

p.330   Judkins, R., *The Art of Creative Thinking* (Sceptre, London 2015)

p.332   'Hieroglyphic Stairway' by Drew Dellinger
https://hellopoetry.com/poem/1336778/
hieroglyphic-stairway-by-drew-dellinger/

p.336   what was clear was Julia's joy in her new role, and at creating a book of daily sketches of their family life in lockdown together, which she described in an article she wrote for *Vogue*
https://www.vogue.co.uk/arts-and-lifestyle/article/
julia-peyton-jones

p.336   Peyton-Jones, J., *Pia's World* (Hurtwood Press, Poole, UK 2021)

p.336   Arthur, K., *Grandma's Locs* (Tate Publishing, London 2024)

p.339   it's important to acknowledge the contribution of people like my parents and lots of parents of migrants who contributed to this country.'
https://www.africanews.com/2022/04/11/
migration-museum-dedicated-to-migrant-entrepreneurs-opens-in-london//

Chapter 18: The Psychedelic Adventure

p.344   Thompson, Hunter S., *Fear and Loathing in Las Vegas*, p.4 (Harper Perennial Modern Classics, London 2005)

p.345   Nutt, Prof. D., *Psychedelics: The revolutionary drugs that could change your life – a guide from the expert* (Yellow Kite, London 2023)

p.346   Furthermore, the size of this effect correlated with volunteers' ratings of complex, dreamlike visions
https://www.imperial.ac.uk/news/171699/
the-brain-lsd-revealed-first-scans/

p.347   in terms of self-reported changes six months later, the psilocybin group did best on social functioning, psychological connectedness and finding meaning in life
https://www.thelancet.com/journals/eclinm/article/
PIIS2589-5370(24)00378-X/fulltext

Notes

p.347   The spiritual element seems significant too: a randomised double-blind trial on fifty-one people where they were given a single high dose of psilocybin (versus a tiny placebo dose) produced substantial and sustained decreases in depression and anxiety in over 80 per cent of patients with life-threatening cancer
https://www.ncbi.nlm.nih.gov/pmc/articles/PMC5367557/

p.348   In 2021 the *New York Times* ran a story on the healing revolution under the headline 'Psilocybin and MDMA are poised to be the hottest new therapeutics since Prozac'
https://www.nytimes.com/2021/05/09/health/psychedelics-mdma-psilocybin-molly-mental-health.html

p.349   the psilocybin-containing magic mushrooms ... have been reclassified as a Class A drug, along with heroin and crystal meth and cocaine, which seems a bit daft, given the mushrooms' much better safety record
https://www.ncbi.nlm.nih.gov/pmc/articles/PMC9353971/

p.349   Imperial Centre for Psychedelic Research said: 'When delivered safely and professionally, psychedelic therapy holds a great deal of promise for treating some very serious mental health conditions.'
https://www.imperial.ac.uk/psychedelic-research-centre/research/
https://www.ncbi.nlm.nih.gov/pmc/articles/PMC9353971/

p.350   Pollan, M., *How to Change Your Mind – The New Science of Psychedelics* (Penguin, London 2019)

p.357   Huxley, A., *The Doors of Perception,* p.26 (Vintage Classics, London 1954, 2004)

p.361   As Huxley says: 'The man who comes back through the Door in the Wall will never be quite the same as the man who went out. He will be wiser but less cocksure, happier but less self-satisfied
Huxley, A., *The Doors of Perception* p.150 (Vintage Classics, London 1954, 2004)

Index

Abaloparatide 222
Accenture 85
ADDitude 70
Addyi (flibanserin) 184
ADHD. *See* Attention
    Deficit Hyperactivity
    Disorder (ADHD)
ADHD Foundation 70
adrenal glands 31, 37, 150,
    154
adrenalin 113
Adult Autism 59
affairs, love 4, 5, 15, 29,
    173, 284, 300–303
Against Violence and
    Abuse 285–6
ageism 71, 72, 77, 78,
    81–3, 148, 155, 293–4
Al Fayed, Mohammed 81
Alba, Bianca 191
alcohol 67, 103, 122, 184,
    242, 245, 249–67, 343,
    352, 353
    advertising, female-
        friendly 251
    Alcoholics
        Anonymous 256,
        260–66, 311
    asthma and 253–4
    binge drinkers 251
    blackouts 259
    brain and 251, 255,
        259, 263
    breast cancer and 259
    'California sober' 257
    Carys (alcohol
        recovery) 262–6
    cortisol/stress levels
        and 259
    cost of 251–2
    dehydrogenase and
        253

depressant 258–9
grey-area drinking 250
hangovers 252, 253,
    263
histamine and 252,
    254
menopause,
    compounds
    physical
    symptoms of 252
metabolise, ability to
    253–4
microbiome and 252
non-alcoholic drinks
    257
osteoporosis and 222
self-medicating with
    5, 250, 256, 352
sobriety as a
    superpower 266
twelve-step
    programmes
    260–66
weight-loss drugs and
    231
Alzheimer's disease 3, 4,
    76, 87–98, 100, 127,
    152, 173
    amyloid plaques and
        88, 93–6, 102,
        160–61, 163
    APOE4 and 91, 94, 96,
        97, 163
    black women and
        88–9
    cold water and 114,
        115
    diet/lifestyle and 50,
        97–8
    as economic and
        public health
        issue 89

Ella Muir and 4, 15,
    30, 87, 90–92, 97,
    100, 103–5, 138,
    152, 202–3, 323,
    352–3, 359, 360
erectile dysfunction
    drugs and 101
hot flushes and 142
HRT and/research into
    the hormonal
    component of 89,
    91–8, 138
leading cause of death
    for women in the
    UK 88
perimenopause 87,
    88, 93
risk begins in midlife
    87, 88
testosterone and 92,
    93, 163
Alzheimer's and Dementia
    96
Alzheimer's Research 95
American diet 50, 241
*American Journal of
    Obstetrics and
    Gynecology, The* 93–4,
    197
amygdala 50–51
amyloid plaques 88, 93–6,
    102, 160–61, 163
Anderson, Gillian: *Want*
    188
Androfeme 157
Angel Yard 318
anger 4, 5, 33, 58, 60, 155,
    284, 285, 303, 334,
    352, 356
anhedonia 18, 230, 275
anti-psychotic medication
    23

anxiety 3, 4
  autism and 54, 57
  'good' anxiety 21
  HRT and 20, 78, 133,
    153, 155
  menopause and 16–25
  perimenopause and
    263, 284
  phone/social media
    and 270, 273
  psychedelics and
    343–4, 347
  weight and 226, 230,
    231
  work and 21, 23, 75,
    77–8
APOE4 91, 94, 96, 97, 163
aromatase inhibitors 161
Arthur, Karen 31–2;
  Grandma's Locs 336–7
'artist dates' 330
Asian women 141, 221
Attention Deficit
  Hyperactivity Disorder
  (ADHD) 53–4, 63–7, 70
Atwood, Margaret: The
  Handmaid's Tale 286
auditory hallucinations 23
autism 53–70
  Autism Spectrum
    Disorder defined
    56–7
  diagnosis 53–70
  meltdown 60–61
Autistica 70
ayahuasca 344, 345,
  346–7, 350

Bader Ginsburg, Ruth 47,
  169
Baker, Hinemoana:
  Perimenopause and
  Libido: A Personal Story
  192
BBC 83
Beagan, Morven 118–19
Beard, Mary 83
Bellevue Law 80
Ben-Ari, Dr Kalanit 27–30,
  34, 35, 185, 226, 298–
  301, 365, 369
Benchley, Robert 308
Berlin, Coco 192
Berry, Professor Sarah 238
Big Pharma 95, 165, 222,
  233
Bijuve 135
'bikini medicine' 38
biopsychosocial chaos 14

bipolar disorder 25–6
Bipolar UK 25
bisphosphonate 216, 222
black women 31–4, 88–9,
  133, 141, 338–40
Blackie, Sharon 142
Blissel gel 146, 181
blood glucose 239–40
blood pressure 97, 98, 99,
  101–2, 109, 110, 138,
  144, 164, 172, 184,
  222, 228, 229, 231, 238
blood tests 22, 133, 152,
  154, 160, 183, 242, 315
Bluetits Chill Swimmers
  108, 123
body shape 4, 225–46
  blood glucose and
    239–40
  blood pressure and
    228, 229, 231
  breast cancer and 227
  bulimia and 226
  cholesterol and 238,
    241, 243, 246
  Continuous Glucose
    Monitor (CGM)
    236–41
  Denby and 244–6
  diet/dieting and 226,
    228, 230–31,
    235–6, 237, 239,
    241, 242, 243,
    244, 246
  estradiol and 227, 238
  estrone and 227
  fat and 225–7, 230–36,
    238, 239, 240–41,
    243, 246
  fibre and 226, 235, 242
  gut microbiome and
    228, 236–9, 241–2,
    246
  insulin resistance and
    227, 228, 238, 239
  Meno Scale calculator
    242
  protein and 226, 233,
    234–5, 240, 241,
    242, 245
  sugar and 231, 233,
    236, 237, 238–41
  Super Size Me 242–3
  teenagers and 226
  ultra-processed food
    (UPF) see ultra-
    processed food
  visceral adipose tissue
    227, 238, 240–41

weight gain and see
  weight
bone. See muscle and
  bone
Boots 146–7
borderline personality
  disorder 65
boredom 8, 71, 155, 273,
  285, 301, 309, 317
Bourgeois, Louise vii
Bournemouth University
  53, 58, 65
brain
  alcohol and 251, 255,
    259, 263
  amygdala 50–51
  'Baby Brain' 39
  brain activity
    reduction during
    menopause 44–5
  brain fog 17, 18–19,
    20, 42–4, 85, 132,
    133, 140–41, 152,
    162, 165, 242, 291
  creativity and 287–8
  dementia and 87–9,
    92–100, 102–3
  energy in 44–5
  estrogen and 42–3
  grey matter 38, 39, 40,
    41, 45–6
  HRT and see hormone
    replacement
    therapy (HRT)
  hypothalamus 42
  meditation/
    mindfulness and
    50–51 see also
    meditation
  Mediterranean diet
    and 50, 97–8
  memory and 44 see
    also memory
  MsBrain study 48,
    93–4
  nerve growth factor
    (NGF) 50, 99
  neurodivergence and
    53, 57, 63, 64, 65,
    67, 70
  neuroscience, women
    and 37–8, 151
  neurotransmitters 17,
    42, 58, 184
  Perimenopause Reboot
    40–43
  phone and 273, 274,
    275, 276–7, 278,
    279

Index

postmenopausal
  renaissance 45–8
postpartum brain 40
Pregnancy Reboot
  39–40
psychedelics and
  345–7, 349
Puberty Reboot 37,
  38–9
rewires during
  menopause/
  Midlife Brain
  Reboot 17–19, 22,
  37–52
scans 44–5, 48, 50, 93,
  114, 117, 151, 346
synaptic pruning 38–9
testosterone and 150,
  151, 152, 158, 162,
  163, 165, 167
wild swimming and
  114–15, 117
workplace and 71, 85
breast cancer
  alcohol and 259
  estrone and 227
  HRT and 109, 128–32,
    135, 136, 139, 143,
    144, 148, 156, 159,
    165, 197, 215
  sex and 179–80
  testosterone and 161–2
Brinton, Professor Roberta
  Diaz 88, 93, 94–5
British Menopause Society
  131, 144, 167, 170,
  203, 215
Brizendine, Dr Louann: The
  Upgrade: How the Female
  Brain Gets Stronger and
  Better in Midlife 47–8
Brouillet, André 26
Brown, Brené 266
Brown, Karen 306
Bruder, Jessica 319
bulimia 226, 355
bullying behaviour 73, 76
Bumble 313
Burney, Fanny 109–10
burnout 58, 60, 71, 74
ByteDance 271

Calvert-Lee, Georgina
  80–82
Cambridge University 96,
  114–16
Cameron (partner of Kate
  Muir) 85, 107, 116,
  236, 237–8, 239, 241,
  256, 268, 312, 330,
  358, 365–6
Cameron, Julia: The
  Artist's Way 330
Can't Buy My Silence 62,
  73, 74
Candy, Lorraine 27, 29
cannabis 5, 366
Cannock Mill eco-village,
  Essex 322
Cardiff University 25, 156
Carhart-Harris, Robin
  346, 351
Carys (alcohol recovery)
  262–6
Casperson, Kelly 128, 150,
  153, 183–4, 185, 267,
  371
cataracts 138
Cave, Nick 106–7
CBD 5, 94
Center for Innovation in
  Brain Science at the
  University of Arizona
  88
Centraal Wonen Delft
  317–18, 321
central nervous system 17
CEOs, FTSE 100
  companies 72
ceremony, psychedelic
  355–9
Charcot, Jean-Martin 26
Chaudhuri, Anita 320–23,
  326–30, 340
Chidwick, Narelle 210,
  216–19
children
  autism and 55, 59,
    62, 66
  'Baby Brain' 39
  divorce and 286–93,
    295, 299, 303
  leaving home 29
  postpartum brain
    and 40
  technology and 270–
    71, 277
  work and 77, 78, 80
cholesterol 99, 100, 103,
  138–9, 222, 238, 241,
  243, 246
Christie, Bridget: The
  Change 43
chronic vulvovaginal pain
  185
Cialis 101, 184
Cleo from 5 to 7 (film) 6,
  7, 367

Climacteric 219–20
Climate Psychology
  Alliance 333
Clitoratti, The 177
clitoris 159, 165, 178–9,
  181, 182, 190, 191, 201
clothes, making 337–8
Clue 166, 192
co-housing 316–25
Cognitive Behavioural
  Therapy (CBT) 35, 94,
  260, 276
cold shock protein 114–15
cold water shock 110–15
comeback, art of the 3, 77–8
communal living 316–25
concentration 16, 31, 53,
  64, 133, 151, 155,
  278–9
Continuous Glucose
  Monitor (CGM)
  236–41
contraception 49, 65,
  135–6, 159, 166, 196,
  211
Cookson, Cath 257
Corryvreckan whirlpool,
  Scotland 13–14, 36
cortisol 31, 37, 41, 58, 113,
  259
Countryfile (TV
  programme) 82–3
couplepause 297–8
couples therapy 29–30,
  185, 297–303
Covid-19 76, 119, 120,
  123, 224, 289, 319–20,
  326, 336, 338
creativity 326–40
  clothes, making 337–8
  'Hieroglyphic
    Stairway' 332
  menopause and 333–40
  motherhood 335–6
  psychotherapy and
    333–4
  photography 326–30
  political awakening
    331–3, 338–9
  The Art of Creative
    Thinking 330–30–1
  The Artist's Way 330
  writing 336–7
Crompton, Siobhan 253
Currie, Dr Heather 170
Cut, The 146

D-Mannose 199
Daily Mail 153, 230–31

Dalton, Dr Katharina 24
Dan the Merman 122
Daswani, Sunita 21–2
dating apps/dating online 207, 302, 310–12, 316–17
Davis, Susan 158, 162
Daye 205
De Beauvoir, Simone 47, 363–4
Deakin, Roger 115–16
default mode network 273, 276
dehydroepiandrosterone (DHEA) 38, 159, 198
Dellinger, Drew: 'Hieroglyphic Stairway' 332
dementia 15, 44, 48, 50, 87–105, 114–15, 123, 127, 137, 139, 156, 167, 175, 201, 203, 204, 227, 316
  Alzheimer's see Alzheimer's
  biggest cause of death for women in the UK 88
  black women and 88–9
  economic and public health issue 89
  vascular dementia 87–8, 98–105
Denby, Nigel 244–6
Dench, Judi 169, 313
Denosumab 222
depression 4, 333, 337, 343
  alcohol and 262, 266
  antidepressants 18, 20, 23–4, 116, 174, 184, 186, 347, 348
  autism and 58
  cold-water swimming and 106, 115, 116–17, 119
  dementia and 97
  diet and 237
  HRT and 127, 132, 133
  menopausal transition and 16–18, 20, 22, 23–6, 32, 33, 40, 42
  post-natal depression 23, 24, 40, 119, 262–3
  psychedelics and 5, 345–50, 353
  testosterone and 157
  workplace and 77

destabilisation 22, 150, 154, 171
DEXA bone scan 210, 211, 213, 222
Di Florio, Professor Arianna 25–7
Diagnostic and Statistical Manual of Mental Disorders (DSM) 18
diagnostic tampon 205–6
diet
  American diet 50, 241
  body shape and 226, 228, 230–31, 235–6, 237, 239, 241, 242, 243, 244, 246
  dementia and 97–8, 102
  depression and 237
  dieting 211, 228, 230, 234–6
  HRT and 50, 139, 140, 144
  muscle/bone and 211, 213, 216–17, 220–21
  Mediterranean diet 50, 97–8, 139
  vagibiome and 198, 200
  weight and see weight
diggersanddreamers.org.uk 317
digital detox 268–82
  addiction and 269, 270, 271, 272, 274–5, 277
  bans 271
  continuous partial attention 278–9
  default mode network 273, 276
  dopamine and 270, 272, 274, 275
  double screen viewing 279
  email 269, 272, 273, 276–8, 280
  mental health and 270–71
  multitasking midlife woman and 276–8
  'nomophobia' (phone deprivation syndrome) 272–3
  notebook and 278
  phantom vibrations 273

phone jail 273–4
phone use 268–81
  senior leaders and 279–80
  sleep and 271, 276, 277, 278
  social role of technology 281–2
  textaphrenia 273
  TikTok 269, 270–73, 277
digital nomads 319–20
disability 68, 78, 135, 228
disappearing at work. See work
divorce 3, 4, 15, 29–30, 51, 62, 66, 155, 178, 192, 284–97, 302–3, 305–7, 309, 324, 364
Dog Blanket, The 324–5
domestic abuse 59, 60, 285–6
donanemab 96
dopamine 17, 37, 58, 114, 230, 250, 270, 272, 274–5
Douyin 271
Doyle, Glennon: Untamed – Stop Pleasing, Start Living 289
dryrobe 111–13, 120–22, 362
dyscalculia 65

economic deprivation 89, 141, 221
Eli Lilly 229, 233
Elizabeth I, Queen 169
Elizabeth II, Queen 49
email 79, 104, 213, 269, 272, 273, 276–8, 280, 312
employment tribunal 80, 82–3
empty nest syndrome 29
endometriosis 143, 155
Ephron, Nora 296–7
erectile dysfunction drugs 101, 157, 158, 168, 183–4, 187, 301
estradiol 134, 145, 227, 238
estriol 145–6
estrogen 4, 14, 284, 285, 315, 345
  alcohol and 251, 252
  brain and 37–43, 45, 47, 57–8
  dementia and 88, 92–5

Index

HRT and 21, 128–38, 144–8
muscle and bone and 214–16, 220, 222
psychosis and 23
sex and 180–83, 192
'sex hormones' and 17
testosterone and 150–52, 154, 156–64, 173–4
The Rage and 4
vaginal microbiome and 196–208
weight/body shape and 227, 228
workplace and 57–8, 84
estrone 227
ethnicity 48, 78, 94, 141, 221, 296
European Association on Urology 199
European Medicines Agency (EMA) 168–9
Evans, Samantha 191
Evvy 206
exercise 3, 50, 87, 139, 140, 144, 148, 153, 161, 163, 164, 180, 191–2, 195, 206–7, 230, 231, 232, 233
exercise snacking 223
high-intensity interval training (HIIT) 99, 218
weight-bearing 97, 98, 153, 213–14, 217–25, 234–5
Extinction Rebellion (XR) 331–2
Extreme Environments Laboratory, University of Portsmouth 110

facial estrogen 145–6
Fair Shares Report 295
Family Law Menopause Project 292, 297
Farideh 155–6
fat 99, 212, 253
body shape and 225–7, 230–36, 238, 239, 240–41, 243, 246
brown fat 113–14
Fawcett Society 18, 71, 77, 157
Feeld 313
fertility 8, 28–9, 31, 83, 148, 150, 155, 184, 192, 202, 210, 361

fibre 139, 220–21, 226, 235, 242
fibroids 135, 140, 143
final salary pension scheme 83
Fiona (journey through marriage and divorce) 286–93, 302–3
flirting 31, 177, 300
Fonda, Jane 47
Food and Drug Administration (FDA), US 157, 168, 169, 184, 202, 213, 346
Forbes '50 Over 50' list 86
Friday, Nancy: My Secret Garden: Women's Sexual Fantasies 188
Friends Co-op 324
friendships 6, 14, 56, 120, 304–10, 325
Frontiers in Aging Neuroscience 92
GABA receptors 17, 42, 58
Gadsby, Hannah 55–7, 68
Gamble-Turner, Professor Julie 53, 65
Garton, Sarah 85
'Gen-M Menopause-Friendly' accreditation tick 147–8
gender bias, medicine and 27, 34, 38, 78, 89, 139, 150, 157, 161, 168–70, 182, 184, 197, 201–2, 206, 209–11
Gendler, Dr Ellen 146
Genitourinary Syndrome of Menopause (GSM) 158–9, 181, 200–201
Gigha, island of 107, 118–19, 121, 122, 123, 320, 358
Glaser, Dr Rebecca 161
Glasgow University 309–10, 312, 320
glaucoma 138
glucose 45, 92, 109, 113, 199, 235, 236, 238–40
Glynne, Dr Sarah 138, 139
Gooding, Dr Charlotte 203–5
Gordon, Bryony 153
Gorman, Heather 119
GP (general practitioner) 20, 24, 58, 60, 72, 75, 78, 132, 134–6,

143–4, 146, 154, 158, 173, 174, 180–83, 197, 203–4, 216, 221–3, 276, 294
Guardian 55, 130, 170, 313–14, 318, 320, 326
Guardian Soulmates 312
gut microbiome 50, 99, 103, 194, 197, 200, 228, 236–9, 241–2, 246, 252
Guy's and St Thomas's Hospital 06

Harding, Professor Chris 198, 199, 203
Harris, Carolyn 132
Harrods 81
Haver, Dr Mary Claire 130, 131, 139, 232
Haward, Mellis 318
heart disease 102, 127, 138–9, 160–61, 228, 231, 241
Heathcote-James, Emma 63–6, 70, 147–8
Hendrix, Harville: Getting the Love You Want 300
Henpicked: Menopause in the Workplace 78, 214, 223
Hinge 310–13
hip replacement 211–12
Hof, Wim 107
honesty 34, 72, 85, 262, 266, 276, 303, 307, 348, 354
Hormonally 166
hormone replacement therapy (HRT) 15, 47, 89, 100–101, 212–16, 265
age-proof yourself with 127–48
Bijuve 135
black women and 33–4
body-identical 49, 93, 101, 127–35, 182–3, 216, 345
brain and 49–50
breast cancer and 128
cataracts and 138
combined patches 136
dementia and 92–8, 100–102
disease protection and 138–9
dosage 135–6

hormone replacement
therapy (HRT) –
continued
economically deprived
and underserved
communities and
141
Gen-M Menopause-
Friendly
accreditation tick
and 147–8
gender bias in
medicine and 139
glaucoma and 138
hysterectomy and/or
ovaries removed
and 135
Jaydess/Kyleena 136
levels of use 139
longevity and 137
menopause movement
and 132
mental health and
136–7
Mirena coil and 135–6
muscle/bone and
212–17, 222–3
neurodivergence and
60, 63, 65
oral combined 128
perimenopause timing
and 133–4
progesterone and
130–31, 134–7
progestin and 93, 101,
128, 129, 130–31,
135–6
Prue Leith and 140
sex and 182, 183, 193
skin and 145–7
testosterone and 135,
153–5, 157–9,
161–2, 165, 166,
171, 173
transdermal 93, 95,
101, 130, 134
urinary tract
infections and
138
vaginal bleeding and
135
vaginal microbiome
and 198, 207
weight and 227, 228,
233, 238–9, 242,
244
wild swimming and
109
Women's Health

Initiative (WHI)
study 129–30, 144
workplace and 75,
78–9
hot flushes 19, 21–2, 28,
42, 48, 85, 94, 132,
133, 135, 140, 142,
148, 171, 242, 253,
265
Hotter Than Ever 310, 364
house millionaires 323
Hunt, Robin 305
Huxley, Aldous: *The Doors
of Perception* 357, 361
Hypoactive Sexual Desire
Disorder (HSDD) 151,
156, 183–4
hypothermia 111, 112, 114
hysterectomy 21, 129, 135,
137, 140, 143, 154, 164
hysteria 26

ikigai ('your reason for
being') 363
Imago Relationship
Therapy 300
immunity 96, 109, 205
Imperial College London
345, 347, 348
Inchauspé, Jessie 239–40
Inside Out (film) 41
Instagram 21, 33, 43, 113,
122, 133, 136, 140, 153,
165, 166, 217, 219, 220,
239, 251, 266, 269–70,
272, 273, 277, 300, 327,
338–9, 350, 371
Institute for
Neurodegenerative
Diseases 96
insulin 37, 113, 114, 227,
228, 238, 239, 259
intentional communities
317
*International Journal of
Circumpolar Health* 117
International Menopause
Society 140–41, 244
Intrarosa 159, 181, 198
Intrinsa 157, 168
irritability 16, 155, 186
Isaacson, Dr Richard 96
isolation 16, 77, 97, 186,
288, 316–17, 319, 334

Jaydess 136
Jo Divine 191
*Journal of the American
Medical Association* 180

*Journal of Women and
Ageing, The* 82
journalling 35–6, 133, 307,
330, 350, 359, 363
photo-journalling
327–9
Judkins, Rod: *The Art
of Creative Thinking*
330–31
July, Miranda: *All Fours* 2,
28, 193, 290

Kamons, Portia 178, 179,
309–10
Karr, Mary: *The Liars' Club*
258
Keating, Erin 310–11, 364
Keats, Paula 143
Khan, Dr Fatima 253
Killing Kittens 176–8, 193,
306
Kulkarni, Jayashri 16,
22–3

lactobacilli 195, 196, 198,
200, 206
Lancet, The 160, 203, 347
Lancet Commission 97
Laneres, Lorraine 152
Langer, Professor Robert
130
Le Week-End (film) 315
lean muscle mass 97, 164,
221
Leary, Dr Timothy 346
lecanemab 96
Leith, Prue 140
Lembke, Dr Anna:
*Dopamine Nation:
Finding Balance in the
Age of Indulgence* 274–5
leqembi 96
lesbians 30, 55, 187, 190,
261, 314
LGBTQI+ 66
Li, Dr William 102
libido 17, 133, 150, 151,
153, 155, 157–8, 166,
168, 170, 174, 176,
182, 184, 192, 285,
301
life expectancy 9, 137
lifestyle changes 34, 50,
89, 94, 97, 98, 100,
139, 180, 213, 217–18,
227, 230
Little Soap Company,
The 64
Live More With Less 217

Index

loneliness 5, 288, 305–6, 316, 318, 322
longevity 3, 9, 34, 50, 128, 137, 149, 153, 156, 166–7, 219, 234, 235, 362
LSD 344, 345, 346
Lyon, Dr Gabrielle 217, 218, 219, 234, 235

Macaulay, Dr Claire 179–80, 186, 187, 189
Magic Medicine (documentary) 348
magic mushrooms 3, 342, 344–5, 346–7, 349
Magnusson, Margareta: *The Gentle Art of Swedish Death Cleaning* 323–4
Mallucci, Professor Giovanna 115
Manyonda, Professor Isaac 154, 155, 165, 173
marriage 4, 14, 15, 30, 62, 66, 69, 177, 187, 192, 256, 264, 283–303, 305, 307, 311, 313, 314, 315, 316, 321
  affairs *see* affairs, love
  couplepause 297–8
  couples therapy 298–303
  divorce *see* divorce
  domestic abuse and 59, 60, 285–6
  Fiona (journey through marriage and divorce) 286–93, 302–3
  Kate Muir remarries 365–7
  mediation 296
  moneypause 292–5
  pensions 293, 295, 316
  renovating relationships *see* relationships, renovating
  same-sex relationships 285
  sex and 285, 300–302
  see also sex
  The Rage and 284–5
Massey, Dr Heather 110, 111, 116, 117
Maté, Dr Gabor 259–60
maternity discrimination 73

Matthews, Rose 58–62, 66, 68–9; 'The Night I Lost My Freedom, and Got It Back Again' 59–60
McCall, Davina 49, 132
McDormand, Frances 319
Mead, Margaret 47
mediation 296
meditation 21–2, 50–51, 75, 255, 262, 276, 278
Mediterranean diet 50, 97–8, 139
#MeToo movement 72
Mehta, Lavina: *The Feel Good Fix* 223–4
memory
  alcohol and 259
  Alzheimer's and 87
  cold shock protein and 115, 117
  estrogen and 17, 93, 202
  high-intensity interval training and 99
  HRT and 345
  loss 4, 39, 42–3, 44, 48, 52, 87, 93, 115, 133, 157
  meditation and 51
  neurons and 38
  psychedelics and 343, 345, 348, 350
  sleep and 39, 94
  testosterone and 151, 155, 162–3, 167, 172
  verbal 48, 163
  visual 95
MENO-D rating 16
menopause 7, 164
  alcohol and *see* alcohol
  body shape and *see* body shape
  brain and *see* brain
  creativity and *see* creativity
  dementia and *see* dementia
  divorce and *see* divorce
  hormone replacement therapy (HRT) and *see* hormone replacement therapy (HRT)
  market 148
  marriage and *see* marriage
  movement 127–8, 131,

132, 172, 174–5, 244
  neurodivergence and *see* neurodivergence
  perimenopause *see* perimenopause
  postmenopausal renaissance 45–8
  psychedelics and *see* psychedelics
  renovating relationships *see* relationships, renovating
  sex and *see* sex
  surgical 21, 40, 137, 154, 159, 168
  technology and *see* digital detox
  testosterone and *see* testosterone
  vaginal microbiome and *see* vaginal microbiome
  weight and *see* weight
  wild swimming and *see* wild swimming
  workplace and *see* workplace
Menopause Charity, The 134, 138, 139, 221
Menopause Mandate 132
Menopause Research and Education 155
@MenopauseWhilstBlack 31, 33, 338–9
@menoscandal Instagram 43, 136, 153
MenoScale calculator 242
MenoWarriors group 85
microaggression 32
Middling Along podcast 85
midlife, definition of 1
midlife crisis
  defined 1
  timing and number of 2
Midlife Sex Festival 187
migraine 44, 65, 75, 78, 133, 156, 328–9
Migration Museum, Lewisham 339–40
mindfulness 50–51, 187, 276
mini-strokes/transient ischemic attacks (TIAs) 98, 100

Mirena coil 135–6
Moggach, Deborah 207, 313–16, 324
Little Black Dress 313
The Best Exotic Marigold Hotel 313, 315–16, 325
Mommunes 318
Monash University 16, 158
moneypause 292–5
mood 16, 17, 24, 37, 41, 50, 60, 109, 117–18, 134, 151, 155, 213, 235, 237, 327, 347
low 18, 20, 42
swings 25, 52, 133, 140, 148, 253
Morse, Emily 189, 190
Mosconi, Dr Lisa 38, 44, 45–7, 163
Brain Food: How to Eat Smart and Sharpen Your Mind 49, 50, 97–8
The Menopause Brain 38, 49, 51, 92–3, 95
Moseley, Dr Rachel 53, 54, 57–8
motherhood 148, 196, 201, 335–6
motivation 17, 77, 151, 153, 163, 244, 260
Mounjaro 228, 232
MsBrain 48, 93–4
Muir, Douglas (father of Kate Muir) 99–100, 205, 342–3, 353, 360, 364
Muir, Ella (mother of Kate Muir) 4, 15, 30, 87, 90–92, 97, 100, 103–5, 138, 152, 202–3, 323, 352–3, 359, 360
multitasking 14, 152, 250, 277, 364
Mumsnet 192
muscle and bone 209–23
Big Pharma and 222
bisphosphonate drugs 216, 222
DEXA bone scan 210, 211, 213, 222
diet and 211, 213, 216–17, 220–21
economic deprivation and 221
ethnicity and 221
exercise and 213, 217–23

fractures 139, 160, 209, 210, 211–14, 220, 222–3
gender bias in medicine and 210–11
hip replacement 211–12
HRT and 212–17, 222–3
muscle mass 97, 144, 156, 157, 164, 175, 191–2, 207, 209, 212–13, 217–21, 223–4, 227, 229, 231–5
osteoporosis *see* osteoporosis
The Musculoskeletal Syndrome of Menopause 219–20
vitamin D 213, 215, 216–17, 221
Muslim women 221, 313

Nadia (pseudonym) (NDA) 78–9
Nagoski, Dr Emily: *Come as You Are* 188
Nanette 55–6
National Autistic Society 70
National Institute for Health and Care Excellence (NICE) 157–8
Nature Mental Health 25
nerve growth factor (NGF) 50, 99
neurodivergence 3, 53–70, 74, 147, 281
ADHD *see* Attention Deficit Hyperactivity Disorder (ADHD)
AuDHD 63–4
autism *see* autism
camouflaging 63–4, 69
defined 53
diagnosis of in late-life 53–70
dyscalculia 65
Emma Heathcote-James 63–6, 70
LGBTQI+ autistic crossover 66
Non-Disclosure Agreements

(NDAs) and 62
perimenopause onset and 65
private healthcare and 67–8
Rose Matthews 58–62
self-diagnosing of neurodivergence on TikTok 54
neurosteroids 17
neurotransmitters 17, 42, 58, 184
New Ground 318, 320
New Scientist 199
Newcastle University 82
Newson Health 24, 251
Newson, Dr Louise 156
NHS (National Health Service) 20, 75, 79, 101, 116, 179, 181, 183, 197, 198, 201, 206, 229, 246, 263, 265
Chelsea and Westminster menopause clinic 130
Fracture Liaison Services (FLS) 214
HRT and 128, 130, 133, 135, 140, 141, 143
muscle and bone health and 210–14, 216, 218, 222, 223
neurodivergence and 60, 67
NHS Sussex 116
talking therapy and 35
testosterone and 151, 154, 156–7, 159, 167–8, 170, 173–4
night sweats 19, 42, 48, 93–4, 133, 157, 265
No7 Menopause Skincare Instant Radiance Serum 146–7
No7 Menopause Skincare Nourishing Overnight Cream 146
Nomadland (film) 319
Non-Disclosure Agreements (NDAs) 7, 62, 72–4, 78, 80–83
noradrenaline 114
Northampton General Hospital 211

Index

Novo Nordisk 233
Nutt, David: *Psychedelics*
345–6

O'Reilly, Miriam 82–3
*Organizational Behavior
and Human Decision
Processes* 84
orgasm 3, 151, 158, 170,
181, 182, 186, 188–90
osteoporosis 3, 138, 139,
141, 156, 159–60,
209–10, 214–15, 217,
218, 221–3, 232, 271
ovaries 21, 37, 38, 40, 89,
135, 137, 140, 143,
150, 154, 159
overwhelm 31, 58, 64, 65,
255, 265, 276, 292, 303
oxytocin 41
Ozempic 174, 228, 230,
231, 233, 235

Panay, Professor Nick 244
panic attacks 19, 276
paranoid thinking 16,
23–4, 263, 307, 350,
356
parents
    death of 5, 29, 30, 305
    dementia and see
        dementia
    divorce and 286–91
    parenting, end of 29,
        335–6
Parker, Dorothy 308,
309–10
part-time work 23, 58, 71,
78, 118, 293, 333
Pearson, Allison 230,
232–3
peeing 195, 197, 199,
206–7, 358
pelvic floor 148, 191–2,
206–7
pensions 8, 79, 83, 85,
233, 293, 295, 316
People, Places and Things
(play) 260–61
Perel, Esther: *Mating in
Captivity* 188
perimenopause 2, 4, 7,
17, 361
    alcohol and 251, 262,
        263, 265
    body shape and 226–7,
        237, 238
    bone and muscle mass
        and 214–16, 220

brain and 37, 40, 41–2,
    43, 44, 45, 46, 51
dementia and 87, 88, 93
Diagnostic and
    Statistical Manual
    of Mental
    Disorders (DSM)
    and 18
divorce and 284, 286,
    292, 294–5, 301
HRT and 20–21, 24,
    128, 129, 133, 134,
    138, 145
mental health and 16,
    24–6, 28, 32
neurodiversity and
    53–4, 57–9, 63,
    65–6
sex and 42, 178, 180,
    187, 192–3, 301
testosterone and 162,
    165
timing of 23, 133–4
vaginal microbiome
    and 196–7
workplace and 75
periods, menstrual 28, 38,
    40, 41–2, 46, 133, 143,
    172, 179, 180, 184–5,
    211, 214
Perkins, Zelda 62, 72–4, 81
Peyton-Jones, Julia 335–6
pheromones 31
phone. *See* digital detox
photography 69, 270, 314,
    317, 326–30
Pleasure Possibility
    coaching programme
    179
PMZ (postmenopausal
    zest) 47
political awakening 331–3
Pollan, Michael: *How to
    Change Your Mind –
    The New Science of
    Psychedelics* 350
polyphenols 102–3
post-traumatic growth
    (PTG) 34, 244
posttraumatic stress
    disorder (PTSD) 31, 79
Postcards from Midlife
    podcast 27, 43
PowerPoint presentation
    19, 363–4
prasterone 159, 188, 198
pregnancy 23, 24, 36, 37, 39,
    73, 113, 143, 156–7, 263
Premarin 146

premature ovarian
    insufficiency (POI) 40
premenstrual dysphoric
    disorder (PMDD) 24
premenstrual syndrome
    41–2
probiotics 198–200, 208,
    241
progesterone 4, 14, 17, 23,
    24, 284
    bone and muscle mass
        and 215, 216, 222
    brain and 37, 39–42
    dementia and 88, 93
    HRT and 128–31,
        134–7, 173, 183,
        222, 345
    neurodivergence and
        57–8
    testosterone and 150–
        52, 156–7, 173
    work and 75, 84
progestin 93, 101, 128, 129,
    130–31, 135–6, 159, 196
protein 50, 99, 114–15, 218,
    220, 226, 233, 234–5,
    240, 241, 242, 245
psilocybin 3, 342, 344,
    345–9, 358, 361
psychedelics 3, 5, 7, 9, 329,
    341–61
    ayahuasca 344, 345,
        346–7, 350
    ceremonies 355–9
    LSD 344, 345, 346
    Magic Medicine
        (documentary) 348
    magic mushrooms 3,
        342, 344–5, 346–7,
        349
    Nutt on 345–6
    psilocybin 3, 342, 344,
        345–9, 358, 361
Psychologies 326, 329
psychosexual 185
psychosis 23
psychotherapists 5, 24,
    27, 33, 34, 35, 61, 66,
    85, 185–6, 226, 312,
    332–4, 342, 365, 369
public speaking 76

Queen's University Belfast
    98

Rachael (menopause)
    19–22, 162
racism 32, 33, 34, 73
    racial weathering 33

405

Rage, The 4, 284–5
Rajpar, Dr Sajjad 146–7
Redfern, Dr Lauren 166–7, 170–72, 174
Redrobe, Dr Sharon 66
Regan, Professor Dame Lesley 49
relationships, renovating 304–25
    communal living/co-housing projects 316–25
    dating online 310–12, 316–17
    decoupling from other couples post-divorce 306–7
    friendships 305–10
    house millionaires 323
    intentional communities 317
    isolation 316–17, 319
    loneliness 305–6, 316, 318, 322
    Moggach and 313–16, 324, 325
    relationship therapy 27, 300
    renting out bedrooms 324
    'snowbirds' 319
    Tiny House Communities 319
    Swedish Death Cleaning 323–4
    vans, living in 319–20
retirement 8, 71, 83, 90, 91, 100, 144, 286–7, 295, 316, 317, 335, 362
retraining 85–6, 211
Robertson-Smith, Dr Bill 211–12, 214, 215
Romosozumab 222
Ross, Deborah 107
Ross, Diana 47
Ross, Jill 85
Ross, Professor Karen 82–3
Royal College of GPs 154
Royal College of Psychiatry 24
Royal Osteoporosis Society 214, 215, 222
Ru, Camilla 337
Rubin, Dr Rachel 168, 181–2, 201

Samuel, Julia 34
Sands, Linda 132
sarcopenia 164, 218

Saxenda 231
Sayle, Emma 176–7, 306
schizophrenia 26
self-compassion 15, 34, 348, 360
self-esteem 16, 62
semaglutides 174, 228–34
serotonin 17, 37, 42, 58, 108, 114, 186, 237, 251, 258, 347, 358
Serpentine Gallery 335–6
sertraline 24, 186
sex 176–93, 301–2
    Addyi (flibanserin) 184
    breast cancer and 179–80
    clitoris 159, 165, 178–9, 181, 182, 190, 191, 201
    communication and 176–7
    erectile dysfunction drugs and 101, 157, 158, 168, 183–4, 187, 301
    Genitourinary Syndrome of Menopause and 158–9, 181, 200–201
    Hypoactive Sexual Desire Disorder 151, 156, 183–4
    Intrarosa 159, 181, 198
    Killing Kittens 176–8, 193, 306
    lesbians and 190
    libido/sex drive see libido
    Midlife Sex Festival online 187
    orgasms see orgasms
    pain and 180–81, 185, 202, 285
    pelvic floor and 191–2
    perimenopausal sex surge 42, 192–3, 301
    'sex hormones' 17, 150
    sex toys 190–91
    sexual visibility 31
    testosterone and 182–3
    The Pleasure Possibility coaching programme 179
    vaginal dryness/vaginal estrogen and 180–82
    vaginismus and 185

Sex with Emily podcast 189
Sex, Myths and the Menopause (documentary) 131, 132, 338
Shahzady, Farhana 285, 291–7
shame 5, 68, 72, 77, 82, 85, 111, 113, 177, 190, 208, 227, 232, 244, 264, 272, 299, 302, 365
sidelined at work 61, 71, 82–3
SilverSingles 313
Silverstone, Anthony 143–4
skin 39, 118, 133, 134, 135, 145–7, 180–81, 196, 216, 231, 242, 252, 256, 269
slavery 318, 339
sleep
    alcohol and 253, 257, 263
    dementia and 93–4, 97, 100, 102
    digital detox and 271, 276, 277, 278
    HRT and 134, 140–41
    menopause and 21–4, 26, 37, 39, 42, 48, 74–5
    progesterone and 17
    wild swimming and 122
smoking 97, 99–100, 129, 229
snake phobia 342–4, 356, 357, 358
Snell, Kristina 66–7
'snowbirds' 319
Søberg, Dr Susanna: Winter Swimming: The Nordic Way Towards a Healthier and Happier Life 114
Spector, Professor Tim 194, 236–7, 241–2
Square Peg Community 70
Srnic, Nikola 243
St George's NHS Hospital London 154
Starmer, Keir 229
Steinke, Darcey: Flash Count Diary 171–2
Stibbe, Eva 314
Stibbe, Nina 312–13, 314,

Index

324; *Went to London,
Took the Dog* 207
Storie, Hannah 118–19
Streeting, Wes 228–9
stress 3, 31, 33, 34, 36, 41,
50, 58, 60, 61, 65, 79,
90, 97, 109, 113, 116,
185, 188, 250, 255,
259, 278, 294, 337
stress incontinence 206
sugar 114, 198, 199, 219,
220, 231, 233, 236,
237, 238–41
suicidal thoughts/suicidal
ideation 20, 25, 32,
58, 348, 350
Super Size Me
(documentary) 242–3
surgical menopause 21, 40,
137, 154, 159, 168
Swedish Death Cleaning
323–4
Swell Sex Symposium,
New York 189

talking therapy 35, 354,
365
tantric sex 187, 188
Tasha (pseudonym) (NDA
agreement) 74–7
tau tangles 88, 93, 96
technology. *See* digital
detox
teenagers 5, 14, 38, 39,
66–7, 226, 270, 271,
308, 353
temper 76, 285
Temple Druid
Community, The 317
testosterone 3, 17, 21, 31,
37–40, 41, 48–9, 78,
83, 92, 93, 101, 128,
135, 149–75, 181,
182–3, 193, 196, 198,
215, 227, 301, 345
access to 173–4
Alzheimer's disease
and 92, 93, 163
breast cancer and
161–2
ESTEEM randomised
controlled trial
156
female body
production of
150–51
gel 135, 149, 156, 157,
162, 182
gendering hormones

and 150–51
GPs and 154
hairiness and 164–5
heart disease and
160–61
libido/sex drive and
151, 155, 157–8
media and 153
medical sexism and
167–73
memory and
cognition and 151,
155, 162–3, 167,
172
muscle mass and 164
NHS cost of for
women 167–8
osteoporosis and
159–60, 215
prescriptions increase
154
Reclaim Testosterone
movement 175
ten things you need
to know about
156–65
trans and non-binary
movement and
150
UTIs and 158–9
vaginal dryness and
158–9
Thatcher, Margaret 49
Theobald, Stephanie 182
Thriving London 277
Thurston, Rebecca 48
TikTok 54, 155–6, 166,
269, 270–73, 277
Times, The 85, 112, 140,
153, 167, 169, 242,
284, 307, 343
Time's Up 73
Tinder 313
Tiny House Communities
319
Top of the Lake (television
series) 319
*Transforming Women's
Long-Term Health* 138,
139
trauma 4, 28, 31–4, 50,
58, 60–62, 68, 185–6,
188, 259, 262, 344,
348, 350, 354–5, 361
post-traumatic growth
(PTG) 34, 244
posttraumatic stress
disorder (PTSD)
31, 79

resurfacing of 4, 31
TriNetX healthcare
database 161

UK Biobank 25–6, 97
UK Cohousing Network
318
UK Dementia Research
Institute 115
Uloko, Dr Maria 168
ultra-processed food (UPF)
50, 139, 233, 237, 274
upcycling 304, 338
urinary tract infections
(UTIs) 91, 127, 133,
138, 158–9, 180,
195–208

Vagifem 181, 204, 207
vaginal bleeding 135
vaginal dryness 133, 138,
145, 158–9, 171, 176,
180–82, 190, 196, 202
vaginal estrogen 21, 146,
148, 158–9, 180–82,
196–207, 285, 315
vaginal microbiome/
vagibiome 3, 159, 190,
194–208
contraceptive pill or
coil and 196
D-Mannose and 199
defined 194–5
gender health gap and
206
Genitourinary
Syndrome of
Menopause (GSM)
and 200–201
lactobacilli and 195,
196, 198, 200, 206
peeing and 195, 197,
199, 206–7
probiotics 199–200,
208
stress incontinence
206
testing 205–6
UTIs and 195–208
vaginal estrogen and
196–207
vaginismus 185
vans, living in 319–20
vascular dementia 87–8,
98–105
Verity, Nicole 331–2
Viagra 101, 183, 315
Victoria, Queen 339
Vidal, Gore 274

Vine, Sarah 230–31
visceral adipose tissue 227, 238, 240–41
vitamins 147, 220
 D 213, 215, 216–17, 221
 E 146
Vohra, Dr Radhika 138, 141, 217–18, 221–2
VolcanicX bracelet 148
vulva 138, 145, 151, 159, 165, 179, 180–82, 185, 195, 196, 198, 201

Walters-James, Leigh 85
wandering womb 26
Ward, Dr Hannah 23–4
warmth, personal 84, 309, 352–3
Watts, Dr Jay 61, 66
#WearYourHappy 338
Webb-Wilson, Dr Gavin 143–4
weddings 258, 338, 365–7
Wegovy 228–30
weight 16, 129, 132, 133, 136, 144, 225, 227–35, 243–6
 weight-loss drugs 174, 228–35
Weill Cornell Medicine, New York 38, 92, 163
Weinstein, Harvey 7, 72–3
Wellcome Foundation 329
wild swimming 106–23
 addictive nature of 109, 115
 afterdrop 111
 benefits 109, 113–14, 116–18, 122–4
 Bluetits Chill Swimmers 108, 123
 cold shock protein 114–15
 cold water shock 110–11
 Deakin on 115–16
 dryrobe/clothing 111–13, 120–22
 Facebook groups 108, 112, 121, 123
 fats and 113–14
 Gigha and 107, 116, 118–19, 121, 122, 123
 hypothermia and 111, 112, 114

immunity and 109
 mental health and 115–17
 MRI brain scans and 117
 neurodegeneration and 114–15
 Nick Cave and 106–7
 Outdoor Swimming Society 111
 OUTSIDE study 116–17
 Parliament Hill Lido, Hampstead 27–8, 107–8
 Spartans and 113
 stress 109, 113, 116
 technique 110
 transcendental experience 117–18
 weather, irrelevance of 108
 Wild Swimming – Scotland 123
Willis, Laura 275–81
Wilson, Bill 260
Winfrey, Oprah 49, 230
Winter, Dr Ashley ('The Angel of Estrogen') 202
Wittenberg-Cox, Avivah 8–9
Women and Hollywood 73
Women's Alzheimer's Movement 95
Women's Brain Initiative, Weill Cornell Medicine 38
Women's Health Initiative (WHI), US 129–30, 144
work, how not to disappear at 71–86
 ageism and 71, 72, 77, 78, 81–3
 boredom and 71
 brain changes and 71, 85
 bullying behaviour 73, 76
 burnout 71, 74
 CEOs, FTSE 100 companies 72
 comebacks and 77–8
 disability and 78
 disappearing, sense of self 76

employment tribunals 80, 82–3
 ethnic minority groups and 78
 final salary pension schemes 83
 Forbes '50 Over 50' list 86
 Henpicked:
  Menopause in the Workplace report 78
 legal equality in 72
 male reaction at work to women who are still fertile, and those who are postmenopausal 83–4
 menopause policies, workplace 78
 motivation and 77
 non-disclosure agreements and 72–4, 78, 80–83
 part-time work 71, 78
 performance management 71
 promotion 71, 74–5
 posttraumatic stress disorder and 79
 private health insurance and 78
 public speaking and 76
 retirement 71, 83
 retraining 85–6
 sackings 7, 71
 shame, culture of 85
 sidelined in favour of younger colleagues 71, 82–3
 temper and 76
 warmth, losing personal 84
Wright, Dr Vonda 210–11, 219–21

yoga 14–15, 50, 75, 119, 192, 262, 342
You Are Not Broken podcast 184, 267

Zepbound 229
Zhao, Chloe 319
Zoe 102, 194, 236–9, 241, 242